Ninja Foodi Cookbook #2019

Delicious, Quick & Easy Ninja Foodi Recipes for Effortless Meals in 2019

550 Recipes

Emma Peterson

Warning-Disclaimer

The purpose of this book is to educate and entertain. The author or publisher does not guarantee that anyone following the techniques, suggestions, tips, ideas, or strategies will become successful. The author and publisher shall have neither liability or responsibility to anyone with respect to any loss or damage caused, or alleged to be caused, directly or indirectly by the information contained in this book.

CONTENTS

Introduction 18

Breakfast

Cheesy Prosciutto Egg Bake 23

Crispy Pancetta Hash with Baked Eggs 23

Strawberry Bread French Toast 24

Raspberry-Cranberry Chia Oatmeal 24

Sausage Wrapped Scotch Eggs 25

Spicy Deviled Eggs 25

Shakshuka with Goat Cheese 26

Kale-Egg Frittata 26

Savory Custards with Ham and Emmental Cheese 27

Butternut Squash Cake Oatmeal 27

Egg Crumpet Sandwich 28

Herbed Homemade Ghee 28

Orange Pepper and Artichoke Frittata 29

Barbecue Chicken Sandwiches 29

Plum Breakfast Clafoutis 30

Chai Latte Steel-Cut Oatmeal 30

French Dip Sandwiches 31

Cheese & Bacon Grits 31

Feta and Poached Egg Heirloom Tomato Topper 32

Maple Giant Pancake with Whipped Cream 32

Sausage and Bacon Cheesecake 33

Veggie Salmon Balls 33

Prosciutto, Mozzarella & Egg in a Cup 34

Onion and Cheese Omelet 34

Ham and Cheese Sandwich 34

Creamy Zucchini Muffins 35

Toasted Herb and Garlic Bagel 35

Raspberry and Vanilla Pancake 36

Paprika Shirred Eggs 36

Three Meat Cheesy Omelet 36

Very Berry Breakfast Puffs 37

Crustless Mediterranean Quiche 37

Sweet Bread Pudding with Raisins 38

Cinnamon Pumpkin Steel Cut Oatmeal 38

Quick Soft-Boiled Eggs 38

Sweet Paprika Hard-Boiled Eggs 39

Lunch Recipes

Egg Rolls 40

Ham & Mozzarella Eggplant Boats 40

Cheat Hawaiian Pizza 41

Italian Sausage Patties 41

Garlicky Chicken on Green Bed 41

Homemade Vegetables Soup 42

Pickle and Potato Salad with Feta 42

Curry Egg Salad 42

Warm Bacon & Potato Salad 43

Quick Chicken Noodle Soup 43

Broccoli and Potato Soup 44

Sweet Potato & Egg Salad 44

Spicy Acorn Squash Soup 45

Minestrone Soup 45

Vegetable Soup 46

Chicken Noodle Soup 46

Homemade Chicken Soup 47

Cream of Pumpkin Chipotle Soup 47

Cauliflower Cheese Soup 48

Cream of Mushroom and Spinach Soup 48

Mexican-Style Chicken Soup 49

Ramen Spicy Soup with Collard Greens 49

Leek and Potato Soup with Sour Cream 50

Tomato Soup with Cheese Croutons 50

Hearty Winter Vegetable Soup 51

Acorn Squash Soup with Coconut Milk 51

Spicy Borscht Soup 52

Two-Bean Zucchini Soup 52

Butternut Squash Curry 52

Creamy Quinoa and Mushroom Pilaf 53

Red Lentils Soup with Tortilla Topping 53

Vegetarian Black Bean Soup 54

Classic French Onion Soup 54

Chicken & Farro Soup 55

Fire-Roasted Tomato and Chorizo Soup 55

Chicken Broth...56

Beef Neck Bone Stock..56

Flavorful Vegetable Stock..56

Perfect Chicken Wings Broth...57

Spicy Beef Broth...57

Basic Applesauce with Cinnamon...58

Ragu Bolognese..58

Snacks, Appetizers & Sides

Tangy Cheesy Arancini...59

Hot Chicken Wings...60

Hot Buttery Chicken Meatballs..60

Cheesy Smashed Sweet Potatoes...61

Fried Beef Dumplings...61

Kale-Artichoke Bites..62

BBQ Chicken Drumsticks...62

Buffalo Chicken Meatballs with Ranch-Style Dip...63

Holiday Egg Brulee...63

Brazilian Cheese Balls..64

Asparagus Wrapped in Prosciutto with Garbanzo Dip...64

Creamy Tomato & parsley Dip...65

Cheese bombs wrapped in Bacon..65

Bacon & Cheese Dip..65

Scrumptious Honey-Mustard Hot Dogs...66

Chicken and Cheese Bake..66

Teriyaki Chicken Wings..66

Green Vegan Dip...67

Homemade Spinach Hummus..67

Sweet-Heat Pickled Cucumbers..68

Crispy Cheesy Straws...68

Crispy Rosemary Potato Fries..68

Cauliflower and Cheddar Tater Tots..69

Eggplant Chips with Honey..69

Wrapped Asparagus in Bacon..70

New York Steak and Minty Cheese..70

Melt-in-the-Middle Meatballs..70

Air Fried Pin Wheels..71

Nutty & Zesty Brussels Sprouts with Raisins..71

Cumin Baby Carrots...72

Garlic and Rosemary Mushrooms..72

Turkey Scotch Eggs 72

Parmesan Cabbage Side Dish 73

Herby Fish Skewers 73

Tomato & Mozzarella Bruschetta 73

Vegetables & Vegan

Sundried Tomatoes, Spinach, and Butternut Squash Stew 74

Swiss Cheese and Mushroom Tarts 74

Rice & Olives Stuffed Mushrooms 75

Sticky Noodles with Tofu and Peanuts 75

Squash Parmesan and Linguine 76

Tangy Risotto and Roasted Bell Peppers 76

Roasted Squash & Rice with Crispy Tofu 77

Rice Stuffed Zucchini Boats 78

Garganelli with Swiss Cheese and Mushrooms 78

Easy Green Squash Gruyere 79

Easy Spanish Rice 79

Cajun Baked Turnips 80

Pesto Minestrone with Cheesy Bread 80

Creamy Cauliflower & Asparagus Farfalle 81

Mushroom Risotto with Swiss Chard 82

Spicy Tangy Salmon with Wild Rice 82

Mashed Broccoli with Cream Cheese 83

Spinach Pesto Spaghetti Squash 83

Cream of Cauliflower & Butternut Squash 84

Crème de la Broc 84

Eggplant Lasagna 85

Buttered Leafy Greens 85

Fall Celeriac Pumpkin Soup 86

Zucchini & Quinoa Stuffed Red Peppers 86

Pine nuts and Steamed Asparagus 87

Bok Choy & Zoddle Soup 87

Mushroom Brown Rice Pilaf 88

Asian-Style Tofu Soup 88

Cheesy Stuffed Mushrooms 89

Vegetarian Minestrone Soup 89

Green Cream Soup 90

Chipotle Chili 90

Vegan Carrot Gazpacho 91

Pesto Quinoa Bowls with Veggies 91

Indian Vegan Curry 92

Green Minestrone 92

Creamy Mashed Potatoes with Spinach 92

Herby-Garlic Potatoes 93

Punjabi Palak Paneer 93

Pilau Rice with Veggies 94

Carrot and Lentil Chili 94

Steamed Artichokes with Lemon Aioli 94

Garlic Veggie Mash with Parmesan 95

Green Beans with Feta and Nuts 95

Mashed Parsnips and Cauliflower 96

Tahini Sweet Potato Mash 96

Aloo Gobi with Cilantro 96

Spicy Cauliflower Rice with Peas 97

Chipotle Vegetarian Chili 97

Thai Vegetable Stew 98

Sweet Carrots with Crumbled Bacon 98

Honey-Glazed Acorn Squash 98

Artichoke with Garlic Mayo 99

Asparagus with Feta 99

Parsley Mashed Cauliflower 100

Turkey Stuffed Potatoes 100

Chorizo Mac and Cheese 100

Winter Minestrone with Pancetta 101

Green Lasagna Soup 101

Italian Sausage with Garlic Mash 102

Rosemary Sweet Potato Medallions 102

Breakfast Burrito Bowls 103

Colorful Vegetable Medley 103

Red Beans and Rice 104

Veggie Skewers 104

Tasty Baby Porcupine Meatballs 105

Grilled Tofu Sandwich 105

Spicy Pepper & Sweet Potato Skewers 106

Pasta with Roasted Veggies 106

Paneer Cutlet 106

Vegetable Tortilla Pizza 107

Poblano & Tomato Stuffed Squash 107

Quinoa and Veggie Stuffed Peppers 108

Avocado Rolls 108

Simple Air Fried Ravioli 108

Crispy Nachos 109

Paneer Cheese Balls 109

Potato Filled Bread Rolls 110

Quick Crispy Kale Chips 110

Roasted Vegetable Salad 110

Quick Crispy Cheese Lings 111

Prawn Toast 111

Pineapple Appetizer Ribs 112

Fish & Seafood Mains

Scottish Seafood Curry 113

Buttery Herb Salmon with Barley Haricot Verts 114

Crispy Cod on Lentils 114

Potato Chowder with Peppery Prawns 115

Traditional Mahi Mahi 115

Mushrooms and Shrimp Egg Wrappers 116

Sausage and Shrimp Paella 117

Chorizo and Shrimp Boil 117

Lemon Cod Goujons & Rosemary Chips 118

Salmon with Dill Chutney 118

Penne all'Arrabbiata with Seafood and Chorizo 119

Spaghetti with Arugula and Scallops 119

Mussel Chowder with Oyster Crackers 120

Tuna Salad with Asparagus & Potatoes 120

Crabmeat with Broccoli Risotto 121

Seafood Gumbo 122

Haddock with Sanfaina 122

Cajun Salmon with Creamy Grits 123

Autumn Succotash with Basil-Crusted Fish 124

Farfalle Tuna Casserole with Cheese 124

Mackerel en Papillote with Vegetables 125

Smoked Salmon Pilaf with Walnuts 126

Italian-Style Flounder 126

Monk Fish with Greens 127

Paprika & Garlic Salmon 127

Alaskan Cod with Fennel & Beans 128

White Wine Black Mussels 128

Parsley Oyster Stew 129

Creamy Crab Soup...129

Paella Señorito..130

Steamed Mediterranean Cod...130

Seared Scallops with Butter-Caper Sauce 131

Steamed Sea Bass with Turnips..131

White Wine Mussels 132

Delicious Coconut Shrimp..132

Fish Finger Sandwich..132

Parmesan Tilapia...133

Crab Cakes..133

Quick and Easy Air Fried Salmon 134

Cajun Salmon with Lemon 134

Tuna Patties..134

Cod Cornflakes Nuggets 135

Pistachio Crusted Salmon 135

Poultry recipes

Lemon Chicken Tenders with Broccoli...136

Garlic Herb Roasted Chicken...136

Sweet Sesame Chicken Wings 137

Crispy Chicken Thighs with Thyme Carrot Roast..138

Quick Chicken Fried Rice...138

Chicken with Crunchy Coconut Dumplings 139

Creamy Turkey Enchilada Casserole 139

Chicken Cassoulet with Frijoles 140

Chicken with Cilantro Rice...140

Black Refried Beans and Chicken Fajitas..141

Chicken Potato Pot Pie 142

Herbed Chicken and Biscuit Chili..142

Hot Crispy Chicken with Carrots and Potatoes...143

Herby Chicken Breasts 143

Herby Dumplings and Italian Season Chicken...144

Tandoori Chicken Thighs..144

Saucy Shredded Chicken...145

Wine Braised Chicken with Mushrooms and Brussel Sprouts 146

Mexican Green Chili Chicken...146

Lemon and Paprika Chicken Thighs 147

BBQ Chicken & Kale Quesadillas...148

Chicken Florentine 148

Chicken Caesar Salad with Salted Croutons 149

Chicken Shawarma Wrap...150

Coq au Vin...151

Cajun Roasted Chicken with Potato Mash..152

Chicken Chili with Cannellini Beans..152

Traditional Chicken Cordon Bleu...153

Pesto Chicken with Roasted Red Pepper Sauce...154

Mexican Chicken & Wild Rice Bowls...154

White Wine Chicken..155

Chicken with Tomato Salsa...156

Cheesy Buffalo Chicken..156

Chicken Noodle Soup with Crispy Bacon...157

Chicken & Green Bean Coconut Curry...157

Chicken & Veggie Tacos with Guacamole..158

Chicken Meatballs Primavera...158

Mediterranean Stuffed Chicken Breasts...159

Sticky Orange Chicken...159

Spinach & Mushroom Chicken Stew..160

BBQ Chicken Drumettes..160

Sage Chicken Thighs...161

Whole Chicken with Lemon & Onion Stuffing...161

Za'atar Chicken with Lemony Couscous...162

Lettuce Carnitas Wraps..162

Lemon Turkey Risotto..163

Thyme Chicken with Veggies..163

Juicy Orange Chicken...164

Beef Congee (Chinese Rice Porridge)...164

Creamy Chicken and Quinoa Soup...164

Creamy Chicken Pasta with Pesto Sauce..165

Chicken and Sweet Potato Corn Chowder..165

Cajun Shredded Chicken and Wild Rice...166

Hawaiian-Style Chicken Sliders with Pineapple Salad.................................166

Asian Turkey Lettuce Cups...167

Honey-Garlic Chicken..167

Pulled Chicken and Peach Salsa...168

Chicken with Beans and Bacon...168

Chicken Cacciatore...169

Vietnamese Pork Soup..169

Tandoori Chicken with Cilantro Sauce...170

Indian Butter Chicken..170

Chicken Chickpea Chili 171

Paprika Buttered Chicken 171

Buffalo Chicken and Navy Bean Chili 172

Chicken in Tikka Masala Sauce..172

Pesto Stuffed Chicken with Green Beans 173

Cajun Chicken with Rice and Peas 173

Spicy Chicken Wings with Lemon..174

Chicken with BBQ Sauce 174

Spicy Salsa Chicken with Feta 174

Chicken and Zucchini Pilaf 175

Chicken in Pineapple Gravy 175

Salsa Verde Chicken with Salsa Verde 176

Chicken Meatballs in Tomato Sauce..176

Honey-Garlic Chicken and Okra 177

Shredded Chicken with Lentils and Rice 177

Saucy Chicken Breasts 178

Chicken with Tomatoes and Capers...178

Winter Chicken Thighs with Cabbage 178

Sriracha Chicken with Black Beans 179

Crunchy Chicken Schnitzels...179

Greek Turkey Meatballs..180

Potato and Ground Turkey Chili 180

Sticky Drumsticks 180

Turkey Meatballs with Rigatoni 181

Spicy Turkey Casserole...181

Chicken Fajitas with Avocado 182

Chicken Burgers with Avocado...182

Hot Chicken Wings...183

Basil & Cheddar Stuffed Chicken 183

Spicy Buttered Turkey...183

Chicken with Prunes 184

Tom Yum Wings...184

Honey-Glazed Chicken Kabobs 184

Cordon Bleu Chicken 185

Rosemary Lemon Chicken 185

Greek-Style Chicken 186

Asian-Style Chicken..186

Crumbed Sage Chicken Scallopini 186

Chicken Tenders with Broccoli & Rice...187

Buttermilk Chicken Thighs...187

Korean-Style Barbecued Satay..187

Sweet Garlicky Chicken Wings..188

Thyme Turkey Nuggets...188

Spicy Chicken Wings...188

Herby Chicken with Asparagus Sauce...189

Greek-Style Chicken with Potatoes 189

Chicken Stroganoff with Fetucini..190

Tuscany-Style Turkey Soup..190

Turkey and Brown Rice Salad with Peanuts...191

Rice, Grains & Pasta

Indian-Style Beef with Rice..192

Creamed Kale Parmesan Farro 192

Veggie Quinoa Bowls with Pesto...193

Shrimp Risotto with Vegetables 193

Baked Garbanzo Beans and Pancetta..194

Black Beans Tacos...194

Herby Millet with Cherry Tomatoes..194

Spicy Lentils with Chorizo...195

Red Lentil and Spinach Dhal...195

Parsley-Lime Bulgur Bowl...196

Spinach and Kidney Bean Stew...196

Tri-Color Quinoa and Pinto Bean Bowl...196

Simple Brown Rice..197

Creamy Grana Padano Risotto..197

Lemony Wild Rice Pilaf..198

Rice Pilaf with Mushrooms..198

Quinoa with Carrots and Onion..198

Three-Bean Veggie Chili..199

Black-Eyed Peas with Kale...199

Easy Vegan Sloppy Joes..200

Indian Yellow Lentils..200

Cherry Tomato-Basil Linguine..200

South American Black Bean Chili 201

Spicy Pinto Bean and Corn Stew...201

Simple Jasmine Rice...202

Chili-Garlic Rice Noodles with Tofu...202

Rigatoni with Sausage and Spinach 202

Chicken and Chickpea Stew...203

Shrimp Lo Mein 203

Beef-Stuffed Pasta Shells..204

Turkey Fajita Tortiglioni...204

Chipotle Mac and Cheese 205

Chicken Ragù Bolognese 205

Pasta Caprese Ricotta-Basil Fusilli...206

Cheese and Spinach Stuffed Shells 206

Pomodoro Sauce with Rigatoni and Kale...207

Pork Spaghetti with Spinach and Tomatoes 207

Beef, Pork & Lamb

Ground Beef Stuffed Empanadas 208

Smoky Horseradish Spare Ribs 208

Teriyaki Pork Noodles 209

Greek Beef Gyros 209

Sweet Gingery Beef and Broccoli 210

Bolognese-Style Pizza 210

Juicy Barbecue Pork Chops...211

Baked Rigatoni with Beef Tomato Sauce..211

Honey Short Ribs with Rosemary Potatoes 212

Thai Roasted Beef..212

Steak and Chips...213

Sticky BBQ Baby Back Ribs 213

Winter Pot Roast with Biscuits...214

Beef Carnitas...214

Classic Carbonnade Flamande 215

Sausage with Noodles and Braised Cabbage 216

Ragu with Pork and Rigatoni..216

Beef and Broccoli Sauce 217

Chorizo Stuffed Yellow Bell Peppers..218

Calzones with Sausage and Mozzarella...218

Sweet Potato Gratin with Peas and Bacon 219

Peanut Sauce Beef Satay 220

Beef and Pepperoncini Peppers...220

Chunky Pork Meatloaf with Mashed Potatoes...221

Short Ribs with Egg Noodles 222

Beef and Cabbage Stew..222

Cheeseburgers in Hoagies..223

Herbed Lamb Chops..223

Beef and Bell Pepper with Onion Sauce...224

Beef Soup with Tortillas 224

Asian Beef Curry 225

Beef and Green Bell Pepper Pot 226

Classic Beef Bourguignon 226

Beef and Cheese Stuffed Mushrooms 227

Pot Roast with Broccoli 227

Beef Stew with Beer 228

Meatballs with Spaqhuetti Sauce 228

Cheddar Cheeseburgers 229

Beef Roast with Peanut Satay Sauce 229

Spiced Beef Chili 230

Beef and Vegetable Stew 230

Beef and Garbanzo Bean Chili 231

Chipotle Beef Brisket 231

Beef Bourguignon 232

Beef and Cherry Tagine 232

Beef and Bacon Chili 233

Beef and Pumpkin Stew 233

Caribbean Ropa Vieja 234

Beef Pho with Swiss Chard 234

Brisket Chili con Carne 235

Meatballs with Marinara Sauce 235

Beer-Braised Short Ribs with Mushrooms 236

Beef and Turnip Chili 236

Italian-Style Pot Roast 237

Mississippi Pot Roast with Potatoes 237

Traditional Beef Stroganoff 238

Beef Stew with Veggies 238

Meatloaf and Cheesy Mashed Potatoes 239

Spiced Beef Shapes 239

BBQ Sticky Baby Back Ribs with 240

Apple and Onion Topped Pork Chops 240

Swedish Meatballs with Mashed Cauliflower 241

Peppercorn Meatloaf 241

Braised Short Ribs with Creamy Sauce 242

Italian Beef Sandwiches with Pesto 242

Short Ribs with Mushroom and Asparagus Sauce 243

The Crispiest Roast Pork 243

Pork Tenderloin with Sweet Pepper Sauce & Potatoes 244

Philippine-Style Pork Chops..244

Honey Barbecue Pork Ribs..245

Char Siew Pork Ribs...245

Crunchy Cashew Lamb Rack...245

Pork Chops with Cremini Mushroom Sauce...246

Ranch Flavored Pork Roast with Gravy..246

Sweet-Garlic Pork Tenderloin...247

Pork Tenderloin with Garlic and Ginger...247

Pork Sandwiches with Slaw...248

BBQ Pork Ribs..248

Italian Sausage with Potato Mash & Onion Gravy..249

Mediterranean Tender Pork Roast...249

Garlicky Braised Pork Neck Bones...250

Hot Pork Carnitas Lettuce Cups...250

Tomatillo & Sweet Potato pork Chili...251

Garlick & Ginger Pork with Coconut Sauce...252

Savory Pork Loin with Carrot & Celery Sauce..252

Spicy Pork Roast with Peanut Sauce..253

Tasty Ham with Collard Greens...253

Pulled Pork Tacos..254

Pork Chops with Broccoli and Gravy...254

Cuban-Style Pork...255

Baby Back Ribs with BBQ Sauce...255

Italian Sausage and Cannellini Stew..256

Red Pork and Chickpea Stew..256

Ranch Pork with Mushroom Sauce..256

Beer-Braised Hot Dogs with Peppers...257

Pork Chops with Plum Sauce..257

Holiday Honey-Glazed Ham...258

Jamaican Pulled Pork with Mango Sauce...258

Crispy Pork Fajitas...259

Sweet and Sour Pork..259

Sausage with Celeriac & Potato Mash..260

Pork Carnitas Wraps..260

Holiday Apricot-Lemon Ham...261

Pork Chops with Squash Purée & Mushroom Gravy...261

Lamb Chops and Creamy Potato Mash..262

Desserts & Beverages

Wheat Flour Cinnamon Balls...263

White Filling Coconut and Oat Cookies..263

Apple Vanilla Hand Pies..264

Raspberry Crumble..264

Simple Vanilla Cheesecake..265

Dark Chocolate Brownies..265

Mixed Berry Cobbler...266

Chocolate Vanilla Swirl Cheesecake...266

Vanilla Hot Lava Cake...267

Raspberry Cream Tart...268

Classic Caramel-Walnut Brownies...268

Tasty Créme Brulee...269

Strawberry & Lemon Ricotta Cheesecake...270

Cheat Apple Pie...270

Berry Vanilla Pudding...271

Cinnamon Apple Crisp..271

New York Cheesecake..272

White Chocolate Chip Cookies...272

Holiday Cranberry Cheesecake...273

Blueberry Muffins...273

Pumpkin Cake...274

Lemon Cheesecake with Strawberries...274

The Most Chocolaty Fudge..275

No Flour Lime Muffins..275

Molten Lava Cake..276

Air Fried Doughnuts...276

Air Fried Snickerdoodle Poppers..276

Pineapple Cake..277

Chocolate Soufflé...277

Cinnamon Mulled Red Wine...277

Homemade Apple Cider..278

Valencian Horchata...278

Moon Milk..278

Almond Milk...279

Tiramisu Cheesecake...279

Chocolate and Banana Squares...280

Coconut Pear Delight..280

Raspberry Cheesecake...280

Lemon & Blueberries Compote 281

Tasty Coconut Cake 281

Brown Sugar & Butter Bars 281

Milk Dumplings in Sweet Sauce 282

Poached Peaches 282

Ninja Pear Wedges 282

Almond and Apple Delight 283

Ninja Cherry Pie 283

Cinnamon Butternut Squash Pie 283

Gingery Chocolate Pudding 284

Orange Banana Bread 284

Delicious Pecan Stuffed Apples 284

Fruity Sauce..285

Savory Peaches with Chocolate Biscuits 285

Vanilla Chocolate Spread 285

Apricots with Honey Sauce 286

Coconut Milk Crème Caramel 286

Chocolate Fondue 286

Homemade Egg Custard 287

Almond Banana Dessert 287

INTRODUCTION

Hello…and welcome to my book about the Ninja Foodi. Let me share all my favorite and amazing recipes with you, so you can make delicious and scrumptious meals for your family and friends. I'll also let you know what the Ninja Foodi is all about, so you can see how easy it is to use.

Let me start by saying that I love the Ninja Foodi! This is the one kitchen tool I can't live without. I used to make meals for my family just because I needed to put something on the table. Now I make great and stunning meals because I'm love in again with cooking for my family.

I've perfected the art of using the Ninja Foodi…and now I'm sharing it all with you in my Ninja Foodi recipe book. The Ninja is a more than just a pressure cooker and air fryer combo. It elevates foods in ways you never imagined.

I've created recipes for every meal and occasion…all the way from breakfast to comforting weeknight dinners to elaborate Sunday dinners when you want to impress family and friends. I've got a recipe for you for all cuisines – fried chicken, stews, soups, and casseroles. And then there's those sweets and desserts that make the perfect finish to any meal. All here for you in one collection of my best recipes.

Just use the Ninja Foodi once and you'll be hooked. You'll never go back to cooking food in the oven or on the stovetop ever again.

Before you get your Ninja ready to start cooking, let's find out what the Ninja Foodi all about. …

MY TOP 5 TIPS AND TRICKS FOR YOUR NINJA FOODI!

1. Anyone can use the Ninja Foodi!

The technology of the Ninja Foodi makes this the perfect appliance for anyone to use…no matter how much you or your family think you can't cook! There are just three little things you need to do:

- Choose one of my amazing recipes.
- Gather the ingredients and get them all prepped.
- Put the ingredients into the Ninja Foodi – choose one of the multiple settings…and walk away until you hear the timer.

2. Forget to take the meat out of the freezer…no problem!

Did you forget to take dinner out of the freezer, so it can thaw in time for tonight's dinner? No problem at all. The Ninja Foodi takes frozen meats, such as chicken, and quickly pressure cooks it to defrost and cook at the same time. Then just use the crisping lid to add a nice brown finish…and dinner is served!

3. Rice is nice

You may think that sticking to your old way of cooking rice on the stovetop is faster and easier than using the Ninja Foodi. You'll want to rethink that old cooking method! Not only is using the Ninja faster and easier on the cleanup, you'll never mess up rice again when you don't get the proportions of rice to water just right. The Ninja cooks rice perfectly each and every time.

4. Read the digital screen

When you're pressure cooking using the Instant Pot, you have to guess at what the pressure level is inside the pot. With the Ninja Foodi, you can use the digital screen so there's no more guessing! Make sure you take advantage of this handy little feature.

5. Use the reversable rack to make baked desserts

The Ninja Foodi is your perfect dessert-maker. Whip up the batter for a cheesecake or brownies…and layer the batter in the same pan you'd pop in the oven. But instead of using the oven, place that pan on the reversible rack that comes with the Ninja, which will hold the pan securely. Set the function to bake, and your cake will be done in no time.

WHAT IS THE NINJA FOODI?

The buzz about the Ninja Foodi is true. It uses cutting edge technology to let you air fry foods as well as get all the benefits of a pressure cooker…all in one! You're probably wondering how that can be possible - to have two very different kitchen appliances in one. It's easy. The Ninja is both because it has two lids.

The lid for the air fryer is attached to the Ninja. Using the air frying function is just as easy as pressure cooking! The lid just swings open and closed. When you're not using it, the air fryer lid is moved out of the way.

The lid of the pressure-cooking side of the Ninja is a completely separate and apart from the rest of appliance. It simply screws on the Ninja when you're using the pressure-cooking function.

It won't take you long to learn how to use the Ninja. I'll let you know how to do that a bit later. But why would you want an air fryer and pressure cooker all in one? Because the Ninja is more than just air fryer and pressure cooker! It can roast, broil, make soups and stews…and it can pressure cook and fry as well.

Having this one amazing appliance means you can get rid of your pressure cooker, instant pot, dehydrator, roasting pan, and slow cooker. Just think of all the kitchen space you'll have when you just have one appliance, the Ninja Foodi, doing all the cooking for you.

Let's look a closer look at all the benefits of owning a Ninja Foodi.

BENEFITS OF USING THE NINJA FOODI

It's a two in one appliance

I can't say it enough, the convenience of having an air fryer and pressure cooker in one appliance makes your life a breeze. And all those added features the Ninja has makes it even better. How many times have you tried to get the Instant Pot of the kitchen appliance cupboard, only to have to move the slow cooker and the pressure cooker out of the way. It's happened to me too many times to count! With the Ninja, you can retire those other appliances and free up valuable space in your kitchen

Get rid of other cookbooks

Meal planning is so much easier with the Ninja Foodi. You don't have to look through three different cookbooks to find the recipe you want to use – Instant Pot, or maybe it's the slow cooker this time? Now you can use just one set of recipes…my own recipes that let you use the Ninja for every meal.

Prepare meals ahead of time

We all lead busy lives. The Ninja Foodi lets you prepare food ahead of time – when you have the time and not when you're under pressure to get dinner on the table. Prep in the morning or the night before. Just follow one of my recipes and get all the ingredients ready to go. If you're using the pressure cooker or slow cooker function, just put the ingredients into the Ninja, set to the right time, and dinner cooks on its own. Or have all the ingredients in the fridge, ready to go for when you arrive home at the end of the day.

Prepare budget-friendly and healthy meals

Eating meat every day can get expensive. When you have the Ninja Foodi, you can make delicious meals using lentil and beans. I use these ingredients in many of my recipes – and my meals are never dull or boring. The Ninja also lets you cook cheaper cuts of meat to perfection. When you pressure cook a beef shank it comes out tender and juicy, cooked with sealed in moisture that you don't get when you cook it any other way.

Skip the fats and oils

It's all about frying with the Ninja Foodi – air frying that is. This means you can enjoy the taste and convenience of fried foods without using all that oil. This is perfect if you're watching what you eat – and trying to eat healthier. Foods are cooked in added liquid, or in their own juices, staying moist and delicious.

Cooks faster than the slow cooker

With the slow cooker, beans take from 4 to 5 hours cook. With the Ninja Foodi, you can get that time down to under 30 with the pressure cooker. And that includes the time it takes for the Ninja to get the pressure up to the right level! What does this mean for you? Simple – you can come home and have a bean soup or stew on the table in no time at all.

Add a crispy finish to pressure cooked foods

One of the biggest benefits of the Ninja Foodi, and one of my personal favorites, the finishing touches you can add to food before you serve it. When you cook some foods in the pressure cooker it can be hard to get a nice crispy finish after it's been cooked. Now, with the Ninja, once you've pressure cooked a whole chicken, you can just remove the liquid and turn on the crisping function. The chicken skin is nicely crisped up, making for a great meal that's sure to impress your family.

USING THE NINJA FOODI

When you first get your Ninja Foodi, it can look a little intimidating with all those functions and buttons to press. I certainly felt that way. But trust me…it won't take you long to get the hang of using the Ninja. Let's take a quick look at the basics of using the Ninja Foodi

Easy to read display

The display on the Ninja Foodi is easy to read. All of the functions are there for you to just press and set. You'll also be able to select temperature and time controls, as well as a start and stop button. As I said, don't let all these buttons make you think you'll never learn how to use the Ninja. The learning curve is fast – after making just one of my recipes you'll know what you're doing.

Pressure cooking

When you use the lid for the pressure cooker, you'll be able to cook all kinds of foods at a low or high pressure. Just set the timer for one minute increments all the way up to one hour. After an hour, you'll be able to up the time in five minute increments and cook all the way to four hours for some foods, such as cheaper cuts of meat. Make sure to try one of my recipes for pressure cooked vegetables…. or for cheesecake!

Air crisping

The air crisp setting uses the lid for air-frying. Set the temperature to cook between 300 to 400 degrees Fahrenheit. For this function, set the timer for two minute increments all the way to one hour. Many of my recipes use this function. You'll be cooking fries and chicken to perfection in no time at all.

Baking and roasting

This is another setting that uses the air-frying lid. And it's just the same as using your oven to bake and roast meats, fish, and any other food that needs baking. I like this setting when I have a bit more time to cook – it's ideal for using on weekends.

Slow cooker

You're never going to use your slow cooker again after you use this function on the Ninja Foodi. After putting all the ingredients in the Ninja, seal the pressure lid in the venting position. Then just use the Ninja the same as you would with the slow cooker, cooking foods for up to 12 hours. I like this function when I want to have the Ninja Foodi cook dinner for me overnight. It's perfect for chili or beef stew.

Steaming

Steaming fish and veggies is a breeze with the Ninja Foodi. And the great thing is that there will be no more over-steaming, causing foods to be limp and tasteless. The Ninja uses the pressure lid to steam veggies and other foods so they're tender, but still crisp and flavorful.

Sauté and sear

I use the sauté and sear function for many of my favorite recipes. This setting lets you brown and sear foods before or after cooking them. After browning foods, you can add a bit of liquid, as per my recipes, and make some great tasting gravies. Sautéing foods in the Ninja Foodi is just like sautéing them on your stovetop.

Easy cleanup

Cleanup takes no time! Once food is cooked, and the Ninja Foodi has cooled down, it's just a matter of cleaning the ceramic, non-stick pot in warm soapy water.

NINJA FOODI RECIPES

The recipes in this book are my absolute favorite…and they're a great introduction to the Ninja Foodi, highlighting just what this amazing kitchen tool can do for you.

Before you start cooking, here's some valuable information for using my recipes in the Ninja Foodi.

Brown and sear some food before putting into the Ninja Foodi

Follow my recipes…in some of them I'll have you brown or sear some of the ingredients, particularly meats, before you start the cooking process. This is so that the juices are sealed into the food, making it cook up that much more tender.

Check some foods to avoid over-cooking

Some foods are easy to over-cook, such as baked foods. In my recipes, I'll remind you if you need to check to avoid over-cooking.

Pat dry some fruits and vegetables

Some foods, such as fruits and vegetables, need to be patted dry before you put them into the Cook and Crisp basket. This is to ensure that they don't get soggy!

Adding Ingredients at the end of cooking time

When layering food in the Ninja Foodi, lay them flat and close together so that you make the most of the space in the pot. I'll guide you in my recipes when there are any foods that shouldn't be stacked or overlapped.

Use hot water when pressure cooking

If you add a tablespoon or two of hot water when you're using the pressure cooker, the pressure will build up faster.

The broil function is great for finishing off meals

Many of my recipes use the broil setting to finish off foods and give them a nice, lovely crispy topping. Remember to check during the cooking process to see how the crisp the food is getting – you don't want to over-crisp!

Adjusting cooking time

If you're using fewer ingredients then my recipe calls for, remember to adjust the cooking time to a little less. The same goes if you're using more ingredients than my recipe calls for…adjust so the Ninja Foodi cooks a little longer. Just be sure to check near the end of cooking time to see if needs to cook longer.

From slow cooker to Ninja Foodi

Foods cooked in a slow cooker for 4 hours on high, can be quickly cooked in the Ninja Foodi for only 25 to 30 minutes! Follow my recipe…I might have you add a bit more liquid than if you were cooking in a slow cooker.

As you can see, the Ninja Foodi is just what you need in your life. You'll be cooking exceptional meals in no time! I hope you enjoy my favorite recipes…these are the ones I make over and over again for my family and friends. It's time to choose your first recipe…and get your Ninja Foodi cooking great food!

BREAKFAST

Cheesy Prosciutto Egg Bake

Servings: 4 | Ready in about: 45 min

INGREDIENTS

4 eggs
1 cup whole milk
1 teaspoon salt
1 teaspoon freshly ground black pepper

1 cup shredded Monterey Jack cheese
1 orange bell pepper, seeded and chopped
8 ounces prosciutto, chopped
1 cup water

DIRECTIONS

Break the eggs into a bowl, pour in the milk, salt, and black pepper and whisk until combined. Stir in the Monterey Jack Cheese.

Put the bell pepper and prosciutto in the cake pan. Then, pour over the egg mixture, cover the pan with aluminum foil and put on the reversible rack.

Put the rack in the pot and pour in the water.

Seal the pressure lid, choose pressure and set to High. Set the time to 20 minutes and choose Start/Stop.

When done cooking, do a quick pressure release and carefully remove the lid that is after the pressure has completely escaped.

When baking is complete, take the pan out of the pot and set it on a heatproof surface, and cool for 5 minutes.

Crispy Pancetta Hash with Baked Eggs

Servings: 4 | Ready in about: 50 min

INGREDIENTS

6 slices pancetta, chopped
1 white onion, diced
2 potatoes, peeled and diced
1 teaspoon sweet paprika

1 teaspoon salt
1 teaspoon freshly ground black pepper
1 teaspoon garlic powder
4 eggs

DIRECTIONS

Choose Sear/Sauté, set to Medium High, and choose Start/Stop to preheat the pot for 5 minutes.

Once heated, lay the pancetta in the pot, and cook, stirring occasionally, for 5 minutes, or until the pancetta is crispy.

Stir in the onion, potatoes, sweet paprika, salt, black pepper, and garlic powder.

Close the crisping lid; choose Bake/Roast, set the temperature to 350°F, and the time to 25 minutes. Cook until the turnips are soft and golden brown while stirring occasionally.

Crack the eggs on top of the hash, close the crisping lid, and choose Bake/Roast. Set the temperature to 350°F, and the time to 10 minutes.

Cook the eggs and check two or three times until your desired crispiness has been achieved. Serve immediately.

Strawberry Bread French Toast

Servings: 4 | Ready in about: 45 min

INGREDIENTS

3 eggs

¼ cup milk

1 tablespoon sugar

1 teaspoon vanilla extract

1 teaspoon cinnamon powder

Cooking spray

6 slices brioche, cubed

3 strawberries, sliced, divided

2 tablespoons brown sugar, divided

¼ cup ricotta cheese, at room temperature

½ cup water

2 tablespoons firm unsalted butter, sliced

¼ cup chopped almonds

2 tablespoons maple syrup

DIRECTIONS

Crack the eggs into a bowl and whisk with the milk, sugar, vanilla, and cinnamon. Set aside.

Grease a baking dish with cooking spray and in a single layer, spread half of the brioche cubes in the pan. Layer half of the strawberry slices on the bread and dust with 1 tablespoon of brown sugar.

Spoon and spread the ricotta cheese on top of the strawberries. Then, make another layer of bread, strawberries, brown sugar, and ricotta cheese.

Pour the egg mixture all over the layered ingredients ensuring to give the bread a good coat.

Next, pour the water into the pot. Fix the pan on the reversible rack, and put the rack with a pan in the pot.

Seal the pressure lid, choose Pressure , set to High, set the timer to 20 minutes, and choose Start/Stop to begin toasting.

Once the timer has read to the end, perform a quick pressure release to let all the pressure out, and carefully open the lid.

Top the French toast with the sliced butter, almonds, and maple syrup. Close the crisping lid; choose Bake/Roast, set the temperature to 390°F, and set the time to 5 minutes.

Check the toast's doneness for your desired crispiness, otherwise, cook for a few more minutes. Serve immediately.

Raspberry-Cranberry Chia Oatmeal

Servings: 4 | Ready in about: 30 min

INGREDIENTS

2 cups old fashioned oatmeal

3¾ cups water

¼ cup plain vinegar

½ teaspoon nutmeg powder

1 tablespoon cinnamon powder

½ teaspoon vanilla extract

½ cup dried cranberries, plus more for garnish

2 raspberries, sliced

⅛ teaspoon salt

Honey, for topping

DIRECTIONS

Combine the oatmeal, water, vinegar, nutmeg, cinnamon, vanilla, cranberries, raspberries, and salt in the pot. Seal the pressure lid, hit Pressure, set to High, and set the timer to 11 minutes. Press Start/Stop to start cooking the oats.

When the timer has ended, perform a natural pressure release for 10 minutes, then a quick pressure release to let off any remaining pressure, and carefully open the lid.

Stir the oatmeal, drizzle with honey and more dried cranberries, and serve immediately.

Sausage Wrapped Scotch Eggs

Servings: 4 | Ready in about: 55 min

INGREDIENTS

1 cup water
4 eggs
Nonstick cooking spray, for preparing the rack

12 ounces Italian sausage patties
1 cup panko bread crumbs
2 tablespoons melted unsalted butter

DIRECTIONS

Pour 1 cup of water into the inner pot. Put the reversible rack in the pot at the bottom, and carefully place the eggs on top.

Seal the pressure lid, choose Pressure, set the pressure to High, and the cook time to 3 minutes. Press Start.

While cooking the eggs, fill half a bowl with cold water and about a cup full of ice cubes to make an ice bath.

After cooking, perform a quick pressure release, and carefully open the lid.

Use tongs to pick up the eggs into the ice bath. Allow cooling for 3 to 4 minutes; peel the eggs.

Pour the water out of the inner pot and return the pot to the base. Grease the reversible rack with cooking spray, fix the rack in the upper position, and place in the pot.

Cover the crisping lid; choose Air Crisp, set the temperature to 360°F and the timer to 4 minutes. Press Start to preheat.

While preheating the pot, place an egg on each sausage patty. Pull the sausage around the egg and seal the edges.

In a small bowl, mix the breadcrumbs with the melted butter. One at a time, dredge the sausage-covered eggs in the crumbs while pressing into the breadcrumbs for a thorough coat.

Open the crisping lid and place the eggs on the rack. Close the crisping lid; choose Air Crisp, adjust the temperature to 360°F, and the cook time to 15 minutes. Press Start.

When the timer has ended, the crumbs should be crisp and a deep golden brown color. Remove the eggs and allow cooling for several minutes. Slice the eggs in half and serve.

Spicy Deviled Eggs

Servings: 6 | Ready in about: 20 min

INGREDIENTS

1 cup water
10 large eggs
¼ cup cream cheese

¼ cup mayonnaise
salt and ground black pepper to taste
¼ tsp chili powder

DIRECTIONS

Add water to the Foodi's pot. Insert the eggs into the steamer basket; place into the pot.

Seal the pressure lid, choose Pressure, set to High, and set the timer to 5 minutes. Press Start.

When ready, release the pressure quickly.

Drop eggs into an ice bath to cool for 5 minutes. Press Start. Peel eggs and halve them.

Transfer yolks to a bowl and use a fork to mash; stir in cream cheese, and mayonnaise. Add pepper and salt for seasoning. Ladle yolk mixture into egg white halves.

Shakshuka with Goat Cheese

Servings: 4 | Ready in about: 50 min

INGREDIENTS

3 tablespoons ghee
1 small red onion, chopped
½ red bell pepper, seeded and chopped
1 medium banana pepper, seeded and minced
2 garlic cloves, chopped
1 teaspoon salt
2 (14.5-ounce) cans diced tomatoes with their juice

½ tsp coriander, ground
½ tsp smoked paprika
½ teaspoon red chili flakes
¼ tsp black pepper, freshly ground
4 eggs
⅓ cup crumbled goat cheese
2 tbsp fresh cilantro, chopped

DIRECTIONS

Choose Sear/Sauté on you Foodi and set on Medium to preheat the inner pot; press Start.

Melt the ghee and sauté the onion, bell pepper, banana pepper, and garlic. Season lightly with salt and cook for 2 minutes until the vegetables are fragrant and beginning to soften.

Then, stir in the tomatoes, coriander, smoked paprika, red chili flakes, and black pepper.

Seal the pressure lid, choose pressure and adjust the pressure to High and the timer to 4 minutes. Press Start to continue cooking.

When the timer has read to the end, perform a quick pressure release. Gently crack the eggs onto the tomato sauce in different areas. Seal the pressure lid again, but with the valve set to Vent. Choose Steam and adjust the cook time to 3 minutes. Press Start to cook the eggs.

When ready, carefully open the pressure lid. Sprinkle with the shakshuka with goat cheese and cilantro. Dish into a serving platter and serve.

Kale-Egg Frittata

Servings: 6 | Ready in about: 20 min

INGREDIENTS

6 large eggs
2 tbsp heavy cream
½ tsp freshly grated nutmeg
Salt and black pepper to taste

1 ½ cups kale, chopped
¼ cup grated Parmesan cheese
cooking spray
1 cup water

DIRECTIONS

In a bowl, beat eggs, nutmeg, pepper, salt, and cream until smooth; stir in Parmesan cheese and kale.

Apply a cooking spray to a cake pan. Wrap aluminum foil around outside of the pan to cover completely.

Place egg mixture into the prepared pan. Add water into the pot of your Foodi. Set your Foodi's reversible rack over the water. Gently lay the pan onto the reversible rack.

Seal the pressure lid, choose Pressure, set to High, and set the timer to 10 minutes. Press Start.

When ready, release the pressure quickly.

Savory Custards with Ham and Emmental Cheese

Servings: 4 | Ready in about: 40 min

INGREDIENTS

2 serrano ham slices, halved widthwise
4 large eggs
1 ounce cottage cheese, at room temperature
¼ cup half and half

¼ teaspoon salt
Ground black pepper to taste
¼ cup grated Emmental cheese
¼ cup caramelized white onions

DIRECTIONS

Preheat the inner pot by choosing Sear/Sauté and adjust to Medium; press Start. Put the serrano ham in the pot and cook for 3 to 4 minutes or until browned, turning occasionally.

Remove the ham onto a paper towel-lined plate. Next, use a brush to coat the inside of four 1- cup ramekins with the ham fat. Set the cups aside, then, empty and wipe out the inner pot with a paper towel, and return the pot to the base.

Crack the eggs into a bowl and add the cottage cheese, half and half, salt, and several grinds of black pepper. Use a hand mixer to whisk the ingredients until co cheese lumps remain.

Stir in the grated emmental cheese and mix again to incorporate the cheese.

Lay a piece of ham in the bottom of each custard cup. Evenly share the onions among the cups as well as the egg mixture. Cover each cup with aluminum foil.

Pour 1 cup of water into the inner pot and fix the reversible rack in the pot. Arrange the ramekins on top. Lock the pressure lid in Seal position; choose Pressure, adjust to High, and set the timer to 7 minutes. Press Start.

After cooking, perform a quick pressure release. Use tongs to remove the custard cups from the pressure cooker. Cool for 1 to 2 minutes before serving.

Butternut Squash Cake Oatmeal

Servings: 4 | Ready in about: 35 min

INGREDIENTS

3 ½ cups coconut milk
1 cup steel-cut oats
1 cup shredded Butternut Squash
½ cup sultanas
⅓ cup honey
1 tsp ground cinnamon

¾ tsp ground ginger
½ tsp salt
½ tsp fresh orange zest
¼ tsp ground nutmeg
¼ cup toasted walnuts, chopped
½ tsp vanilla extract

DIRECTIONS

In the pressure cooker, mix sultanas, orange zest, ginger, milk, honey, squash, salt, oats, and nutmeg.

Seal the pressure lid, choose Pressure, set to High, and set the timer to 12 minutes; press Start. When ready, do a natural pressure release for 10 minutes.

Into the oatmeal, stir in the vanilla extract and sugar.

Top with walnuts and serve.

Egg Crumpet Sandwich

Servings: 2 | Ready in about: 25 min

INGREDIENTS

2 tablespoons butter
2 tablespoons chopped bacon
2 eggs, large
¼ tsp salt

Black pepper to taste
2 tbsp Monterey Jack cheese, grated
2 crumpets, split

DIRECTIONS

Brush two cups with 1 tbsp of butter. Share the bacon into the cups, crack an egg into each one, and prick the egg yolks with a toothpick in different places.

Sprinkle the top with salt and black pepper and divide the cheese on top to cover the eggs. Cover the cups with aluminium foil and crimp the sides down.

Pour 1 cup of water into the pot, fix the reversible rack at the bottom the pot, and arrange the cups on top.

Seal the pressure lid, select Pressure; adjust the pressure to High, and the cook time to 1 minute; press Start.

When done cooking, perform a quick pressure release, and carefully open the lid. Remove the rack and cups without taking off the foil.

Empty the water from the inner pot and return the pot to the base. Use tongs to lift the cups into the bottom of the pot and fix the reversible rack in the upper position of the pot.

Cover the crisping lid, choose Broil and adjust the time to 2 minutes; press Start.

While heating, spread the remaining butter over the crumpet halves.

Open the crisping lid, arrange the crumpet halves on the rack with the buttered-side up, and close the lid. Choose Broil again and adjust the cooking time to 4 minutes; press Start

When the crumpets are ready, transfer to a cutting board, and remove the cups with tongs.

Run a butter knife in and around the cups and turn out each egg onto the lower half of each crumpet. Top with the other half and serve.

Herbed Homemade Ghee

Servings: 10 | Ready in about: 17 min

INGREDIENTS

8 ounces unsalted butter, softened
2 tbsp parsley, minced

1tbsp fresh chives, chopped
Sea salt to taste

DIRECTIONS

Set your Foodi to Sear/Sauté, set to Medium High, and choose Start/Stop to preheat the pot. Melt butter and cook for 7 to 9 minutes as you stir in cycles of 3 minutes until browning.

Select Start/Stop and allow the butter to slightly cool.

Use cheesecloth to strain the butter into a sealable container. Add the parsley, chives, and salt and combine thoroughly.

Let cool before closing the lid. Keep in the fridge until ready to use.

Orange Pepper and Artichoke Frittata

Servings: 4 | Ready in about: 60 min

INGREDIENTS

2 tablespoons unsalted butter
½ small red onion, chopped
¼ large orange bell pepper, chopped
1 cup coarsely chopped artichoke hearts
8 large eggs

½ teaspoon salt
¼ cup full cream milk
¾ cup shredded Colby cheese, divided
¼ cup grated Pecorino Romano or similar cheese
¼ teaspoon freshly ground black pepper

DIRECTIONS

On your Foodi, press Sear/Sauté and adjust to Medium-High; press Start. Melt the butter and sauté the onion, bell pepper, and artichoke hearts in the butter. Cook for 5 minutes or until the onion and pepper are soft.

While the vegetables soften, whisk the eggs with salt and allow sitting for 1 minute. Pour the milk into the eggs and whisk again then stir ½ cup of colby cheese into the mixture.

When the vegetables are cooked, pour the egg mixture into the pot. Gently stir to distribute the vegetables evenly. Reduce the heat to Medium and cook the eggs, undisturbed, until the edges are set about 7 to 9 minutes.

Press Stop to cancel the Sear/Sauté function. Then, run a silicone spatula around the edges of the frittata to loosen from the side of the pot.

Close the crisping lid; choose Bake/Roast and set the temperature to 370 F, and the cook time to 3 minutes. Press Start to begin baking.

After 1 minute, open the lid and sprinkle the remaining ¼ cup of Colby and the Pecorino Romano cheese over the frittata. Close the lid and cook for the remaining 2 minutes.

Open the lid by which time the cheese should have melted and the top not browned, but set. Sprinkle the frittata with black pepper, let rest for 2 minutes, and slice into wedges, to serve.

Barbecue Chicken Sandwiches

Servings: 4 | Ready in about: 45 min

INGREDIENTS

4 chicken thighs, boneless and skinless
Salt to taste
2 cups barbecue sauce
1 onion, minced
2 garlic cloves, minced

2 tbsp minced fresh parsley
1 tbsp lemon juice
1 tbsp mayonnaise
1½ cups iceberg lettuce, shredded
4 burger buns

DIRECTIONS

Season the chicken with salt, and transfer into the inner pot. Add in garlic, onion and barbeque sauce. Coat the chicken by turning in the sauce.

Seal the pressure lid, choose Pressure, set to High, and set the timer to 15 minutes. Press Start.

When ready, do a natural pressure release for 10 minutes. Use two forks to shred the chicken and mix into the sauce. Press Sear/Sauté and let the mixture to simmer for 15 minutes to thicken the sauce, until desired consistency.

Meanwhile, using a large bowl, mix the lemon juice, mayonnaise, salt, and parsley; toss lettuce into the mixture to coat. Separate the chicken in equal parts to match the sandwich buns; apply lettuce for topping and complete the sandwiches.

Plum Breakfast Clafoutis

Servings: 4 | Ready in about: 60 min

INGREDIENTS

2 teaspoons butter, softened
1 cup plums, chopped
⅔ cup whole milk
⅓ cup half and half
⅓ cup sugar
½ cup flour

2 large eggs
¼ teaspoon cinnamon
½ teaspoon vanilla extract
A pinch of salt
2 tablespoons confectioners' sugar

DIRECTIONS

Grease four ramekins with the butter and divide the plums into each cup.

Pour the milk, half and half, sugar, flour, eggs, cinnamon, vanilla, and salt in a bowl and use a hand mixer to whisk the ingredients on medium speed until the batter is smooth, about 2 minutes. Pour the batter over the plums two-third way up.

Pour 1 cup of water into the inner pot. Fix the reversible rack at the bottom of the pot and put the ramekins on the rack. Lay a square of aluminium foil on the ramekins but don't crimp.

Put the pressure lid together and lock in Seal position. Choose Pressure, set to high, and set the time to 11 minutes; press Start.

When ready, perform a quick pressure release and carefully open the lid. Use tongs to remove the foil. Close the crisping lid and choose Bake/Roast. Adjust the temperature to 400°F and the time to 6 minutes. Press Start to brown the top of the clafoutis.

Check after about 4 minutes to ensure the clafoutis are lightly browned; otherwise bake for a few more minutes. Remove the ramekins onto a flat surface. Cool for 5 minutes, and then dust with the confectioners' sugar. Serve warm.

Chai Latte Steel-Cut Oatmeal

Servings: 4 | Ready in about: 20 min

INGREDIENTS

3 ½ cups milk
½ cup raw peanuts
1 cup steel-cut oats
¼ cup agave syrup
1 tsp coffee
1½ tsp ground ginger

1¼ tsp ground cinnamon
½ tsp salt
¼ tsp ground allspice
¼ tsp ground cardamom
1 tsp vanilla extract

DIRECTIONS

Using an immersion blender, puree peanuts and milk to obtain smooth consistency; transfer into the cooker pot.

To the peanuts-milk mixture, add agave syrup, oats, ginger, allspice, cinnamon, salt, cardamom, tea leaves, and cloves to mix well. Seal the pressure lid, choose Pressure, set to High, and set the timer to 12 minutes. Press Start.

Let pressure to release naturally on completing the cooking cycle. Add vanilla extract to the oatmeal and stir well before serving.

French Dip Sandwiches

Servings: 8 | Ready in about: 1 hr 35 min

INGREDIENTS

2 ½ pounds beef roast
2 tbsp olive oil
1 onion, chopped
4 garlic cloves, sliced
½ cup dry red wine

2 cups beef broth stock
1 tsp dried oregano
16 slices Fontina cheese
8 split hoagie rolls

DIRECTIONS

Generously apply pepper and salt to the beef for seasoning.

Warm oil on Sear/Sauté and brown the beef for 2 to 3 minutes per side. Set aside on a plate.

Add onions and cook for 3 minutes, until translucent. Mix in garlic and cook for one a minute until soft.

To the Foodi, add red wine to deglaze. Scrape the cooking surface to remove any browned sections of the food using a wooden spoon's flat edge; mix in beef broth and take back the juices and beef to your pressure cooker. Over the meat, scatter some oregano.

Seal the pressure lid, choose Pressure, set to High, and set the timer to 50 minutes; press Start. Release pressure naturally for around 10 minutes. Transfer the beef to a cutting board and slice.

Roll the sliced beef and add a topping of onions. Each sandwich should be topped with 2 slices fontina cheese.

Place the sandwiches in the pot, close the crisping lid and select Air Crisp. Adjust the temperature to 360°F and the time to 3 minutes. Press Start.

When cooking is complete, the cheese should be cheese melt.

Cheese & Bacon Grits

Servings: 4 | Ready in about: 20 min

Ingredients:

3 slices smoked bacon, diced
1 ½ cups grated Cheddar cheese
1 cup ground Grits
2 tsp butter

Salt and black pepper
½ cup water
½ cup milk

Directions:

To preheat the Ninja Foodi, select Sear/Sauté mode and set to HIGH pressure. Cook bacon until crispy, about 5 minutes. Set aside.

Add the grits, butter, milk, water, salt, and pepper to the pot and stir using a spoon. Close the pressure lid and secure the pressure valve.

Choose the Pressure mode and cook for 3 minutes on High. Press Start/Stop.

Once the timer has ended, turn the vent handle and do a quick pressure release. Add in cheddar cheese and give the pudding a good stir with the same spoon.

Close crisping lid, press BAKE/ROAST button and cook for 8 minutes on 370 degrees F. Press Start key.

When ready, dish the cheesy grits into serving bowls and spoon over the crisped bacon.

Serve right away with toasted bread.

Feta and Poached Egg Heirloom Tomato Topper

Servings: 4 | Ready in about: 10 min

Ingredients:

4 large eggs
4 small slices feta cheese
1 cup water
2 large Heirloom ripe tomatoes, halved crosswise

Salt and black pepper to taste
1 tsp chopped fresh herbs, of your choice
2 tbsp grated Parmesan cheese
Cooking spray

Directions:

Pour the water into the Ninja Foodi and fit the reversible rack.

Grease the ramekins with the cooking spray and crack each egg into them.

Season with salt and pepper. Cover the ramekins with aluminum foil.

Place the cups on the trivet. Seal the lid.

Select Steam mode for 3 minutes on High pressure. Press Start/Stop.

Once the timer goes off, do a quick pressure release.

Use a napkin to remove the ramekins onto a flat surface.

In serving plates, share the halved tomatoes, feta slices, and toss the eggs in the ramekin over on each tomato half.

Sprinkle with salt and pepper, parmesan, and garnish with chopped herbs.

Maple Giant Pancake with Whipped Cream

Servings: 6 | Ready in about: 30 min

Ingredients:

3 cups flour
¾ cup sugar
5 eggs
⅓ cup olive oil
⅓ cup sparkling water

⅓ tsp salt
1 ½ tsp baking soda
2 tbsp maple syrup
A dollop of whipped cream to serve

Directions:

Start by pouring the flour, sugar, eggs, olive oil, sparkling water, salt, and baking soda into a food processor and blend until smooth.

Pour the batter into the Ninja Foodi and let it sit in there for 15 minutes. Close the lid and secure the pressure valve.

Select the Pressure mode on Low pressure for 10 minutes. Press Start/Stop.

Once the timer goes off, press Start/Stop, quick-release the pressure valve to let out any steam and open the lid.

Gently run a spatula around the pancake to let loose any sticking.

Once ready, slide the pancake onto a serving plate and drizzle with maple syrup. Top with the whipped cream to serve.

Sausage and Bacon Cheesecake

Servings: 6 | Ready in about: 25 min

Ingredients:

8 eggs, cracked into a bowl
8 oz breakfast sau sage, chopped
3 bacon slices, chopped
1 large green bell pepper, chopped
1 large red bell pepper, chopped
1 cup chopped green onion

1 cup grated Cheddar cheese
1 tsp red chili flakes
Salt and black pepper to taste
½ cup milk
4 slices bread, cut into ½ -inch cubes
2 cups water

Directions:

Add the eggs, sausage chorizo, bacon slices, green and red bell peppers, green onion, chili flakes, cheddar cheese, salt, pepper, and milk to a bowl and use a whisk to beat them together.

Grease a bundt pan with cooking spray and pour the egg mixture into it. After, drop the bread slices in the egg mixture all around while using a spoon to push them into the mixture.

Open the Ninja Foodi, pour in water, and fit the rack at the center of the pot. Place bundt pan on the rack and seal the pressure lid.

Select Pressure mode on High pressure for 6 minutes, and press Start/Stop.

Once the timer goes off, press Start/Stop, do a quick pressure release. Run a knife around the egg in the bundt pan, close the crisping lid and cook for another 4 minutes on Bake/Roast on 380 degrees F.

When ready, place a serving plate on the bundt pan, and then, turn the egg bundt over. Use a knife to cut the egg into slices. Serve with a sauce of your choice.

Veggie Salmon Balls

Servings: 4 | Ready in about: 40 min

Ingredients:

2 (5 oz) packs steamed salmon flakes
1 Red onion, chopped
Salt and black pepper to taste
1 tsp garlic powder
2 tbsp olive oil
1 red bell pepper, seeded and chopped
4 tbsp butter, divided

3 eggs, cracked into a bowl
1 cup breadcrumbs
4 tbsp mayonnaise
2 tsp Worcestershire sauce
¼ cup chopped parsley
3 large potatoes, cut into chips

Directions:

Turn on the Ninja Foodi and select Sear/Sauté mode on High pressure.

Heat the oil and add half of the butter. Once it has melted, add the onions and the chopped red bell peppers. Cook for 6 minutes while stirring occasionally. Press Start/Stop.

In a mixing bowl, add salmon flakes, sautéed red bell pepper and onion, breadcrumbs, eggs, mayonnaise, Worcestershire sauce, garlic powder, salt, pepper, and parsley.

Use a spoon to mix well while breaking the salmon into the tiny pieces. Use your hands to mold 4 patties out of the mixture. Add the remaining butter to melt, and when melted, add the patties. Fry for 4 minutes, flipping once.

Then, close the crisping lid, select Bake/Roast mode and bake for 4 minutes on 320 degrees F. Remove them onto a wire rack to rest. Serve the cakes with a side of lettuce and potato salad with a mild drizzle of herb vinaigrette.

Prosciutto, Mozzarella & Egg in a Cup

Servings: 2 | Ready in about: 20 min

INGREDIENTS:

2 slices bread

2 prosciutto slices, chopped

2 eggs

4 tomato slices

2 tbsp grated mozzarella

2 tbsp mayonnaise

Salt and pepper, to taste

Cooking spray

DIRECTIONS:

Preheat the Ninja Foodi to 320 degrees F. Grease two large ramekins with cooking spray.

Place one bread slice in the bottom of each ramekin. Arrange 1 prosciutto slice and 2 tomato slices on top of each bread slice. Divide the mozzarella between the ramekins.

Crack the eggs over the mozzarella. Season with salt and pepper. Close the crisping lid and cook for 10 minutes on Air Crisp mode. Top with mayonnaise.

Onion and Cheese Omelet

Servings: 1 | Ready in about: 10 min

INGREDIENTS:

2 eggs

2 tbsp grated cheddar cheese

1 tsp soy sauce

½ onion, sliced

¼ tsp pepper

1 tbsp olive oil

DIRECTIONS:

Whisk the eggs along with the pepper, onion, and soy sauce, in a bowl, until well-combined.

Grease a baking tray with olive oil and pour in the egg mixture. Close the crisping lid and cook for 5-6 minutes on Air Crisp mode at 350 F. Once the timer beeps, check to ensure the eggs have set.

Top with the grated cheddar cheese. Fold the omelet in half and serve with a green salad.

Ham and Cheese Sandwich

Servings: 1 | Ready in about: 10 min

INGREDIENTS:

2 tsp butter

2 slices of bread

2 slices of American cheese

1 slice of ham

DIRECTIONS:

Spread one teaspoon of butter on the outside of each of the bread slices.

Place one cheese slice on the inside of one bread slice, top with ham slice and another cheese slice. Cover with the second bread slice to create the sandwich.

Place into the Ninja Foodi basket, close the crisping lid and cook for 4 minutes on Air Crisp mode at 370 F. Flip the sandwich and cook for an additional 4 minutes. When the timer beeps, remove the sandwich, cut diagonally and serve immediately with ketchup or chutney.

Creamy Zucchini Muffins

Servings: 4 | Ready in about: 20 min

INGREDIENTS:

1 ½ cups flour
1 tsp cinnamon
3 eggs
2 tsp baking powder
2 tbsp sugar

1 cup milk
2 tbsp butter, melted
1 tbsp yogurt
½ cup shredded zucchini
2 tbsp cream cheese

DIRECTIONS:

In a bowl, whisk the eggs along with the sugar, a pinch of salt, cinnamon, cream cheese, sifted flour, and baking powder.

In another bowl, combine all liquid ingredients. Gently mix the dry and liquid mixtures. Stir in zucchini.

Line the muffin tins and pour in the batter. Close the crisping lid and cook for 12 minutes on Air Crisp mode at 350 F.

Once the timer beeps, check with a toothpick to ensure the muffins are set. If necessary, return them to the Ninja Foodi, and cook for 2-3 more minutes. Transfer to a cooling rack before serving. Serve with a scraping of butter.

Toasted Herb and Garlic Bagel

Servings: 1 | Ready in about: 6 min

INGREDIENTS:

2 tbsp butter, softened
1 tsp dried basil
1 tsp dried parsley
1 tsp garlic powder

1 tbsp Parmesan cheese
Salt and pepper, to taste
1 bagel

DIRECTIONS:

Cut the bagel in half.

Place in the Ninja Foodi, close the crisping lid and cook for 3 minutes on Air Crisp mode at 370 F .

Combine the butter, Parmesan, garlic, basil, and parsley, in a small bowl.

Season with salt and pepper, to taste.

Spread the mixture onto the toasted bagel.

Return the bagel to the Ninja Foodi, and cook for an additional 3 minutes on Roast mode. Serve with tangy tomato relish on the side.

Raspberry and Vanilla Pancake

Servings: 4 | Ready in about: 15 min

INGREDIENTS:

2 cups all-purpose flour
1 cup milk
3 eggs, beaten
1 tsp baking powder
1 cup brown sugar

1 ½ tsp vanilla extract
½ cup frozen raspberries, thawed
2 tbsp maple syrup
Pinch of salt
Cooking spray

DIRECTIONS:

In a bowl, mix the sifted flour, baking powder, salt, milk, eggs, vanilla extract, sugar, and maple syrup, until smooth. Gently stir in the raspberries.

Grease the basket of your Ninja Foodi with cooking spray.

Drop the batter into the basket. Close the crisping lid and cook for 10 minutes on Air Crisp mode at 390 F. Serve the pancake right away.

Paprika Shirred Eggs

Servings: 2 | Ready in about: 20 min

INGREDIENTS:

2 tsp butter, for greasing
4 eggs, divided
2 tbsp heavy cream
4 slices of ham

3 tbsp Parmesan cheese
¼ tsp paprika
¼ tsp pepper
2 tsp chopped chives

DIRECTIONS:

Grease a pie pan with the butter.

Arrange the ham slices on the bottom of the pan to cover it completely. Use more slices if needed.

Whisk one egg along with the heavy cream, salt, and pepper, in a small bowl.

Pour the mixture over the ham slices. Crack the other eggs over the ham.

Scatter Parmesan cheese over, close the crisping lid and cook for 14 minutes on Air Crisp mode at 320 F. Sprinkle with paprika and garnish with chives.

Three Meat Cheesy Omelet

Servings: 2 | Ready in about: 20 min

INGREDIENTS:

1 beef sausage, chopped
4 slices prosciutto, chopped
3 oz salami, chopped
1 cup grated mozzarella cheese
4 eggs

1 tbsp chopped onion
1 tbsp ketchup

DIRECTIONS:

Preheat the Ninja Foodi to 350 degrees F on Air Crisp mode.

Whisk the eggs with the ketchup, in a bowl. Stir in the onion.

Spritz the inside of the Ninja Foodi basket with a cooking spray. Add and brown the sausage for about 2 minutes.

Meanwhile, combine the egg mixture, mozzarella cheese, salami and prosciutto.

Pour the egg mixture over the sausage and stir it. Close the crisping lid and cook for 10 minutes. Once the timer beeps, ensure the omelet is just set. Serve immediately.

Very Berry Breakfast Puffs

Servings: 3 | Ready in about: 20 min

INGREDIENTS:

3 pastry dough sheets
2 tbsp mashed strawberries
2 tbsp mashed raspberries

¼ tsp vanilla extract
2 cups cream cheese
1 tbsp honey

DIRECTIONS:

Divide the cream cheese between the dough sheets and spread it evenly.

In a small bowl, combine the berries, honey, and vanilla.

Divide the mixture between the pastry sheets.

Pinch the ends of the sheets, to form puff.

You can seal them by brushing some water onto the edges, or even better, use egg wash. Lay the puffs into a lined baking dish.

Place the dish into the Ninja Foodi, close the crisping lid and cook for 15 minutes on Air Crisp mode at 370 F.

Once the timer beeps, check the puffs to ensure they're puffed and golden.

Serve warm.

Crustless Mediterranean Quiche

Servings: 2 | Ready in about: 40 min

INGREDIENTS:

4 eggs
½ cup chopped tomatoes
1 cup crumbled feta cheese
1 tbsp chopped basil
1 tbsp chopped oregano

¼ cup chopped kalamata olives
¼ cup chopped onion
2 tbsp olive oil
½ cup milk
Salt and pepper to taste

DIRECTIONS:

Brush a pie pan with the olive oil.

Beat the eggs along with the milk, salt, and pepper. Stir in all of the remaining ingredients.

Pour the egg mixture into the pan. Close the crisping lid and cook for 30 minutes on Air Crisp mode at 340 F. Leave to cool before serving.

Sweet Bread Pudding with Raisins

Servings: 3 | Ready in about: 45 min

INGREDIENTS:

8 slices of bread
½ cup buttermilk
¼ cup honey
1 cup milk
2 eggs
½ tsp vanilla extract

2 tbsp butter, softened
¼ cup sugar
4 tbsp raisins
2 tbsp chopped hazelnuts
Cinnamon for garnish

DIRECTIONS:

Beat the eggs along with the buttermilk, honey, milk, vanilla, sugar, and butter. Stir in raisins and hazelnuts. Cut the bread into cubes and place it in a bowl. Pour the milk mixture over the bread. Let soak for about 10 minutes.

Close the crisping lid and cook the bread pudding for 25 minutes on Roast mode. Leave the dessert to cool for 5 minutes, then invert onto a plate and sprinkle with cinnamon to serve.

Cinnamon Pumpkin Steel Cut Oatmeal

Servings: 4 | Ready in about: 25 min

INGREDIENTS

1 tbsp butter
2 cups steel cut oats
¼ tsp cinnamon
3 cups water

1 cup pumpkin puree
½ tsp salt
3 tbsp maple syrup
½ cup pumpkin seeds, toasted

DIRECTIONS

Melt butter on Sear/Sauté. Add in cinnamon, oats, salt, pumpkin puree and water.

Seal the pressure lid, choose Pressure, set to High, and set the timer to 10 minutes; press Start. When cooking is complete, do a quick release.

Open the lid and stir in maple syrup and top with toasted pumpkin seeds to serve.

Quick Soft-Boiled Eggs

Servings: 4 | Ready in about: 15 min

INGREDIENTS

4 large eggs
1 cups water

Salt and ground black pepper, to taste

DIRECTIONS

To the pressure cooker pot, add water and place a reversible rack. Carefully place eggs on it.

Seal the pressure lid, choose Pressure, set to High, and set the timer to 3 minutes. Press Start.

When cooking is complete, do a quick pressure release.

Allow cooling completely in an ice bath. Peel the eggs and season with salt and pepper before serving.

Sweet Paprika Hard-Boiled Eggs

Servings: 3 | Ready in about: 25 min

INGREDIENTS

1 cup water
6 eggs

Salt and ground black pepper, to taste
1 tsp sweet paprika

DIRECTIONS

In the Foodi, add water and place a reversible rack on top. Lay your eggs on the rack.

Seal the pressure lid, choose Pressure, set to High, and set the timer to 5 minutes. Press Start.

Once ready, do a natural release for 10 minutes. Transfer the eggs to ice cold water to cool completely. When cooled, peel and slice. Season with salt and pepper. Sprinkle with sweet paprika before serving.

LUNCH RECIPES

Egg Rolls

Servings: 3 | Ready in about: 18 min

INGREDIENTS:

1 package egg roll wrappers (12 wrappers)
1 cup ground beef
2 garlic cloves, minced
½ onion, chopped
1 large grated carrot

1 cup grated mozzarella cheese
2 tsp olive oil
¼ tsp salt
¼ tsp pepper

DIRECTIONS:

Place the onion, garlic, carrot, and beef in a saucepan over medium heat, and cook for 6-7 minutes. Take the pan off the heat.

Leave to cool for a few minutes, then mix in the mozzarella. Season to taste with salt, and pepper.

Grease the Ninja Foodi cooking basket with 1 tsp of the olive oil and set aside.

Lay the egg roll sheets onto a dry and clean surface; divide the mixture between them.

Roll the egg rolls and tuck the corners and edges in to create secure rolls.

Lower the rolls into the Ninja Foodi cooking basket and brush them with the remaining olive oil. Close the crisping lid and cook for 13 minutes on Air Crisp mode at 370 F.

Once ready, check if the rolls are golden and crispy. Serve with green salad.

Ham & Mozzarella Eggplant Boats

Servings: 2 | Ready in about: 17 min

INGREDIENTS:

2 eggplants
6 ham slices, chopped
1 cup mozzarella cheese, shredded

1 tsp dried parsley
Salt and pepper, to taste
Cooking spray

DIRECTIONS:

Grease the Ninja Foodi basket with cooking spray; set aside.

Cut the eggplants lengthwise in half and scoop some of the flesh out, leaving the skin intact. Season with salt and pepper.

Chop the scooped flesh and mix with mozzarella cheese, salt, and pepper.

Divide the cheese mixture between the eggplant halves. Cover with ham slices, and sprinkle with parsley.

Put the eggplant in the greased basket, close the crisping lid and cook for 12 minutes on Air Crisp mode at 350 F.

Serve with a fresh salad.

Cheat Hawaiian Pizza

Servings: 2 | Ready in about: 15 min

INGREDIENTS:

2 tortillas
8 ham slices
8 mozzarella slices

8 thin pineapple slices
2 tbsp tomato sauce
Fresh basil leaves, chopped

DIRECTIONS:

Spread each tortilla with tomato sauce. Scatter over the ham, pineapple, and mozzarella.

Place the pizza into your Ninja Foodi basket, close the crisping lid and cook for 10 minutes on Air Crisp mode.

When the timer beeps, remove and allow to sit for 2 minutes before slicing. Sprinkle the basil over and serve with napkins.

Italian Sausage Patties

Servings: 4 | Ready in about: 20 min

INGREDIENTS:

1 lb ground Italian sausage
¼ cup breadcrumbs
1 tsp dried parsley
1 tsp red pepper Flakes

½ tsp salt
¼ tsp black pepper
¼ tsp garlic powder
1 egg, beaten

DIRECTIONS:

Line the basket with parchment paper; set aside.

Combine all ingredients in a large bowl. Use your hands (clean!) to combine the mixture thoroughly. Make patties out of the sausage mixture and arrange them on the basket. Close the crisping lid and cook for 14 minutes on Air Crisp at 350 F. After 7 minutes, flip each patty. Once ready, remove and serve with tzatziki sauce.

Garlicky Chicken on Green Bed

Servings: 1 | Ready in about: 20 min

INGREDIENTS:

½ cup baby spinach leaves
½ cup shredded romaine lettuce
3 large kale leaves, chopped
4 oz chicken breasts, cubed

3 tbsp olive oil, divided
1 tsp balsamic vinegar
1 garlic clove, minced
Salt and pepper, to taste

DIRECTIONS:

Place the chicken in a bowl along with 1 tbsp olive oil and garlic. Season with salt and pepper; toss to combine.

Place on a lined baking dish and cook for 14 minutes on Roast mode in your Ninja Foodi at 390 F.

Add the greens in a large bowl. Pour the remaining olive oil, balsamic vinegar, salt, and pepper, and toss to combine. When the timer rings out, remove the chicken from the Ninja Foodi. Arrange the greens on a serving platter and top with the chicken, to serve.

Homemade Vegetables Soup

Servings: 5 | Ready in about: 40 min

INGREDIENTS

2 tbsp olive oil
1 leek, sliced
2 cloves garlic, minced
2 carrots, diced
1 celery stalk, chopped
4 potatoes, quartered

1 red bell pepper, diced
1/4 tsp red pepper flakes
Salt and pepper to taste
1 ½ cups vegetable stock
2 tbsp parsley

DIRECTIONS

Heat olive oil on Sear/Sauté. Add garlic and leek and cook for 5 minutes. Add in red bell pepper, carrots, salt, potatoes, red pepper flakes, and pepper. Mix in vegetable stock.

Seal the pressure lid, choose Pressure, set to High, and set the timer to 15 minutes. Press Start.

When ready, allow the pressure to release naturally for 10 minutes. Add cilantro and coconut milk to the soup. Use an immersion blender to blend the soup until smooth.

Pickle and Potato Salad with Feta

Serves: 12 | Ready in about about: 30 min

INGREDIENTS

3 pounds potatoes, peeled and chopped
3 cups water
1 tsp salt
1 cup mayonnaise
¼ cup mustard

¼ cup pickle
¼ cup diced white onion, chopped
2 tbsp salt
1 cup feta cheese, crumbled
Salt to taste

DIRECTIONS

In the pot, mix 1 tsp salt, water, and potatoes. Seal the pressure lid, select Pressure and cook for 6 minutes on High. Press Start.

Once ready, do a natural release for 10 minutes. Drain the potatoes and allow to cool. Chop into smaller pieces.

In a bowl, mix salt, pickles, mayonnaise, potatoes, mustard, and onion to get the desired consistency. Chill for one hour while covered. Top with feta cheese to serve.

Curry Egg Salad

Servings: 6 | Ready in about: 10 min

INGREDIENTS

2 cups water
Cooking spray
6 eggs
¼ cup crème frâiche
2 spring onions, minced

1 tbsp dill, minced
1 tbsp curry paste
2 tsp mustard
Salt and black pepper to taste

DIRECTIONS

Grease a cake pan with cooking spray. Carefully crack in the eggs.

To the inner pot, add water. Set the pan with the eggs on a reversible rack.

Seal the pressure lid, choose Pressure, set to High, and the timer to 5 minutes; press Start.

Once ready, do a quick release. Drain any water from the eggs in the pan. Loosen the eggs on the edges with a knife. Transfer to a cutting board and chop into smaller sizes.

Transfer the chopped eggs to a bowl. Add in onion, mustard, salt, dill, crème frâiche, curry powder, and black pepper.

Warm Bacon & Potato Salad

Servings: 6 | Ready in about: 19 min

INGREDIENTS

6 slices smoked bacon, chopped
½ cup apple cider vinegar
½ cup water
3 tbsp honey
2 tsp mustard

1 tsp fresh flat-leaf parsley, chopped
1 tsp salt
1/3 tsp black pepper
6 red potatoes, peeled and quartered
2 red onions, sliced

DIRECTIONS

On Sear/Sauté, set to Medium High, and choose Start/Stop to preheat the pot. Brown the bacon for 2 minutes per side. Set aside.

In a bowl, mix honey, salt, mustard, vinegar, water, and black pepper. In the inner pot, add potatoes, chopped bacon, and onions and top with vinegar mixture.

Seal the pressure lid, choose Pressure, set to High, and set the timer to 6 minutes. Press Start.

When ready, allow the pressure to release naturally for 10 minutes. Place on serving plate and add fresh parsley for garnishing.

Quick Chicken Noodle Soup

Servings: 6 | Ready in about: 15 min

INGREDIENTS

1 tbsp canola oil
6 spring onions, chopped
2 garlic cloves, finely diced
1 carrot, chopped
2 celery stalks, chopped finely

2 chicken breasts, boneless, skinless, cut into bite-size chunks
6 cups chicken broth
8 ounces dry egg noodles
Salt and ground black pepper, to taste
2 tbsp chopped fresh parsley leaves

DIRECTIONS

Heat oil on Sear/Sauté. Add in celery, spring onion, garlic, and carrots. Cook for 5 minutes until tender.

Add in chicken, egg noodles, 1 tsp salt, chicken broth, and black pepper. Seal the pressure lid, choose Pressure, set to High, and set the timer to 15 minutes. Press Start.

When ready, do a quick release, open the lid and add in parsley. Taste and adjust the seasoning before serving.

Broccoli and Potato Soup

Servings: 4 | Ready in about: 35 min

INGREDIENTS

⅓ cup butter
1 head broccoli, cut into florets
2 cloves garlic, minced
1 onion, chopped
2 ½ pounds potatoes, peeled and chopped

4 cups vegetable broth
½ cup heavy cream
Salt and black pepper to taste
Cheddar cheese, grated for garnish
½ cup fresh chopped scallions, for garnish

DIRECTIONS

Melt the butter on Sear/Sauté. Add onion and garlic and cook for 5 minutes. Add in broth, potatoes, and broccoli, and mix well. Press the Start/Stop button.

Seal the pressure lid, choose Pressure, set to High, and set the timer to 5 minutes. Press Start.

When ready, allow the pressure to release naturally for 10 minutes. Transfer the potato mixture in an immersion blender and puree until smooth.

Add in heavy cream and season with pepper and salt as desired. Divide among bowls and top with cheese and scallions.

Sweet Potato & Egg Salad

Servings: 8 | Ready in about: 20 min

INGREDIENTS

1 ½ cups water
6 sweet potatoes, peeled and diced
4 large eggs
2 ½ cups mayonnaise

¼ cup dill, chopped
⅓ cup Greek yogurt
Salt and ground black pepper to taste
½ cup Arugula

DIRECTIONS

In your Foodi, add water. Place eggs and potatoes into the reversible rack; transfer to the pot and seal the pressure lid.

Choose Pressure, and set timer to 4 minutes; press Start.

After cooking has completed, release pressure quickly. Open the lid.

Take out the eggs and place in a bowl of ice-cold water for purposes of cooling.

In a large bowl, combine yogurt, mayonnaise, and dill.

In a separate bowl, mash potatoes using a potato masher; mix with mayonnaise mixture to coat. Skin and dice the eggs; transfer to the potato salad and mix.

Add pepper and salt to the salad before serving.

Spicy Acorn Squash Soup

Servings: 4 | Ready in about: 25 min

INGREDIENTS

4 cups vegetable broth
2 tbsp butter
1 onion, diced
1 (2 pounds) acorn squash, peeled, seeded, chopped
2 carrots, peeled and diced

½ tsp ground cinnamon
¼ tsp chili pepper
A pinch of salt
½ cup coconut milk
1/3 cup sour cream

DIRECTIONS

Set Foodi to Sear/Sauté, set to Medium High, and choose Start/Stop to preheat. Melt butter; add onion and cook for 3 minutes until soft. Add in carrots, cinnamon, squash, salt, and chili pepper and stir-fry for 2 minutes until fragrant.

Add the stock to the vegetable mixture. Seal the pressure lid, choose Pressure, set to High, and set the timer to 12 minutes; press Start.

Quick-release the pressure.

Add soup to a food processor and puree to obtain a smooth consistency. Take the soup back To the Foodi, stir in coconut milk until you get a consistent color.

Divide into serving bowls. Serve hot with a dollop of sour cream.

Minestrone Soup

Servings: 6 | Ready in about: 25 min

INGREDIENTS

2 tbsp olive oil
1 yellow onion, diced
1 cup celery, chopped
1 carrot, peeled and diced
1 green bell pepper, chopped
2 cloves garlic, minced
3 cups chicken broth
½ tsp dried parsley
½ tsp dried thyme
½ tsp dried oregano

½ tsp salt
¼ tsp ground black pepper
2 bay leaves
1 (28 ounces) can diced tomatoes
1 (6 ounces) can tomato paste
2 cups kale
1 (14 ounces) can Navy beans, rinsed and drained
½ cup white rice
¼ cup Parmesan cheese

DIRECTIONS

Warm olive oil on Sear/Sauté. Stir in carrot, celery and onion and cook for 5 to 6 minutes until soft. Add garlic and bell pepper and cook for 2 minutes as you stir until aromatic.

Stir in pepper, thyme, stock, salt, parsley, oregano, tomatoes, bay leaves, and tomato paste to dissolve; mix in rice.

Seal the pressure lid, choose Pressure, set to High, and set the timer to 15 minutes; press Start. Once ready, do a quick pressure release.

Add kale to the liquid and stir. Use residual heat in slightly wilting the greens. Get rid of bay leaves. Stir in navy beans. Serve topped with parmesan cheese.

Vegetable Soup

Servings: 8 | Ready in about: 42 min

INGREDIENTS

2 tbsp olive oil
1 cup leeks, chopped
2 garlic cloves, minced
4 cups vegetable stock
1 carrot, diced
1 parsnip, diced
1 celery stalk, diced
1 cup sliced mushrooms
1 cup broccoli florets

1 cup cauliflower florets
½ red bell pepper, diced
1/4 head green cabbage, chopped
½ cup green beans
2 tbsp nutritional yeast
½ tsp dried thyme
½ salt, or more to taste
½ tsp ground black pepper
½ cup fresh parsley, chopped

DIRECTIONS

Heat oil on Sear/Sauté on Medium High. Add in garlic and onion and cook for 6 minutes until slightly browned.

Add in vegetable stock, carrot, celery, broccoli, bell pepper, green beans, salt, nutritional yeast, cabbage, cauliflower, mushrooms, potato, thyme, and pepper.

Seal the pressure lid, choose Pressure, set to High, and set the timer to 25 minutes; press Start. When ready, release pressure naturally, for about 5 minutes. Stir in parsley and serve.

Chicken Noodle Soup

Servings: 6 | Ready in about: 40 min

INGREDIENTS

1 tbsp olive oil
1 onion, minced
3 cloves garlic, minced
1 turnip, chopped
1 cup celery rib, chopped
1 tbsp dry basil

1 bay leaf
6 cups chicken broth
1 pound chicken breasts, bone-in, skin-on
8 ounces extra-wide dry egg noodles
Salt and ground black pepper to taste

DIRECTIONS

Set your Foodi to Sear/Sauté, set to Medium High, and choose Start/Stop to preheat the pot. Warm olive oil; stir in garlic and onion and cook for 3 minutes until soft. Mix in celery, bay leaf, basil, and turnip.

Add 3 cups chicken broth to the pot and deglaze. Scrape any brown bits from the pan's bottom and add chicken.

Seal the pressure lid, choose Pressure, set to High, and set the timer to 10 minutes; press Start. When ready, naturally release the pressure for about 7 minutes.

Transfer chicken breasts to another bowl. Do away with the skin and bones. Using two forks, shred the meat.

Set the cooker to Sear/Sauté. Transfer the chicken back to the pot; add the noodles and the remaining chicken stock.

Simmer the stock and cook for 10 minutes until noodles are done. Add pepper and salt for seasoning.

Homemade Chicken Soup

Servings: 8 | Ready in about: 1 hr 10 min

INGREDIENTS

1 ½ pounds chicken drumsticks, boneless
4 celery stalks 1 cup fennel bulb, chopped
2 onions, diced
2 carrots, diced
2 garlic cloves
3 parsley, chopped

2 bay leaves
Salt and ground black pepper to taste
½ cup matzo meal
2 eggs, beaten
2 tbsp canola oil
1 tsp baking powder

DIRECTIONS

In your pressure cooker, add chicken drumsticks, bay leaves, onion, carrots, pepper, garlic, parsley, salt, and fennel. Add enough water such that ingredients are covered by 2 inches.

Seal the pressure lid, choose Pressure, set to High, and set the timer to 30 minutes; press Start. Release pressure naturally, for about 10 minutes.

Meanwhile, mix baking powder, eggs, oil, pepper, salt and matzo meal in a small bowl. Use a plastic wrap to close the bowl and place in a refrigerator for 10 minutes.

Get rid of celery stalks from the pressure cooker. Transfer chicken to a cutting board and strip and shred it from the bones. Take back to the pot.

Select Sear/Sauté and boil the soup. Roll matzo mixture into 1-inch balls and place in the boiling soup. Cook for 3 mins to heat through as you gently stir.

Cream of Pumpkin Chipotle Soup

Servings: 4 | Ready in about: 25 min

INGREDIENTS

1 tbsp olive oil
1 onion, chopped
2 chipotle peppers, seeded and finely minced
1 tsp ground black pepper
¼ tsp grated nutmeg
¼ tsp ground cloves

1 pinch ground cinnamon
1 large butternut pumpkin, cut into small pieces
4 cups vegetable broth
1 tsp salt
1 cup half-and-half

DIRECTIONS

Warm oil on Sear/Sauté and sauté nutmeg, pepper, clove, cinnamon, and onion for 3 to 5 minutes until translucent.

Add pumpkin and cook for 5 minutes as you stir infrequently.

Pour in the broth and add chipotle peppers and any remaining pumpkin.

Seal the pressure lid, choose Pressure, set to High, and set the timer to 10 minutes; press Start. When ready, release pressure quickly.

Stir in half-and-half and transfer to a blender to purée until you obtain a smooth consistency.

Cauliflower Cheese Soup

Servings: 5 | Ready in about: 20 min

INGREDIENTS

2 tbsp butter
½ tbsp olive oil
1 onion, chopped
2 stalks celery, chopped
1 large head cauliflower, cut into florets

1 potato, peeled and finely diced
3 cups vegetable broth
2 cups milk
1 bay leaf
4 ounces blue cheese

DIRECTIONS

Set your Foodi to Sear/Sauté, set to Medium High, and choose Start/Stop to preheat the pot. Warm oil and butter.

Add celery and onion and sauté for 3 to 5 minutes until onion becomes fragrant; stir in half the cauliflower and cook for 5 minutes until golden brown. Add in stock, bay leaf and the remaining cauliflower.

Seal the pressure lid, choose Pressure, set to High, and set the timer to 5 minutes; press Start. When ready, release the pressure quickly. Remove the bay leaf and discard.

Place the soup in an immersion blender, add in the milk and puree until smooth.

Spoon the soup into serving bowls and top with blue cheese before serving.

Cream of Mushroom and Spinach Soup

Servings: 4 | Ready in about: 25 min

INGREDIENTS

1 tbsp olive oil
8 Button Mushrooms, sliced
1 cup spinach, chopped
1 red onion, chopped
4 cups vegetable stock
2 sweet potatoes, peeled and chopped

2 tbsp white wine
1 tbsp dry Porcini mushrooms, soaked and drained
½ tsp sea salt
1 cup creme fraiche
½ tsp black pepper

DIRECTIONS

Set your Foodi to Sear/Sauté, set to Medium High, and choose Start/Stop to preheat the pot. Press Start. Add in olive oil and sliced mushrooms and cook for 3 to 5 minutes until browning on both sides; set aside.

Add onion and spinach, and cook for 3 to 5 minutes until onion is translucent.

Stir in chopped mushrooms, and cook for a further 5 minutes as you stir occasionally until golden brown.

Pour in wine to deglaze the bottom of the pot, scrape the bottom to remove browned bits. Cook for 5 minutes until all the wine evaporates.

Mix in the remaining chopped fresh mushrooms, potatoes, soaked mushrooms, wine, vegetable stock, and salt.

Seal the pressure lid, choose Pressure, set to High, and set the timer to 5 minutes. Press Start. Once cooking is complete, do a quick release.

Add in pepper and creme fraiche to mix. Using an immersion blender, whizz the mixture until smooth. Stir in the sautéed mushrooms.

Add reserved mushrooms for garnish before serving.

Mexican-Style Chicken Soup

Servings: 5 | Ready in about: 35 min

INGREDIENTS

5 boneless, skinless chicken thighs
5 cups chicken broth
14 ounces canned whole tomatoes, chopped
2 jalapeno peppers, stemmed, cored, and chopped
2 tbsp tomato puree
3 cloves garlic, minced
1 tbsp chili powder

1 tbsp ground cumin
½ tsp dried oregano
1 (14.5 ounces) can black beans, rinsed and drained
2 cups frozen corn kernels, thawed
Crushed tortilla chips for garnish
¼ cup Cheddar cheese, shredded for garnish
Fresh cilantro, chopped for garnish

DIRECTIONS

Place the chicken in your pressure cooker; add oregano, garlic, tomato puree, chicken stock, cumin, tomatoes, chili powder, and jalapeno peppers.

Seal the pressure lid, choose Pressure, set to High, and set the timer to 10 minutes; press Start. When ready, release pressure quickly. Transfer the chicken to a large plate.

On Sear/Sauté cook corn and black beans. Shred the chicken with a pair of forks, and return to the pot, stirring well. Simmer the soup for 5 minutes until heated through.

Divide in serving plates; add a topping of cilantro, shredded cheese and crushed tortilla chips.

Ramen Spicy Soup with Collard Greens

Servings: 4 | Ready in about: 20 min

INGREDIENTS

1 tbsp olive oil
½ tsp ground ginger
2 tbsp garlic, minced
6 cups chicken broth stock
2 tbsp soy sauce
1 tbsp chili powder

1 cup mushrooms, sliced
10 ounces ramen noodles
1 (1-pound) package fresh collard greens, trimmed
A bunch of fresh cilantro, chopped to serve
1 red chilli, sliced to serve

DIRECTIONS

Set your Foodi to Sear/Sauté, set to Medium High, and choose Start/Stop to preheat the pot. Warm oil; stir in garlic and ginger and cook for 2 minutes until soft.

Add vegetable stock to the pot. Mix in chili powder, ramen noodles and soy sauce.

Seal the pressure lid, press Pressure, set to High, and set the timer to 10 minutes; press Start.

When ready, release pressure quickly. Stir in collard greens until wilted. Ladle the soup into serving bowls and add red chili and cilantro to serve.

Leek and Potato Soup with Sour Cream

Servings: 5 | Ready in about: 30 min

INGREDIENTS

2 tbsp butter
3 leeks, white part only, thinly sliced
2 cloves garlic, minced
4 cups vegetable broth
3 potatoes, peeled and cubed

½ cup sour cream
2 tbsp rosemary
2 bay leaves
salt and ground black pepper to taste
2 tbsp fresh chives, to garnish

DIRECTIONS

Melt the butter on Sear/Sauté. Stir in garlic and leeks and cook for 3 to 4 minutes until soft. Stir in bay leaves, potatoes, and broth.

Seal the pressure lid, press Pressure, set to High, and set the timer to 15 minutes; press Start.

When ready, release pressure quickly. Remove the bay leaves and cobs and discard.

Transfer soup to immersion blender and puree soup to obtain a smooth consistency. Add pepper and salt for seasoning. Apply a topping of and freshly diced chives. Serve with sour cream.

Tomato Soup with Cheese Croutons

Servings: 6 | Ready in about: 1 hr

INGREDIENTS

2 tbsp olive oil
1 onion, chopped
1 carrot, peeled and chopped
1 garlic clove, minced
Salt and ground black pepper to taste
1 cup vegetable stock
28 ounces canned tomatoes

1 cup heavy cream
4 Monterey Jack cheese, sliced
4 slices of bread
2 Gouda cheese, sliced
4 tbsp butter, at room temperature
2 tbsp parsley, finely chopped

DIRECTIONS

Warm oil on Sear/Sauté. Add in garlic, onion, carrot, pepper and salt and sauté for 6 minutes until soft. In the pot, add vegetable stock to deglaze. Scrape any brown bits from the pot.

Mix the stock with tomatoes. Seal the pressure lid, choose Pressure, set to High, and set the timer to 30 minutes; press Start. When the cooking is over, let naturally release pressure, for about 10 minutes.

Transfer soup to immersion blender and process to get a smooth consistency. Add in heavy cream and stir; add pepper and salt for seasoning.

Place 2 slices Monterey Jack cheese onto 1 bread slice and cover with 1 Gouda cheese slice, and the second slice of bread. Spread a tbsp of butter and parsley over the top. Do the same with the rest of the cheese, bread, parsley, and butter.

Place the sandwiches on the crisping basket. Spread 1 tbsp butter on top of each sandwich. Close the crisping lid, choose Air Crisp, set the temperature to 390°F, and set the time to 5 minutes. After 3 minutes, flip the sandwiches and cook for 2 more minutes.

When cooking ended, the sandwiches should be browned and all the cheese melt. Transfer sandwiches to a cutting board and chop into bite-sized cubes. Divide the soup into serving plates and apply a topping of parsley cheese croutons before serving.

Hearty Winter Vegetable Soup

Servings: 5 | Ready in about: 30 min

INGREDIENTS

2 tbsp olive oil
1 onion, chopped
2 carrots, peeled and chopped
1 cup celery, chopped
2 cloves garlic, minced
5 cups chicken broth
2 turnips, peeled and chopped

28 ounces canned tomatoes
15 ounces canned garbanzo beans, rinsed and drained
1 cup frozen green peas
2 bay leaves
1 sprig fresh sage
salt and ground black pepper to taste
¼ cup parmesan cheese, grated

DIRECTIONS

Set your Foodi to Sear/Sauté, set to Medium High, and choose Start/Stop to preheat the pot. Warm oil; stir in celery, carrots, and onion and cook for 4 minutes until soft. Add in garlic and cook for 30 seconds until crispy.

InTo the Foodi, add vegetable broth, parsnip, garbanzo beans, bay leaves, tomatoes, pepper, salt, peas, and sage.

Seal the pressure lid, press Pressure, set to High, and set the timer to 12 minutes; press Start.

Once done, release remaining pressure quickly. Serve topped with parmesan cheese.

Acorn Squash Soup with Coconut Milk

Servings: 6 | Ready in about: 1 hr PREP TIME: 25 min COOK TIME: 25 min

INGREDIENTS

1 tbsp olive oil
1 onion, diced
1 stalk celery, diced
1 large carrot, diced
½ tsp salt
2 garlic cloves, minced

1 pound acorn squash, peeled diced
6 cups chicken stock
Juice from 1 lemon
1 cup coconut milk
Salt and freshly ground black pepper
2 tbsp cilantro leaves, chopped

DIRECTIONS

Heat oil on Sear/Sauté and stir-fry carrot, celery, garlic, salt and onion, for 4 to 5 minutes until soft. Mix acorn squash with the vegetables; cook for 1 more minute until tender. Pour in chicken broth.

Seal the pressure lid, press Pressure, set to High, and set the timer to 20 minutes; press Start.

Release pressure naturally for about 10 minutes. Add in lemon juice and coconut milk and stir.

Transfer the soup to an immersion blender and process to obtain a smooth consistency. You may add pepper and salt if desired. Divide soup into serving plates. Garnish with cilantro and black pepper to serve.

Spicy Borscht Soup

Servings: 4 | Ready in about: 30 min

INGREDIENTS

2 tbsp olive oil
1 cup leeks, chopped
1 tsp garlic, smashed
2 beets, peeled and diced
1 tbsp cayenne pepper, finely minced
1 dried habanero pepper, crushed

4 cups beef stock
3 cups white cabbage, shredded
1 tsp salt
2 tsp red wine apple cider vinegar
¼ tsp paprika
Greek yogurt for garnish

DIRECTIONS

Set your Foodi to Sear/Sauté, set to Medium High, and choose Start/Stop to preheat the pot. Warm the oil; stir in garlic and leeks and cook for 5 minutes until soft. Mix in, stock, paprika, salt, peppers, vinegar, beets, white cabbage, cayenne pepper, and crushed red pepper.

Seal the pressure lid, choose Pressure, set to High, and set the timer to 20 minutes; press Start. When ready, do a quick pressure release. Place in serving bowls and apply a topping of Greek yogurt before serving.

Two-Bean Zucchini Soup

Servings: 5 | Ready in about: 35 min

INGREDIENTS

1 tbsp olive oil
1 onion, chopped
2 cloves garlic, minced
5 cups vegetable broth
1 cup dried chickpeas
½ cup dried pinto beans, soaked overnight

½ cup dried navy beans, soaked overnight
3 carrots, chopped
1 large celery stalk, chopped
1 tsp dried thyme
16 oz zucchini noodles
Sea salt and ground black pepper, to taste

DIRECTIONS

Set your Foogi to Sear/Sauté, set to Medium High, and choose Start/Stop to preheat the pot. Warm oil; stir in garlic and onion and cook for 5 minutes until golden brown. Mix in pepper, vegetable broth, carrots, salt, celery, beans, and thyme.

Seal the pressure lid, choose Pressure, set to High, and set the timer to 15 minutes; press Start. Once ready, naturally pressure release for about 10 minutes. Mix zucchini noodles into the soup and stir until wilted. Taste and adjust the seasoning.

Butternut Squash Curry

Servings: 5 | Ready in about: 30 min

INGREDIENTS

1½ pounds butternut squash, roughly chopped
4 cups chicken stock
½ cup buttermilk
4 spring onions, chopped into lengths
2 tbsp curry powder
1½ tsp ground turmeric

1½ tsp ground cumin
¼ tsp cayenne pepper, or more to taste
2 bay leaves
salt and ground black pepper, to taste
A bunch of cilantro leaves, chopped

DIRECTIONS

In your pressure cooker's pot, stir in squash, buttermilk, curry powder, turmeric, spring onions, stock, cumin, and cayenne pepper. Apply pepper and salt for seasoning. Add bay leaves to the liquid and ensure they are submerged.

Seal the pressure lid, choose Pressure, set to High, and set the timer to 10 minutes.

When ready, naturally release the pressure for 10 minutes. Discard bay leaves.

Transfer the soup to a blender and process until smooth. Use a fine-mesh strainer to strain the soup. Divide into plates and garnish with cilantro before serving.

Creamy Quinoa and Mushroom Pilaf

Servings: 4 | Ready in about: 20 min

INGREDIENTS

4 cups vegetable broth
1 carrot, peeled and chopped
1 stalk celery, diced
2 cups quinoa, rinsed
1 cup mushrooms, sliced
1 onion, chopped

2 garlic cloves, smashed
1 tsp salt
½ tsp dried thyme
3 tbsp butter
½ cup heavy cream

DIRECTIONS

Melt the butter on Sear/Sauté. Add onion, garlic, celery, and carrot, and cook for 8 minutes until tender. Mix in broth, thyme, quinoa, mushrooms, and salt.

Seal the pressure lid, choose Pressure, set to High, and set the timer to 10 minutes; press Start. When ready, release pressure quickly.

Carefully open the lid and stir in heavy cream. Cook for 2 minutes to obtain a creamy consistency. Serve warm.

Red Lentils Soup with Tortilla Topping

Servings: 6 | Ready in about: 50 min

INGREDIENTS

2 ½ cups vegetable broth
1 ½ cups tomato sauce
1 onion, chopped
1 cup dry red lentils
½ cup prepared salsa verde
2 garlic cloves, minced

1 tbsp smoked paprika
2 tsp ground cumin
1 tsp chili powder
¼ tsp cayenne pepper
Salt and ground black pepper to taste
Crushed tortilla chips for garnish

DIRECTIONS

To the Foodi, add in tomato sauce and vegetable broth. Stir in onion, salsa verde, cumin, cayenne pepper, chili powder, garlic, red lentils, and paprika. Season with salt and pepper.

Seal the pressure lid, press Pressure, set to High, and set the timer to 20 minutes; press Start.

Once ready, release pressure naturally for 10 minutes. Divide into serving bowls and add crushed tortilla topping.

Vegetarian Black Bean Soup

Servings: 6 | Ready in about: 30 min

INGREDIENTS

1 tsp olive oil
1 onion, chopped
2 celery stalks, chopped
3 carrots, chopped
2 serrano peppers, deseeded and chopped
5 cups vegetable broth

30 ounces canned diced tomatoes
1 (14 ounces) can black beans, rinsed and drained
¼ cup chopped fresh cilantro
2 tsp ground cumin
1 tsp fine sea salt
Black pepper to taste

DIRECTIONS

Set your Foodi to Sear/Sauté, set to Medium High, and choose Start/Stop to preheat the pot. Warm oil; add in carrots, onion, jalapeño peppers and celery and cook for 6 to 7 minutes until soft. Mix in broth, sea salt, black beans, cumin, tomatoes, and cilantro.

Seal the pressure lid, press Pressure, set to High, and set the timer to 8 minutes; press Start.

Once ready, release pressure naturally for 10 minutes. Season with pepper before serving.

Classic French Onion Soup

Servings: 8 | Ready in about: 45 min

INGREDIENTS

2 tbsp butter
8 cups thinly sliced onions
½ cup water
2 tsp sugar
1 tsp salt
½ tsp ground black pepper

½ cup dry white wine
4 cups beef stock
2 sprigs fresh thyme
2 bay leaves
4 baguette slices
1 cup Swiss cheese, shredded

DIRECTIONS

Melt butter on Sear/Sauté. Add in onions and cook for 3 to 5 minutes until soft. To the onions, add water, pepper, sugar, and salt, and pepper as you stir.

Seal the pressure lid, press Pressure, set to High, and set the timer to 15 minutes; press Start.

Once ready, do a quick release. Add beef stock, bay leaves and thyme sprigs into the pot.

Seal the pressure lid again, choose Pressure, set to High, and set the timer to 4 minutes; press Start. Quick-release pressure. Remove the bay leaves and thyme and discard. Preheat the oven's broiler.

Divide into four soup bowls. Top with ¼ cup swiss cheese and 1 baguette slice. Transfer the bowls to a baking sheet and cook for 2 to 4 minutes under the broiler until golden brown.

Chicken & Farro Soup

Servings: 6 | Ready in about: 1 hr

INGREDIENTS

1 tbsp olive oil
4 boneless, skinless chicken thighs
¼ cup white wine
1 cup farro
1 large onion, sliced
2 celery stalks, cut into squares

3 large carrots, sliced
1 tsp garlic powder
1 tsp ground cumin
1 bay leaf
6 cups chicken broth
2 tsp fresh parsley leaves to garnish

DIRECTIONS

Warm oil on Sear/Sauté. Brown the chicken on all sides, approximately 6 minutes. Transfer the chicken to a bowl.

Into the pot, add wine to deglaze, scraping any brown bits present at the bottom of the cooker.

Mix the wine with farro, cumin, stock, onion, carrots, celery, garlic powder, and bay leaf.

Close the lid and turn steam vent to sealing. Seal the pressure lid, choose Pressure, set to High, and set the timer to 20 minutes; press Start.

When cooking is done, naturally release the pressure for about 10 minutes.

Divide between serving bowls and add parsley for garnish.

Fire-Roasted Tomato and Chorizo Soup

Servings: 6 | Ready in about: 30 min PREP TIME: 5 min COOK TIME: 23 min

INGREDIENTS

1 tbsp olive oil
2 shallots, sliced
3 cloves garlic, minced
1 tsp salt
4 cups beef broth
28 ounces fire-roasted diced tomatoes

½ cup fresh ripe tomatoes
½ cup raw cashews
1 tbsp red wine vinegar
3 chorizo sausage, chopped
½ tsp ground black pepper
½ cup thinly sliced fresh basil

DIRECTIONS

Warn oil on Sear/Sauté and cook chorizo until crispy. Remove to a to a plate lined with paper towel. To the pot, add in garlic and onion and cook for 5 minutes until soft. Season with salt.

Stir in red wine vinegar, broth, diced tomatoes, cashews, tomatoes, and black pepper.

Seal the pressure lid, choose Pressure, set to High, and set the timer to 8 minutes. Press Start. When ready, release pressure quickly.

Pour the soup into an immersion blender and process to obtain a smooth consistency.

Divide into deep bowls, top with crispy chorizo and decorate with basil. Serve and enjoy!

Chicken Broth

Servings: 16 | Ready in about: 50 min

INGREDIENTS

2 pounds chicken carcasses
4 carrots, cut into chunks
1 cup leeks, chopped
1 onion, quartered
1 cup celery, chopped
2 large garlic cloves

1 sprig fresh thyme
1 bunch fresh parsley
Salt to taste
10 peppercorns
2 bay leaves

DIRECTIONS

To your Foodi, add chicken carcasses, onion, pepper, thyme, celery, carrots, garlic, parsley, and bay leaves; top with enough water.

Seal the pressure lid, press Pressure, set to High, and set the timer to 30 minutes; press Start.

When ready, release the pressure quickly. Use a colander to drain the broth and do away with solids. Allow the broth to cool for about 1 hour.

Beef Neck Bone Stock

Servings: 8 | Ready in about: 2 hr 10 min

INGREDIENTS

1 carrot, chopped
2 onions, chopped
2 cups celery, chopped
2 pounds Beef Neck Bones
12 cups water, or more

1 tsp cider vinegar
2 bay leaves
10 peppercorns
Salt to taste

DIRECTIONS

In the pot, add carrot, ginger, vinegar, onion, and beef bones. Add enough water to cover ingredients.

Seal the pressure lid, press Pressure, set to High, and set the timer to 120 minutes; press Start. Release pressure naturally for about 20 minutes. Remove the bones and bay leaves, and discard.

Use a fine-mesh strainer to strain the liquid. Allow the broth to cool. From the surface, skim fat and throw away. Refrigerate for a maximum of 7 days.

Flavorful Vegetable Stock

Servings: 10 | Ready in about: 55 min

INGREDIENTS

2 onions, chopped
2 cups celery, chopped
2 carrots, chopped
4 garlic cloves
1 cup kale
1 cup bell pepper, chopped

A handful of rosemary
A handful of parsley
10 peppercorns
2 bay leaves
Salt to taste
8 cups cold water, filtered

DIRECTIONS

In the pot, add onions, carrots, parsley, bay leaves, garlic, kale, celery, rosemary, and peppercorns; top with cold water.

Seal the pressure lid, press Pressure, set to High, and set the timer to 15 minutes; press Start.

Release pressure naturally for 15 minutes, then release the remaining pressure quickly.

Use a wide and shallow bowl to hold the stock you strain through a fine-mesh strainer.

Allow cool to room temperature. Seal into jars and place in the refrigerator for a maximum of 2 weeks.

Perfect Chicken Wings Broth

Servings: 8 | Ready in about: 1 hr 30 min

INGREDIENTS

2 pounds chicken wings
4 spring onions, diced
2 large carrots, diced
4 cloves garlic

1 small handful fresh parsley
1 small handful fresh thyme
1 bay leaf
6 cups water

DIRECTIONS

In the Foodi, add chicken, carrots, parsley, thyme, onions, garlic, and bay leaf. Pour in water.

Seal the pressure lid, choose Pressure, set to High, and set the timer to 45 minutes. Press Start.

Release pressure naturally for about 10 minutes. Use a fine-mesh strainer to strain the broth and Allow cooling to room temperature. Transfer the broth to containers and seal. Place in the refrigerator for a maximum of one week.

Spicy Beef Broth

Servings: 8 | Ready in about: 1 hr 10 min

INGREDIENTS

2 pounds beef stew meat
2 leeks, chopped
1 onion, chopped
2 cups celery, chopped
2 red chilies, deseeded and chopped
2 carrots, chopped

1 tsp fresh ginger, grated
4 garlic cloves
8 cups water
1 tsp cider vinegar
salt to taste

DIRECTIONS

In the Foodi, mix meat, celery, garlic carrots, leeks, onion, red chilies, and ginger. Top with vinegar and water.

Seal the pressure lid, choose Pressure, set to High, and set the timer to 45 minutes. Press Start. Release pressure naturally for 10 minutes, then release the remaining pressure quickly.

Use a fine-mesh strainer to strain the broth into a bowl; add salt for seasoning.

Serve or refrigerate using sealable containers.

Basic Applesauce with Cinnamon

Servings: 4 | Ready in about: 45 min

INGREDIENTS

4 apples, cored, sliced
½ cup water

1 tsp ground cinnamon
1 tsp honey

DIRECTIONS

Add apples, cinnamon, water, and honey to your Foodi.

Seal the pressure lid, choose Pressure, set to High, and set the timer to 4 minutes; press Start. Once ready, release pressure naturally for 10 minutes.

If you desire a chunky blend, stir vigorously. For smooth applesauce, puree the mixture in a blender. Allow cooling before transferring in containers for storage.

Ragu Bolognese

Servings: 10 | Ready in about: 45 min

INGREDIENTS

4 ounces bacon, chopped
1 tbsp butter
1 large onion, minced
2 celery stalks, minced
2 large carrots, minced
2 pounds ground beef
3 tbsp dry white wine

2 (28 ounces) cans crushed tomatoes
3 bay leaves
1 tsp salt
½ tsp black pepper
½ cup yogurt
1/4 cup chopped fresh basil

DIRECTIONS

Set your Foodi on Sear/Sauté, set to Medium High, and choose Start/Stop to preheat the pot. Place in bacon and cook until crispy for 4 to 5 minutes.

Mix in celery, butter, carrots, and onion, and continue cooking for about 5 minutes until vegetables are softened. Mix in ¼ tsp pepper, ½ tsp salt, and beef, and cook for 4 minutes until golden brown.

Stir in the wine and allow to soak, approximately 4 more minutes. Add in bay leaves, tomatoes, and remaining pepper and salt.

Seal the pressure lid, choose Pressure, set to High, and set the timer to 15 minutes. Press Start. Once ready, release pressure naturally for 10 minutes.

Add yogurt and stir. Serve alongside noodles and use basil to garnish.

Tangy Cheesy Arancini

Servings: 6 | Ready in about: 105 min

INGREDIENTS

½ cup olive oil, plus 1 tablespoon
1 small white onion, diced
2 garlic cloves, minced
5 cups chicken stock
½ cup apple cider vinegar
2 cups short grain rice

1½ cups grated Parmesan cheese, plus more for garnish
1 cup chopped green beans
1 teaspoon salt
1teaspoon freshly ground black pepper
2 cups fresh panko bread crumbs
2 large eggs

DIRECTIONS

Choose Sear/Sauté on the pot and set to Medium High. Choose Start/Stop to preheat the pot.

Add 1 tablespoon of oil and the onion, cook the onion until translucent, add the garlic and cook further for 2 minutes or until the garlic starts getting fragrant.

Stir in the stock, vinegar, and rice. Seal the pressure lid, choose pressure, set to High, and set the time to 7 minutes; press Start.

After cooking, perform a natural pressure release for 10 minutes, then a quick pressure release and carefully open the pressure lid.

Stir in the Parmesan cheese, green beans, salt, and pepper to mash the rice until a risotto forms. Spoon the mixture into a bowl and set aside to cool completely.

Clean the pot and in a bowl, combine the breadcrumbs and the remaining olive oil. In another bowl, lightly beat the eggs.

Form 12 balls out of the risotto or as many as you can get. Dip each into the beaten eggs, and coat in the breadcrumb mixture.

Put half of the rice balls in the Crisping Basket in a single layer.

Close the crisping lid, hit Air Crisp, set the temperature to 400°F, and set the time to 10 minutes; press Start. Leave to cool before serving.

Hot Chicken Wings

Servings: 4 | Ready in about: 60 min

INGREDIENTS

½ cup water

½ cup sriracha sauce

2 tbsp butter, melted

1 tbsp lemon juice

2 lb chicken wings, frozen

½ (1-ounce) ranch salad mix

½ teaspoon paprika

Non-stick cooking spray

DIRECTIONS

Mix the water, sriracha, butter and lemon juice or vinegar in the pot. In the Crisping Basket, put the wings, and then the basket into the pot.

Seal the pressure lid, choose Pressure, set to High, set the timer at 5 minutes, and press Start. When the timer is done reading, perform a quick pressure release, and carefully open the lid.

Pour the paprika and ranch dressing all over the chicken and oil with cooking spray.

Cover the crisping lid. Choose Air Crisp, set the temperature to 370 F, and the timer to 15 minutes. Choose Start to commence frying.

After half the cooking time, open the lid, remove the basket and shake the wings. Oil the chicken again with cooking spray and return the basket to the pot.

Close the lid and continue cooking until the wings are crispy to your desire.

Hot Buttery Chicken Meatballs

Servings: 6 | Ready in about: 90 min

INGREDIENTS

1 pound ground chicken

1 green bell pepper, minced

2 celery stalks, minced

¼ cup crumbled queso fresco

¼ cup hot sauce

¼ cup panko bread crumbs

1 egg

2 tablespoons melted butter

½ cup water

DIRECTIONS

Choose Sear/Sauté on the pot and set to High. Choose Start/Stop to preheat the pot. Meanwhile, in a bowl, evenly combine the chicken, bell pepper, celery, queso fresco, hot sauce, breadcrumbs, and egg. Form meatballs out of the mixture.

Then, pour the melted butter into the pot and fry the meatballs in batches until lightly browned on all sides. Use a slotted spoon to remove the meatballs onto a plate.

Put the Crisping Basket in the pot. Pour in the water and put all the meatballs in the basket.

Seal the pressure lid, choose Pressure, set to High, and set the timer to 5 minutes. Choose Start/Stop to begin cooking.

When done cooking, perform a quick pressure release and carefully open the lid.

Close the crisping lid. Choose Air Crisp, set the temperature to 360°F, and set the time to 10 minutes; press Start.

After 5 minutes, open the lid, lift the basket and shake the meatballs. Return the basket to the pot and close the lid to continue cooking until the meatballs are crispy.

Cheesy Smashed Sweet Potatoes

Servings: 4 | Ready in about: 70 min

INGREDIENTS

12 ounces baby sweet potatoes
1 teaspoon melted butter
¼ cup shredded Monterey Jack cheese
¼ cup sour cream

2 slices bacon, cooked and crumbled
1 tablespoon chopped scallions
Salt to taste

DIRECTIONS

Put the Crisping Basket in the pot and close the crisping lid. Choose Air Crisp, set the temperature to 350°F, and the time to 5 minutes. Press Start/Stop to begin preheating.

Meanwhile, toss the sweet potatoes with the melted butter until evenly coated.

Once the pot and basket have preheated, open the lid and add the sweet potatoes to the basket. Close the lid, Choose Air Crisp, set the temperature to 350°F, and set the time to 30 minutes; press Start.

After 15 minutes, open the lid, pull out the basket and shake the sweet potatoes. Return the basket to the pot and close the lid to continue cooking.

When ended, check the sweet potatoes for your desired crispiness, which should also be fork tender.

Take out the sweet potatoes from the basket and use a large spoon to crush the soft potatoes just to split lightly. Top with the cheese, sour cream, bacon, and scallions, and season with salt.

Fried Beef Dumplings

Servings: 8 | Ready in about: 45 min

INGREDIENTS

8 ounces ground beef
½ cup grated cabbage
1 carrot, grated
1 large egg, beaten
1 garlic clove, minced
2 tablespoons coconut aminos

½ tablespoon melted ghee
½ tablespoon ginger powder
½ teaspoon salt
½ teaspoon freshly ground black pepper
20 wonton wrappers
2 tablespoons olive oil

DIRECTIONS

Put the Crisping Basket in the pot. Close the crisping lid, choose Air Crisp, set the temperature to 400°F, and the time to 5 minutes; press Start/Stop.

In a large bowl, mix the beef, cabbage, carrot, egg, garlic, coconut aminos, ghee, ginger, salt, and black pepper.

Put the wonton wrappers on a clean flat surface and spoon 1 tablespoon of the beef mixture into the middle of each wrapper. Run the edges of the wrapper with a little water; fold the wrapper to cover the filling into a semi-circle shape and pinch the edges to seal. Brush the dumplings with olive oil.

Lay the dumplings in the preheated basket, choose Air Crisp, set the temperature to 400°F, and set the time to 12 minutes. Choose Start/Stop to begin frying.

After 6 minutes, open the lid, pull out the basket and shake the dumplings. Return the basket to the pot and close the lid to continue frying until the dumplings are crispy to your desire.

Kale-Artichoke Bites

Servings: 8 | Ready in about: 70 min

INGREDIENTS

¼ cup frozen chopped kale
¼ cup finely chopped artichoke hearts
¼ cup ricotta cheese
2 tablespoons grated Parmesan cheese
¼ cup goat cheese
1 large egg white

1 teaspoon dried basil
1 lemon, zested
½ teaspoon salt
½ teaspoon freshly ground black pepper
4 (13-by-18-inch) sheets frozen phyllo dough, thawed
1 tablespoon olive oil

DIRECTIONS

In a bowl, mix the kale, artichoke hearts, ricotta cheese, parmesan cheese, goat cheese, egg white, basil, lemon zest, salt, and pepper.

Put the Crisping Basket in the pot. Close the crisping lid, choose Air Crisp, set the temperature to 375°F, and the time to 5 minutes; press Start/Stop.

Then, place a phyllo sheet on a clean flat surface. Brush with olive oil, place a second phyllo sheet on the first, and brush with oil. Continue layering to form a pile of four oiled sheets.

Working from the short side, cut the phyllo sheets into 8 strips. Cut the strips in half to form 16 strips.

Spoon 1 tablespoon of filling onto one short side of every strip. Fold a corner to cover the filling to make a triangle; continue repeatedly folding to the end of the strip, creating a triangle-shaped phyllo packet. Repeat the process with the other phyllo bites.

Open the crisping lid and place half of the pastry in the basket in a single layer. Close the lid, Choose Air Crisp, set the temperature to 350°F, and the timer to 12 minutes; press Start/Stop.

After 6 minutes, open the lid, and flip the bites. Return the basket to the pot and close the lid to continue baking. When ready, take out the bites into a plate. Serve warm.

BBQ Chicken Drumsticks

Servings: 6 | Ready in about: 30 min

Ingredients:

3 lb chicken drumsticks
3 tbsp garlic powder
Salt to taste

1 cup Barbecue sauce
¼ cup butter, melted
½ cup water

Directions:

Season drumsticks with garlic powder and salt.

Open the Ninja Foodi, pour in the water, and fit in the reversible rack. Arrange the drumsticks on top, close the lid, secure the pressure valve, and select Pressure mode for 5 minutes. Press Start/Stop to start cooking.

Once the timer has ended, do a natural pressure release for 10 minutes, and then a quick pressure release to let out any more steam. Open the lid.

Remove the drumsticks to a crisp basket and add the butter and half of the barbecue sauce. Stir the chicken until well coated in the sauce. Insert the basket in the pot and close the crisping lid. Select Air Crisp, set to 380 degrees F, and cook for 10 minutes. Select Start/Stop.

Once nice and crispy, remove drumsticks to a bowl, and top with the remaining barbecue sauces. Stir and serve the chicken with a cheese dip.

Buffalo Chicken Meatballs with Ranch-Style Dip

Servings: 4 | Ready in about: 34 min

Ingredients:

5 tbsp Hot sauce
2 tbsp Buffalo wing sauce
1 lb ground chicken
1 egg, beaten
2 tbsp minced garlic

2 tbsp olive oil
2 tbsp chopped green onions
Green onions for garnish
Salt and pepper, to taste

For the dip:
½ cup Roquefort cheese, crumbled
¼ tbsp heavy cream
2 tbsp mayonnaise

Juice from ½ lemon
2 tbsp olive oil

Directions:

Mix all salsa ingredients in a bowl until uniform and creamy, and refrigerate.

Add the ground chicken, salt, garlic, and two tablespoons of green onions. Mix well with your hands.

Rub your hands with some oil and form bite-size balls out of the mixture.

Lay onto your crisp basket fryer basket. Spray with cooking spray.

Select Air Crisp, set the temperature to 385 degrees F and the time to 14

minutes. At the 7-minute mark, turn the meatballs.

Meanwhile, add the hot sauce and butter to a bowl and microwave them until the butter melts. Mix the sauce with a spoon.

Pour the hot sauce mixture and a half cup of water over the meatballs.

Close the lid, secure the pressure valve, and select Sear/Sauté mode on High Pressure for 10 minutes. Press Start/Stop.

Once the timer has ended, do a quick pressure release. Dish the meatballs.

Garnish with green onions, and serve with Roquefort sauce.

Holiday Egg Brulee

Servings: 8 | Ready in about: 12 min

Ingredients:

8 large eggs
Salt to taste

1 cup water
Ice bath

Directions:

Open the Ninja Foodi, pour the water in, and fit the reversible rack in it. Put the eggs on the rack in a single layer, close the lid, secure the pressure valve, and select Pressure on High Pressure for 5 minutes. Press Start/Stop. Once the timer has ended, do a quick pressure release, and open the pot.

Remove the eggs into the ice bath and peel the eggs. Put the peeled eggs in a plate and slice them in half.

Sprinkle a bit of salt on them and then followed by the sugar. Lay onto your crisp basket fryer basket. Select Air Crisp mode, set the temperature to 390 degrees F and the time to 3 minutes.

Brazilian Cheese Balls

Servings: 4 | Ready in about: 35 min

Ingredients:

2 cups flour

1 cup milk

A pinch of salt

2 eggs, cracked into a bowl

2 cups grated mozzarella cheese

½ cup olive oil

Directions:

Grease the crisp basket with cooking spray and set aside.

Put the Ninja Foodi on Medium and select Sear/Sauté mode.

Add the milk, oil, and salt, and let boil. Add the flour and mix it vigorously with a spoon.

Let the mixture cool. Once cooled, use a hand mixer to mix the dough well, and add the eggs and cheese while still mixing. The dough should be thick and sticky.

Use your hands to make 14 balls out of the mixture, and put them in the greased basket. Put the basket in the pot and close the crisping lid.

Select Air Crisp, set the temperature to 380 degrees F and set the timer to 15 minutes.

At the 7-minute mark, shake the balls.

Serve with lemon aioli, garlic mayo or ketchup.

Asparagus Wrapped in Prosciutto with Garbanzo Dip

Servings: 6 | Ready in about: 15 min

Ingredients:

1 lb asparagus, stalks trimmed

10 oz Prosciutto, thinly sliced

Cooking spray

For the Dip:

1 cup canned garbanzo beans

1 medium onion, diced

2 cloves of garlic, minced

2 medium jalapeños, chopped

1 cup crushed tomatoes

1 cup vegetable broth

1 ½ tbsp olive oil

1 tsp. paprika

¾ tsp. sea salt

½ tsp. chili powder

Directions:

Open the Ninja Foodi and add the garbanzo beans, onion, jalapeños, garlic, tomatoes, broth, oil, paprika, chili powder, and salt.

Close the lid, secure the pressure valve, and select Pressure mode on High for 8 minutes. Press Start/Stop.

Once the timer has ended, do a quick pressure release, and open the pot.

Transfer the ingredients to a food processor, and blend until creamy and smooth. Set aside. Wrap each asparagus with a slice of prosciutto from top to bottom.

Grease the crisp basket with cooking spray, and add in the wrapped asparagus. Close the crisping lid, select Air Crisp mode at 370 degrees F and set the time to 8 minutes. Press Start/Stop. At the 4-minute mark, turn the bombs. Remove the wrapped asparagus onto a plate and serve with bean dip.

Creamy Tomato & parsley Dip

Servings: 6 | Ready in about: 18 min

Ingredients:

1 cup chopped tomatoes

10 oz shredded Parmesan cheese

¼ cup chopped parsley

10 oz cream cheese

½ cup heavy cream

1 cup water

Directions:

Open the Ninja Foodi and pour in the tomatoes, parsley, heavy cream, cream cheese, and water.

Close the lid, secure the pressure valve, and select Pressure for 3 minutes at High. Press Start/Stop.

Once the timer has ended, do a natural pressure release for 10 minutes.

Stir the mixture with a spoon while mashing the tomatoes with the back of the spoon. Add the parmesan cheese and Close the crisping lid.

Select Bake/Roast mode, set the temperature to 370 degrees F and the time to 3 minutes. Dish the dip into a bowl and serve with chips or veggie bites.

Cheese bombs wrapped in Bacon

Servings: 8 | Ready in about: 20 min

Ingredients:

16 oz Mozzarella cheese, cut into 8 pieces

8 bacon slices, cut in half

3 tbsp butter, melted

Directions:

Wrap each cheese string with a slice of bacon and secure the ends with toothpicks. Set aside.

Grease the crisp basket with the melted butter and add in the bombs. Close the crisping lid, select Air Crisp mode, and set the temperature to 370 degrees F and set the time to 10 minutes.

At the 5-minute mark, turn the bombs. When ready, remove to a paper-lined plate to drain the excess oil. Serve on a platter with toothpicks and tomato dip.

Bacon & Cheese Dip

Servings: 10 | Ready in about: 10 min

Ingredients:

4 chopped tomatoes

1¼ cup shredded Monterey Jack cheese

1¼ cup cream cheese

10 bacon slices, chopped roughly

1 cup water

Directions:

Turn on the Ninja Foodi and select Air Crisp mode. Set the temperature to 370 degrees F and the time to 8 minutes. Add the bacon pieces and close the crisping lid. Press Start/Stop.

When ready, open the lid and add the water, cream cheese, and tomatoes. Do Not Stir. Close the lid, secure the pressure valve, and select Pressure mode on High for 5 minutes. Press Start/Stop.

Once the timer has ended, do a quick pressure release, and open the lid. Stir in the cheddar cheese and mix to combine. Serve with a side of chips.

Scrumptious Honey-Mustard Hot Dogs

Servings: 4 | Ready in about: 22 min

Ingredients:

20 Hot Dogs, cut into 4 pieces
1 tsp Dijon mustard
1½ tsp soy sauce
¼ cup honey

¼ cup red wine vinegar
Salt and black pepper to taste
½ cup tomato puree
¼ cup water

Directions:

Add the tomato puree, red wine vinegar, honey, soy sauce, Dijon mustard, salt, and black pepper in a medium bowl. Mix them with a spoon.

Put sausage weenies in the crisp basket, and close the crisping lid.

Select Air Crisp mode. Set the temperature to 370 degrees F and the timer to 4 minutes. Press Start/Stop. At the 2-minute mark, turn the sausages.

Once ready, open the lid and pour the sweet sauce over the sausage weenies.

Close the pressure lid, secure the pressure valve, and select Pressure mode on High for 3 minutes. Press Start/Stop.

Once the timer has ended, do a quick pressure release. Serve and enjoy.

Chicken and Cheese Bake

Servings: 6 | Ready in about: 1 hour 18 min

Ingredients:

1 lb chicken breast
½ cup breadcrumbs
10 oz Cheddar cheese

½ cup sour cream
10 oz cream cheese
½ cup water

Directions:

Open the Ninja Foodi and add the chicken, water, and cream cheese.

Close the lid, secure the pressure valve, and select Pressure mode on High for 10 minutes. Press Start/Stop.

Once the timer has ended, do a quick pressure release, and open the pot.

Shred the chicken with two forks and add the cheddar cheese. Sprinkle with breadcrumbs, and close the crisping lid. Select Bake/Roast, set the temperature to 380 degrees F and the timer to 3 minutes.

Serve warm with veggie bites.

Teriyaki Chicken Wings

Servings: 6 | Ready in about: 30 min

INGREDIENTS

1 tbsp honey
1 cup teriyaki sauce
1 tsp finely ground black pepper
2 lb chicken wings

2 tbsp. cornstarch
2 tbsp. cold water
1 tsp sesame seeds

DIRECTIONS

In the pot, combine honey, teriyaki sauce and black pepper until the honey dissolves completely; toss in chicken to coat. Seal the pressure lid, choose Pressure, set to High, and set the timer to 10 minutes. Press Start.

When ready, release the pressure quickly.

Transfer chicken wings to a platter. Mix cold water with the cornstarch.

Press Sear/Sauté and stir in cornstarch slurry into the sauce and cook for 3 to 5 minutes until thickened.

Top the chicken with thickened sauce. Add a garnish of sesame seeds, and serve.

Green Vegan Dip

Servings: 4 | Ready in about: 20 min

INGREDIENTS

2 cups broccoli florets
1 cup water
¾ cup green bell pepper, chopped
¼ cup raw cashews
10 ounces canned green chiles, drained with liquid reserved

¼ cup soy sauce
½ tsp sea salt
¼ tsp chili powder
¼ tsp garlic powder

DIRECTIONS

In the cooker, add cashews, broccoli, green bell pepper, and water.

Seal the pressure lid, choose Pressure, set to High, and set the timer to 5 minutes. Press Start.

When ready, release the pressure quickly.

Drain water from the pot; add reserved liquid from canned green chilies, sea salt, garlic powder, chili powder, soy sauce, and cumin. Use an immersion blender to blend the mixture until smooth; set aside in a mixing bowl. Stir green chilies through the dip; add your desired optional additions.

Homemade Spinach Hummus

Servings: 12 | Ready in about: 1 hr 10 min

INGREDIENTS

8 cups water
2 cups dried chickpeas
5 tbsp grapeseed oil
2 tsp salt, divided

½ cup tahini
5 tbsp lemon juice
2 cups spinach, chopped
5 garlic cloves, crushed

DIRECTIONS

In the pressure cooker, mix 2 tbsp oil, water, 1 tsp salt, and chickpeas. Seal the pressure lid, choose Pressure, set to High, and set the timer to 35 minutes. Press Start.

When ready, release the pressure quickly.

In a small bowl, reserve ½ cup of the cooking liquid and drain chickpeas.

Mix half the reserved cooking liquid and chickpeas in a food processor and puree until no large chickpeas remain; add remaining cooking liquid, spinach, lemon juice, remaining tsp salt, garlic, and tahini. Process hummus for 8 minutes until smooth. Stir in the remaining 3 tbsp of olive oil before serving.

Sweet-Heat Pickled Cucumbers

Servings: 6 | Ready in about: 5 min

INGREDIENTS

1 pound small cucumbers, sliced into rings
2 cups white vinegar
1 cup water
1 cup sugar

1/4 cup green garlic, minced
2 tbsp Dill Pickle Seasoning
2 tsp salt
1 tsp cumin

DIRECTIONS

Into the pot, add sliced cucumber, vinegar and pour water on top. Sprinkle sugar over cucumbers. Add cumin, dill pickle seasoning, and salt. Stir well to dissolve the sugar. Seal the pressure lid, choose Pressure, set to High, and set the timer to 4 minutes. Press Start.

When ready, release the pressure quickly.

Ladle cucumbers into a large storage container and pour cooking liquid over the top. Chill for 1 hour.

Crispy Cheesy Straws

Servings: 8 | Ready in about: 45 min

INGREDIENTS:

2 cups cauliflower florets, steamed
1 egg
3 ½ oz oats
1 red onion, diced

1 tsp mustard
5 oz cheddar cheese
Salt and pepper, to taste

DIRECTIONS:

Add the oats in a food processor and process until they resemble breadcrumbs.

Place the steamed florets in a cheesecloth and squeeze out the excess liquid.

Put the florets in a large bowl, and add the rest of the ingredients to the bowl.

Mix well with your hands, to combine the ingredients thoroughly.

Take a little bit of the mixture and twist it into a straw.

Place in the lined Ninja Foodi basket; repeat with the rest of the mixture.

Close the crisping lid and cook for 10 minutes on Air Crisp mode at 350 F.

After 5 minutes, turn them over and cook for an additional 10 minutes.

Crispy Rosemary Potato Fries

Servings: 4 | Ready in about: 30 min

INGREDIENTS:

4 russet potatoes, cut into sticks
2 tbsp butter, melted
2 garlic cloves, crushed

1 tsp fresh rosemary, chopped
Salt and pepper, to taste

DIRECTIONS:

Add butter, garlic, salt, and pepper to a bowl; toss until the sticks are well-coated.

Lay the potato sticks into the Ninja Foodi's basket. Close the crisping lid and cook for 15 minutes at 370 F.

Shake the potatoes every 5 minutes.

Once ready, check to ensure the fries are golden and crispy all over if not, return them to cook for a few minutes.

Divide standing up between metal cups lined with nonstick baking paper, and serve sprinkled with rosemary.

Cauliflower and Cheddar Tater Tots

Servings: 10 | Ready in about: 35 min

INGREDIENTS:

2 lb cauliflower florets, steamed
5 oz cheddar cheese
1 onion, diced
1 cup breadcrumbs
1 egg, beaten

1 tsp chopped parsley
1 tsp chopped oregano
1 tsp chopped chives
1 tsp garlic powder
Salt and pepper, to taste

DIRECTIONS:

Mash the cauliflower and place it in a large bowl.

Add the onion, parsley, oregano, chives, garlic powder, salt, and pepper, and cheddar cheese. Mix with hands until thoroughly combined.

Form 12 balls out of the mixture. Line a baking sheet with paper.

Dip half of the tater tots into the egg and then coat with breadcrumbs.

Arrange them on the baking sheet, close the crisping lid and cook in the Ninja Foodi at 350 F for 15 minutes on Air Crisp mode. Repeat with the other half.

Eggplant Chips with Honey

Servings: 4 | Ready in about: 20 min

INGREDIENTS:

2 eggplants
2 tsp honey
⅓ cup olive oil
⅓ cup cornstarch

½ cup water
1 tsp dry thyme
A pinch of salt

DIRECTIONS:

Cut the eggplants in slices of ½ -inch each.

In a big bowl, mix the cornstarch, water, olive oil, and eggplant slices, until evenly coated.

Line the Ninja Foodi basket with baking paper and spray with olive oil. Place the eggplants in the basket, scatter with thyme and cook for 15 minutes on Air Crisp mode, shaking every 5 minutes at 370 F.

When ready, transfer the eggplants to a serving platter and drizzle with honey.

Serve with yogurt dip.

Wrapped Asparagus in Bacon

Servings: 6 | Ready in about: 30 min

INGREDIENTS:

1 lb asparagus spears, trimmed
1 lb bacon, sliced
½ cup Parmesan cheese, grated

Cooking spray
Salt and pepper, to taste

DIRECTIONS:

Place the bacon slices out on a work surface, top each one with one asparagus spear and half of the cheese. Wrap the bacon around the asparagus.

Line the Ninja Foodi basket with parchment paper.

Arrange the wraps into the basket, scatter over the remaining cheese, season with salt and black pepper, and spray with cooking spray.

Close the crisping lid and cook for 8 to 10 minutes on Roast mode at 370 F. If necessary work in batches. Serve hot!

New York Steak and Minty Cheese

Servings: 4 | Ready in about: 15 min

INGREDIENTS:

2 New York strip steaks
12 kalamata olives
8 oz halloumi cheese
2 tbsp chopped parsley

2 tbsp chopped mint
Juice and zest of 1 lemon
Salt and pepper, to taste
Olive oil

DIRECTIONS:

Season the steaks with salt and pepper, and gently brush with olive oil.

Place into the Ninja Foodi, close the crisping lid and cook for 6 minutes (for medium rare) on Air Crisp mode at 350 F. When ready, remove to a plate and set aside.

Drizzle the cheese with olive oil and place it in the Ninja Foodi; cook for 4 minutes.

Remove to a serving platter and serve with sliced steaks and olives, sprinkled with herbs, and lemon zest and juice.

Melt-in-the-Middle Meatballs

Servings: 6 | Ready in about: 30 min

INGREDIENTS:

2 lb ground beef
1 potato, shredded
2 eggs, beaten
2 tbsp chopped chives
¼ tsp pepper
½ tsp garlic powder

½ tsp salt
Cooking spray
½ cup Parmesan cheese, grated
1 package cooked spaghetti to serve
2 cups tomato sauce to serve
Basil leaves to serve

DIRECTIONS:

In a large bowl, combine the potato, salt, pepper, garlic powder, eggs, and chives.

Form 12 balls out of the mixture. Spray with cooking spray.

Arrange half of the balls onto a lined Ninja Foodi basket.

Close the crisping lid and cook for 14 minutes on Air Crisp mode at 330 F. After 7 minutes, turn the meatballs.

Repeat with the other half. Serve over cooked spaghetti mixed with tomato sauce, sprinkled with Parmesan cheese and basil leaves.

Air Fried Pin Wheels

Servings: 6 | Ready in about: 50 min

INGREDIENTS:

1 sheet puff pastry

8 ham slices

1 ½ cups Gruyere cheese, grated

4 tsp Dijon mustard

DIRECTIONS:

Place the pastry on a lightly floured flat surface.

Brush the mustard over and arrange the ham slices; top with cheese.

Start at the shorter edge and roll up the pastry.

Wrap it in a plastic foil and place in the freezer for about half an hour, until it becomes firm and comfortable to cut.

Meanwhile, slice the pastry into 6 rounds.

Line the Ninja Foodi basket with parchment paper, and arrange the pinwheels on top. Close the crisping lid and cook for 10 minutes on Air Crisp mode at 370 F.

Leave to cool on a wire rack before serving.

Nutty & Zesty Brussels Sprouts with Raisins

Servings: 4 | Ready in about: 45 min

INGREDIENTS:

14 oz Brussels sprouts, steamed

2 oz raisins

1 tbsp olive oil

Juice and zest of 1 orange

2 oz toasted pine nuts

DIRECTIONS:

Soak the raisins in the orange juice and let sit for about 20 minutes.

Drizzle the Brussels sprouts with the olive oil, and place them in the basket of the Ninja Foodi.

Close the crisping lid and cook for 15 minutes on Air Crisp mode at 370 F.

Remove to a bowl and top with pine nuts, raisins, and orange zest.

Cumin Baby Carrots

Servings: 4 | Ready in about: 25 min

INGREDIENTS:

1 ¼ lb baby carrots

2 tbsp olive oil

1 tsp cumin seeds

½ tsp cumin powder

½ tsp garlic powder

1 handful cilantro, chopped

1 tsp salt

½ tsp black pepper

DIRECTIONS:

Place the baby carrots in a large bowl. Add cumin seeds, cumin, olive oil, salt, garlic powder, and pepper, and stir to coat them well.

Put the carrots in the Ninja Foodi's basket, close the crisping lid and cook for 20 minutes on Roast mode at 370 F. Remove to a platter and sprinkle with chopped cilantro, to serve.

Garlic and Rosemary Mushrooms

Servings: 4 | Ready in about: 20 min

INGREDIENTS:

2 rosemary sprigs

12 oz button mushrooms

¼ cup melted butter

½ tsp salt

¼ tsp black pepper

3 garlic cloves, minced

DIRECTIONS:

Wash and pat dry the mushrooms and cut them in half. Place in a large bowl. Add the remaining ingredients to the bowl and toss well to combine.

Transfer the mushrooms to the basket of the Ninja Foodi. Close the crisping lid and cook for 12 minutes on Air Crisp mode, shaking once halfway through, at 350 F.

Turkey Scotch Eggs

Servings: 6 | Ready in about: 20 min

INGREDIENTS:

10 oz ground turkey

4 eggs, soft boiled, peeled

1 white onion, chopped

½ cup flour

2 garlic cloves, minced

2 eggs, lightly beaten

Salt and pepper to taste

½ cup breadcrumbs

1 tsp dried mixed herbs

Cooking spray

DIRECTIONS:

Mix together the onion, garlic, salt, and pepper. Shape into 4 balls. Wrap the turkey mixture around each egg, and ensure the eggs are well covered.

Dust each egg ball in flour, then dip in the beaten eggs and finally roll in the crumbs, until coated. Spray with cooking spray. Lay the eggs into your Ninja Foodi's basket. Set the temperature to 390 degrees F, close the crisping lid and cook for 15 minutes. After 8 minutes, turn the eggs. Slice in half and serve warm.

Parmesan Cabbage Side Dish

Servings: 4 | Ready in about: 30 min

INGREDIENTS:

½ head of cabbage, cut into 4 wedges
4 tbsp butter, melted
2 cup Parmesan cheese

Salt and pepper, to taste
1 tsp smoked paprika

DIRECTIONS:

Line the basket with parchment paper. Brush the butter over the cabbage wedges; season with salt and pepper.

Coat the cabbage with the Parmesan cheese. Arrange in the basket and sprinkle with paprika.

Close the crisping lid and cook for 15 minutes on Air Crisp mode, flip over and cook for an additional 10 minutes, at 330 F.

Herby Fish Skewers

Servings: 4 | Ready in about: 75 min

INGREDIENTS

3 tbsp olive oil
2 garlic cloves, grated
1 tsp dill, chopped
1 tsp parsley, chopped

Salt to taste
1 lemon, juiced and zested
1 lemon, cut in wedges to serve
1 pound cod loin, boneless, skinless, cubed

DIRECTIONS:

In a bowl, combine the olive oil, garlic, dill, parsley, salt, and lemon juice. Stir in the cod and place in the fridge to marinate for 1 hour. Thread the cod pieces onto halved skewers.

Arrange into the oiled Ninja Foodi basket; close the crisping lid and cook for 10 minutes at 390 F. Flip them over halfway through cooking. When ready, remove to a serving platter, scatter lemon zest and serve with wedges.

Tomato & Mozzarella Bruschetta

Servings: 2 | Ready in about: 15 min

INGREDIENTS:

1 Italian Ciabatta Sandwich Bread
Olive oil to brush
2 tomatoes, chopped
2 garlic cloves, minced

1 cup grated mozzarella cheese
Basil leaves, chopped
Salt and pepper to taste

DIRECTIONS:

Cut the bread in half, lengthways, then each piece again in half. Drizzle each bit with olive oil and sprinkle with garlic. Top with the grated cheese, salt, and pepper.

Place the bruschetta pieces into the Ninja Foodi basket, close the crisping lid and cook for 12 minutes on Air Crisp mode at 380 F. At 6 minutes, check for doneness.

Once the Ninja Foodi beeps, remove the bruschetta to a serving platter, spoon over the tomatoes and chopped basil to serve.

VEGETABLES & VEGAN

Sundried Tomatoes, Spinach, and Butternut Squash Stew

Servings: 6 | Ready in about: 65 min

INGREDIENTS

1 tablespoon butter
1 white onion, diced
4 garlic cloves, minced
2 lb butternut squash, peeled and cubed
4 cups vegetable broth
1 (15-ounce) can sundried tomatoes, undrained
2 (15-ounce) cans chickpeas, drained

1½ teaspoons cumin powder
½ teaspoon smoked paprika
1 teaspoon coriander powder
½ teaspoon salt
½ teaspoon freshly ground black pepper
4 cups baby spinach

DIRECTIONS

Choose Sear/Sauté, set to Medium High, and the timer to 5 minutes; press Start/Stop to preheat the pot. Combine the butter, onion, and garlic in the pot. Cook, stirring occasionally, for 5 minutes or until soft and fragrant.

Add the butternut squash, vegetable broth, tomatoes, chickpeas, cumin, paprika, coriander, salt, and black pepper to the pot. Put the pressure lid together and lock in the Seal position.

Choose Pressure, set to High, and set the time to 8 minutes; press Start/Stop. When the timer is done reading, perform a quick pressure release. Stir in the spinach to wilt, adjust the taste with salt and black pepper, and serve warm.

Swiss Cheese and Mushroom Tarts

Servings: 4 | Ready in about: 75 min

INGREDIENTS

2 tablespoons melted butter, divided
1 small white onion, sliced
5 ounces oyster mushrooms, sliced
¼ teaspoon salt
¼ teaspoon freshly ground black pepper

¼ cup dry white wine
1 sheet puff pastry, thawed
1 cup shredded Swiss cheese
1 tablespoon thinly sliced fresh green onions

DIRECTIONS

Choose Sear/Sauté, set to High, and set the time to 5 minutes. Choose Start/Stop to preheat the pot.

Add 1 tablespoon of butter, the onion, and mushrooms to the pot. Sauté for 5 minutes or until the vegetables are tender and browned.

Season with salt and black pepper, pour in the white wine, and cook until evaporated, about 2 minutes. Spoon the vegetables into a bowl and set aside.

Unwrap the puff pastry and cut into 4 squares. Pierce the dough with a fork and brush both sides with the remaining oil. Share half of the cheese evenly over the puff pastry squares, leaving a ½- inch border around the edges. Also, share the mushroom mixture over the pastry squares and top with the remaining cheese.

Put the Crisping Basket in the pot. Close the crisping lid, choose Air Crisp, set the temperature to 400°F, and the time to 5 minutes.

Once the pot has preheated, put 1 tart in the Crisping Basket. Close the crisping lid, choose Air Crisp, set the temperature to 360°F, and set the time to 6 minutes; press Start.

After 6 minutes, check the tart for your preferred brownness. Take the tart out of the basket and transfer to a plate. Repeat the process with the remaining tarts. Garnish with the green onions and serve.

Rice & Olives Stuffed Mushrooms

Servings: 4 | Ready in about: 70 min

INGREDIENTS

4 large Portobello mushrooms, stems and gills removed
2 tablespoons melted butter
½ cup brown rice, cooked
1 tomato, seed removed and chopped
¼ cup black olives, pitted and chopped
1 green bell pepper, seeded and diced
½ cup feta cheese, crumbled
1 lemon, juiced
½ teaspoon salt
½ teaspoon ground black pepper
Minced fresh cilantro, for garnish

DIRECTIONS

Put the Crisping Basket in the pot. Close the crisping lid, choose Air Crisp, setting the temperature to 375°F, and setting the time to 5 minutes. Press Start/Stop to preheat the pot.

Brush the mushrooms with the melted butter. Open the crisping lid and arrange the mushrooms, open-side up and in a single layer in the preheated basket.

Close the crisping lid. Choose Air Crisp, set the temperature to 375°F, and set the time to 20 minutes. Choose Start/Stop. In a bowl, combine the brown rice, tomato, olives, bell pepper, feta cheese, lemon juice, salt, and black pepper.

Open the crisping lid and spoon the rice mixture equally into the 4 mushrooms. Close the lid. Choose Air Crisp, set the temperature to 350°F, and set the time to 8 minutes. Press Start/Stop to commence cooking.

When the mushrooms are ready, remove to a plate, garnish with fresh cilantro and serve immediately.

Sticky Noodles with Tofu and Peanuts

Servings: 4 | Ready in about: 20 min

INGREDIENTS

1 package tofu, cubed
8 ounces egg noodles
2 bell peppers, sliced
¼ cup soy sauce
¼ cup orange juice
1 tbsp fresh ginger, peeled and minced
2 tbsp vinegar
1 tbsp sesame oil
1 tbsp sriracha
¼ cup roasted peanuts
3 scallions, thinly sliced

DIRECTIONS

In the pressure cooker, mix tofu, bell peppers, orange juice, sesame oil, ginger, egg noodles, soy sauce, vinegar, and sriracha; cover with enough water. Seal the pressure lid, choose Pressure, set to High, and set the timer to 2 minutes. Press Start. When ready, release the pressure quickly.

Place the mixture into four plates; apply a topping of scallions and peanuts before serving.

Squash Parmesan and Linguine

Servings: 4 | Ready in about: 75 min

INGREDIENTS

1 pound linguine
2 teaspoons salt
4 cups water + 2 tbsp
1 cup flour
2 eggs
1 cup seasoned panko breadcrumbs

½ cup grated Parmesan cheese + more for garnish
1 yellow squash, peeled and sliced
1 (24-ounce) tomato sauce
2 tablespoons olive oil
1 cup shredded mozzarella cheese
Minced fresh cilantro, for garnish

DIRECTIONS

Break the spaghetti in half and place in the pot. Pour 4 cups of water and 1 teaspoon of salt.

Seal the pressure lid, choose Pressure, set to High, and set the time to 2 minutes; press Start.

In a bowl, combine the flour and the remaining salt evenly. In another bowl, whisk the eggs and 2 tablespoons of water. In a third bowl, mix the breadcrumbs and Parmesan cheese.

Coat each squash slice in the flour. Shake off the excess flour, dip the slice in the egg wash, and then dredge in the breadcrumbs. Place in a plate and set aside.

When ready, perform a quick pressure release. Drain the pasta through a colander and transfer to the pot. Pour all but ¼ cup of the tomato sauce over the linguine; mix gently.

Fix the reversible rack inside the pot over the linguine. Place the breaded squash on the rack and lightly brush with oil.

Close the crisping lid. Choose Air Crisp, set the temperature to 350°F, and set the time to 15 minutes. Press Start/Stop to cook.

When done cooking, spread the remaining tomato sauce on top of the squash, and sprinkle with the mozzarella cheese.

Close the crisping lid again, choose Broil, and set the time to 3 minutes; press Start/Stop.

When ready, spoon the pasta into plates, place the breaded squash to the side, and garnish with fresh cilantro.

Tangy Risotto and Roasted Bell Peppers

Servings: 4 | Ready in about: 80 min

INGREDIENTS

2 tablespoons ghee, divided
1 garlic clove, minced
5 cups vegetable stock
¼ cup freshly squeezed lemon juice
1 teaspoon grated lemon zest
2 cups carnaroli rice

2 teaspoons salt, divided
4 mixed bell peppers, seeds removed and chopped diagonally
1 teaspoon freshly ground black pepper
2 tablespoons unsalted butter
1½ cups grated Parmesan cheese, plus more for garnish

DIRECTIONS

On the pot, choose Sear/Sauté and set to Medium High. Choose Start/Stop to preheat the pot. Melt the ghee and cook the garlic until fragrant, about 1 minute. Then, pour the stock, lemon juice, lemon zest, and rice into the pot. Sprinkle with 1 teaspoon of salt and stir to combine well.

Seal the pressure lid, hit Pressure, set to High, and the timer to 7 minutes; press Start. While the rice cooks, in a bowl, toss the peppers with the remaining ghee, salt, and black pepper.

When the timer has ended, do a natural pressure release for 10 minutes, then a quick pressure release. Stir the butter into the rice until properly mixed.

Then, put the reversible rack inside the pot in the higher position, which will be over the risotto. Arrange the bell peppers on the rack.

Close the crisping lid. Choose Broil and set the time to 8 minutes; press Start/Stop.

When done cooking, take out the rack from the pot. Stir the Parmesan cheese into the risotto.

To serve, spoon the risotto into serving plates, top with the bell peppers and garnish with extra Parmesan. Serve immediately.

Roasted Squash & Rice with Crispy Tofu

Servings: 4 | Ready in about: 70 min

INGREDIENTS

¾ cup water

1 small butternut squash, peeled and diced

2 tablespoons melted butter, divided

1 teaspoon salt

1 teaspoon freshly ground black pepper

1 tablespoon coconut aminos

1 (15-ounce) block extra-firm tofu, drained and cubed

2 teaspoons arrowroot starch

1 cup jasmine rice, cooked

DIRECTIONS

Pour the rice and water into the pot and mix with a spoon. Seal the pressure lid, choose Pressure, set to High and set the time to 2 minutes. Choose Start/Stop to boil the rice.

in a bowl, toss the butternut squash with 1 tablespoon of melted butter and season with the salt and black pepper. Set aside.

In another bowl, mix the remaining butter with the coconut aminos, and toss the tofu in the mixture. Pour the arrowroot starch over the tofu and toss again to combine well.

When done cooking the rice, perform a quick pressure release, and carefully open the pressure lid.

Put the reversible rack in the pot in the higher position and line with aluminum foil. Arrange the tofu and butternut squash on the rack.

Close the crisping lid. Choose Air Crisp, set the temperature to 400°F, and set the time to 20 minutes. Choose Start/Stop to begin cooking. After 10 minutes, use tongs to turn the butternut squash and tofu.

When done cooking, check for your desired crispiness and serve the tofu and squash with the rice.

Rice Stuffed Zucchini Boats

Servings: 4 | Ready in about: 55 min

INGREDIENTS

2 small zucchini
½ cup cooked white short grain rice
½ cup canned white beans, drained and rinsed
½ cup chopped tomatoes
½ cup chopped toasted cashew nuts

½ cup grated Parmesan cheese, divided
2 tablespoons melted butter, divided
½ teaspoon salt
½ teaspoon freshly ground black pepper

DIRECTIONS

Cut each zucchini in half and then, cut in half lengthwise and scoop out the pulp. Chop the pulp roughly and place in a medium bowl.

In the bowl, add the rice, beans, tomatoes, cashew nuts, ¼ cup of Parmesan cheese, 1 tablespoon of melted butter, the salt, and black pepper. Combine the mixture well but not to break the beans.

Put the Crisping Basket in the pot. Close the crisping lid, choose Air Crisp, set the temperature to 400°F, and the time to 5 minutes.

Spoon the mixed ingredients into the zucchini boats and arrange the stuffed zucchinis in a single layer in the preheated basket. Close the crisping lid. Choose Air Crisp, set the temperature to 400°F, and the time to 15 minutes. Choose Start/Stop to begin cooking.

After 15 minutes, sprinkle the zucchini boats with the remaining Parmesan cheese and butter.

Close the crisping lid. Choose Broil, set the time to 5 minutes, and choose Start/Stop to broil.

When done cooking, ensure it is as crisp as you desire, otherwise broil for a few more minutes.

Remove the zucchinis onto a plate, allow cooling for about a minute, and serve.

Garganelli with Swiss Cheese and Mushrooms

Servings: 4 | Ready in about: 60 min

INGREDIENTS

8 ounces garganelli
1 (12–fluid ounce) can full fat evaporated milk
1¼ cups water
1½ teaspoons salt
1 large egg
1½ teaspoons arrowroot starch
8 ounces Swiss cheese, shredded

1 recipe sautéed mushrooms
2 tablespoons chopped fresh cilantro
3 tablespoons sour cream
1½ cups panko breadcrumbs
3 tablespoons melted unsalted butter
3 tablespoons grated Cheddar cheese

DIRECTIONS

Pour the garganelli into the inner pot, add half of the evaporated milk, the water, and salt.

Seal the pressure lid, choose Pressure, set to High and the time to 4 minutes. Press Start.

In a bowl, whisk the remaining milk with the egg. In another bowl, combine the arrowroot starch with the Swiss cheese.

When the pasta has cooked, perform a natural pressure release for 3 minutes, then a quick pressure release and carefully open the lid. Pour in the milk-egg mixture and a large handful of the starch mixture. Stir to melt the cheese and then add the remaining cheese in 3 or 4 batches while stirring to melt. Mix in the mushrooms, cilantro, and sour cream.

In a bowl, mix the breadcrumbs, melted butter, and cheddar cheese. Then, sprinkle the mixture evenly over the pasta. Close the crisping lid. Choose Broil and adjust the time to 5 minutes. Press Start to begin crisping.

When done, the top should be brown and crispy, otherwise broil further for 3 minutes, and serve immediately.

Easy Green Squash Gruyere

Servings: 4 | Ready in about: 70 min

INGREDIENTS

1 large green squash, sliced
2 teaspoons salt
3 tablespoons melted unsalted butter
1½ cups panko breadcrumbs

⅓ cup grated Gruyere cheese
2 cups tomato sauce
1 cup shredded mozzarella cheese

DIRECTIONS

Season the squash slices on both sides with salt and place the slices on a wire rack to drain liquid for 5 to 10 minutes.

In a bowl, combine the melted butter, breadcrumbs, and Gruyere cheese and set aside.

Rinse the squash slices with water and blot dry with paper towel. After, arrange the squash in the inner pot in a single layer as much as possible and pour the tomato sauce over the slices.

Seal the pressure lid, choose Pressure, set to High, and the time to 5 minutes. Press Start to commence cooking. When the timer has read to the end, perform a quick pressure release. Sprinkle the squash slices with the mozzarella cheese.

Close the crisping lid. Choose Bake/Roast; adjust the temperature to 375°F and the cook time to 2 minutes. Press Start to broil.

After, carefully open the lid and sprinkle the squash with the breadcrumb mixture. Close the crisping lid again, choose Bake/Roast, adjust the temperature to 375°F, and the cook time to 8 minutes. Press Start to continue broiling. Serve immediately.

Easy Spanish Rice

Servings: 4 | Ready in about: 50 min

INGREDIENTS

3 tablespoons ghee
1 small onion, chopped
2 garlic cloves, minced
1 banana pepper, seeded and chopped
1 cup jasmine rice
⅓ cup red salsa

¼ cup stewed tomatoes
½ cup vegetable stock
1 teaspoon Mexican Seasoning Mix
1 (16-ounce) can pinto beans, drained and rinsed
1 teaspoon salt
1 tablespoon chopped fresh parsley

DIRECTIONS

On your Foodi, choose Sear/Sauté and adjust to Medium. Press Start to preheat the inner pot.

Add the ghee to melt until no longer foaming and cook the onion, garlic, and banana pepper in the ghee. Cook for 2 minutes or until fragrant. Stir in the rice, salsa, tomato sauce, vegetable stock, Mexican seasoning, pinto beans, and salt. Seal the pressure lid, choose Pressure and adjust the pressure to High and the cook time to 6 minutes; press Start. After cooking, do a natural pressure release for 10 minutes. Stir in the parsley, dish the rice, and serve.

Cajun Baked Turnips

Servings: 4 | Ready in about: 85 min

INGREDIENTS

4 small turnips, scrubbed clean
¼ cup whipping cream
¼ cup sour cream
½ cup chopped roasted red bell pepper

1 teaspoon Cajun seasoning mix
1½ cups shredded Monterey Jack cheese
4 green onions, chopped, divided
⅓ cup grated Parmesan cheese

DIRECTIONS

Pour 1 cup of water into the inner pot. Put the reversible rack in the pot and place the turnips on top.

Seal the pressure lid, choose Pressure, adjust the pressure to High, and the cook time to 10 minutes; press Start. After cooking, perform a natural pressure release for 5 minutes.

Remove the turnips to a cutting board and allow cooling. Slice off a ½-inch piece from the top and the longer side of each turnip. Scoop the pulp into a bowl, including the flesh from the sliced tops making sure not to rip the skin of the turnip apart.

In the bowl with the pulp, add the whipping cream and sour cream and use a potato mash to break the pulp and mix the ingredients until fairly smooth. Stir in the roasted bell pepper, Cajun seasoning, and Monterey Jack cheese. Fetch out 2 tablespoons of green onions and stir the remaining into the mashed turnips.

Next, fill the turnip skins with the mashed mixture and sprinkle with the Parmesan. Pour the water into the inner pot and return the pot to the base.

Put the Crisping basket into the pot. Close the crisping lid; choose Air Crisp, adjust the temperature to 375°F, and the time to 2 minutes. Press Start.

When the timer is done, open the lid and put the turnips in the basket. Close the crisping lid; choose Air Crisp, adjust the temperature to 375°F, and the cook time to 15 minutes. Press Start. Cool for a few minutes and garnish with the reserved onions.

Pesto Minestrone with Cheesy Bread

Servings: 4 | Ready in about: 60 min

INGREDIENTS

3 tablespoons ghee
1 medium red onion, diced
1 celery stalk, diced
1 large carrot, peeled and diced
1 small yellow squash, diced
1 (14-ounce) can chopped tomatoes
1 (27-ounce) can cannellini beans, rinsed and drained
3 cups water
1 cup chopped zucchini
1 bay leaf

1 teaspoon mixed herbs
¼ teaspoon cayenne pepper
½ teaspoon salt
1 Pecorino Romano rind
3 tablespoons butter, at room temperature
¼ cup shredded Pecorino Romano cheese
1 garlic clove, minced
4 slices white bread
⅓ cup olive oil based pesto

DIRECTIONS

On your Foodi, choose Sear/Sauté, and adjust to Medium to preheat the inner pot. Press Start. Add the ghee to the pot to melt and sauté the onion, celery, and carrot for 3 minutes or until the vegetables start to soften.

Stir in the yellow squash, tomatoes, beans, water, zucchini, bay leaf, mixed herbs, cayenne pepper, salt, and Pecorino Romano rind.

Seal the pressure lid, choose Pressure, adjust to High, and set the time to 4 minutes. Press Start. In a bowl, mix the butter, shredded cheese, and garlic. Spread the mixture on the bread slices.

After cooking the soup, perform a natural pressure release for 2 minutes, then a quick pressure release and carefully open the lid.

Adjust the taste of the soup with salt and black pepper, and remove the bay leaf.

Put the reversible rack in the upper position of the pot and lay the bread slices in the rack with the buttered-side up.

Close the crisping lid. Choose Broil; adjust the cook time to 5 minutes, and Press Start/Stop to begin broiling.

When the bread is crispy, carefully remove the rack, and set aside.

Ladle the soup into serving bowls and drizzle the pesto over. Serve with the garlic toasts.

Creamy Cauliflower & Asparagus Farfalle

Servings: 4 | Ready in about: 60 min

INGREDIENTS

1 bunch asparagus, trimmed, cut into 1-inch pieces
2 cups cauliflower florets
3 tablespoons melted butter, divided
3 teaspoons salt, divided
10 ounces farfalle
3 garlic cloves, minced

2½ cups vegetable stock
½ cup heavy cream
1 cup cherry tomatoes, halved
¼ cup chopped basil
½ cup grated Parmesan cheese

DIRECTIONS

Put the Crisping Basket in the Foodi. Close the crisping lid, choose Air Crisp; adjust the temperature to 375°F and the time to 2 minutes; press Start.

Pour the asparagus, and cauliflower, in a large bowl and drizzle with 1 tablespoon of melted butter. Season with ½ teaspoon of salt and toss. Open the cooker and transfer the vegetables to the basket.

Close the crisping lid; choose Air Crisp, adjust the temperature to 375°F, and set the timer to 10 minutes. Press Start to begin roasting. After 5 minutes, carefully open the lid and mix the vegetables. Close the lid and continue cooking.

When done roasting, take out the basket, and cover the top with aluminum foil; set aside.

Place the farfalle into the inner pot and add the remaining butter. Using tongs, toss the farfalle to coat, and add the remaining salt, garlic, and water. Stir to combine.

Seal the pressure lid, choose Pressure; adjust the pressure to High and the cook time to 5 minutes; press Start. After cooking, do a quick pressure release and carefully open the lid.

Stir the heavy cream and tomatoes into the pasta, tossing well.

Choose Sear/Sauté and adjust to Medium. Press Start to simmer the cream until the sauce has your desired consistency.

Gently mix in the asparagus, and cauliflower. Allow warming to soften the vegetables, then stir in the basil and Parmesan cheese. Dish the creamy farfalle and serve warm.

Mushroom Risotto with Swiss Chard

Servings: 4 | Ready in about: 60 min

INGREDIENTS

3 tablespoons ghee, divided
1 small bunch Swiss chard, chopped
1 cup short grain rice
⅓ cup white wine
2 cups vegetable stock

½ teaspoon salt
½ cup sautéed mushrooms
½ cup caramelized onions
⅓ cup grated Pecorino Romano cheese

DIRECTIONS

Press Sear/Sauté and adjust to Medium. Press Start to preheat the inner pot. Melt 2 tablespoons of ghee and sauté the Swiss chard for 5 minutes until wilted. Spoon into a bowl and set aside.

Use a paper towel to wipe out any remaining liquid in the pot and melt the remaining ghee. Stir in the rice and cook for about 1 minute. Add the white wine and cook for 2 to 3 minutes, with occasional stirring until the wine has evaporated. Add in stock and salt; stir to combine.

Seal the pressure lid, choose Pressure; adjust the pressure to High and the cook time to 8 minutes; press Start. When the timer is done reading, perform a quick pressure release and carefully open the lid.

Stir in the mushrooms, swiss chard, and onions and let the risotto heat for 1 minute. Mix the cheese into the rice to melt, and adjust the taste with salt.

Spoon the risotto into serving bowls and serve immediately.

Spicy Tangy Salmon with Wild Rice

Servings: 4 | Ready in about: 50 min

INGREDIENTS

1 cup wild rice
1 cup vegetable stock
4 skinless salmon fillets
A bunch of asparagus, trimmed and cut diagonally
3 tablespoons olive oil, divided
1 teaspoon salt
1 teaspoon freshly ground black pepper

2 limes, juiced
2 tablespoons honey
1 teaspoon sweet paprika
2 jalapeño peppers, seeded and diced
4 garlic cloves, minced
2 tablespoons chopped fresh parsley

DIRECTIONS

Pour the brown rice and vegetable stock in the pot; stir to combine. Put the reversible rack in the pot in the higher position and lay the salmon fillets on the rack.

Seal the pressure lid, choose Pressure, set to High, and set the time to 2 minutes; press Start.

In a bowl, toss the broccoli with 1 tablespoon of olive oil and season with the salt and black pepper. In another bowl, evenly combine the remaining oil, the lime juice, honey, paprika, jalapeño, garlic, and parsley.

When done cooking, do a quick pressure release, and carefully open the pressure lid.

Pat the salmon dry with a paper towel and coat the fish with the honey sauce while reserving a little for garnishing.

Arrange the asparagus around the salmon. Close the crisping lid; choose Broil and set the time to 7 minutes. Choose Start/Stop.

When ready, remove the salmon from the rack. Dish the salmon with asparagus and rice. Garnish with parsley and remaining sauce. Serve immediately.

Mashed Broccoli with Cream Cheese

Servings: 4 | Ready in about: 12 min

Ingredients:

3 heads broccoli, chopped
6 oz cream cheese
2 cloves garlic, crushed

2 tbsp butter, unsalted
Salt and black pepper to taste
2 cups water

Directions:

Turn on the Ninja Foodi and select Sear/Sauté mode, adjust to High.

Drop in the butter, once it melts add the garlic and cook for 30 seconds while stirring frequently to prevent the garlic from burning.

Then, add the broccoli, water, salt, and pepper.

Close the lid, secure the pressure valve, and select Pressure mode on High pressure for 5 minutes. Press Start/Stop.

Once the timer has ended, do a quick pressure release and use a stick blender to mash the ingredients until smooth to your desired consistency and well combined.

Stir in Cream cheese. Adjust the taste with salt and pepper. Close the crisping lid and cook for 2 minutes on Broil mode.

Serve warm.

Spinach Pesto Spaghetti Squash

Servings: 4 | Ready in about: 11 min

Ingredients:

4 lb spaghetti squash

1 cup water

For the Pesto
½ cup spinach, chopped
2 tbsp walnuts
2 garlic cloves, minced

Zest and juice from ½ lemon
Salt and ground pepper, to taste
⅓ cup extra virgin olive oil

Directions:

In a food processor put all the pesto ingredients and blend until everything is well incorporated. Season to taste and set aside.

Put the squash on a flat surface and use a knife to slice in half lengthwise. Scoop out all seeds and discard them.

Next, open the Ninja Foodi, pour the water into it and fit the reversible rack at the bottom. Place the squash halves on the rack, close the lid, secure the pressure valve, and select Steam on High pressure for 5 minutes. Press Start/Stop.

Once the timer has ended, do a quick pressure release, and open the lid.

Remove the squash halves onto a cutting board and use a fork to separate the pulp strands into spaghetti-like pieces. Return to the pot and close the crisping lid. Cook for 2 minutes on Broil mode.

Scoop the spaghetti squash into serving plates and drizzle over the spinach pesto.

Cream of Cauliflower & Butternut Squash

Servings: 4 | Ready in about: 32 min

Ingredients:

2 tsp olive oil

1 large white onion, chopped

4 cloves garlic, minced

1 (2 pounds) butternut squash, peeled, seeded, and cubed

2 heads cauliflower, cut in florets

3 cups chicken broth

3 tsp paprika

Salt and black pepper to taste

1 cup milk, full fat

Topping:

Grated Cheddar cheese, crumbled bacon, chopped chives, pumpkin seeds

Directions:

Select Sear/Sauté mode and set to High. Heat olive oil, add the white onion and garlic and sauté for 3 minutes.

Next, pour in the butternut squash, cauliflower florets, broth, paprika, pepper, and salt (if needed because of the broth). Stir the ingredients with a spoon.

Close the lid, secure the pressure valve, select Pressure mode on High pressure and adjust the time for 8 minutes. Press Start button.

Once the timer has ended, do a quick pressure release, and open the lid. Stir in the milk and use a stick blender to puree the soup. Adjust the seasoning.

Stir in cheese, close the crisping lid and cook for 2 minutes on Broil mode.

Dish the soup into serving bowls. Add the remaining toppings on the soup and serve warm.

Crème de la Broc

Servings: 6 | Ready in about: 25 min

Ingredients:

3 cups heavy cream

3 cups vegetable broth

4 tbsp butter

4 tbsp flour

4 cups chopped broccoli florets, only the bushy tops

1 medium Red onion, chopped

3 cloves garlic, minced

1 tsp Italian Seasoning

Salt and black pepper to taste

1 ½ oz cream cheese

1 ½ cups grated yellow and white Cheddar cheese + extra for topping

Directions:

Select Sear/Sauté mode, adjust to High and melt the butter once the pot is ready. Add the flour and use a spoon to stir until it clumps up. Gradually pour in the heavy cream while stirring until white sauce forms.

Fetch out the butter sauce into a bowl and set aside.

Press Stop and add the onions, garlic, broth, broccoli, Italian seasoning, and cream cheese. Use a wooden spoon to stir the mixture.

Seal the lid, and select Pressure mode on High pressure for 12 minutes. Press Start/Stop. Once the timer has ended, do a quick pressure release.

Add in butter sauce and cheddar cheese, salt, and pepper. Close the crisping lid and cook on Broil mode for 3 minutes.

Dish the soup into serving bowls, top it with extra cheese, to serve.

Eggplant Lasagna

Servings: 4 | Ready in about: 25 min

Ingredients:

3 large eggplants, sliced in uniform ¼ inches
4 ¼ cups Marinara sauce
1 ½ cups shredded Mozzarella cheese

Cooking spray
Chopped fresh basil to garnish
¼ cup Parmesan cheese, grated

Directions:

Open the pot and grease it with cooking spray. Arrange the eggplant slices in a single layer on the bottom of the pot and sprinkle some cheese all over it.

Arrange another layer of eggplant slices on the cheese, sprinkle this layer with cheese also, and repeat the layering of eggplant and cheese until both ingredients are exhausted.

Lightly spray the eggplant with cooking spray and pour the marinara sauce all over it.

Close the lid and pressure valve, and select Pressure mode on High pressure for 8 minutes. Press Start/Stop.

Once the timer has stopped, do a quick pressure release, and open the lid. Sprinkle with grated parmesan cheese, close the crisping lid and cook for 10 minutes on Bake/Roast mode on 380 degrees F.

With two napkins in hand, gently remove the inner pot. Allow cooling for 10 minutes before serving.

Garnish the lasagna with basil and serve warm as a side dish.

Buttered Leafy Greens

Servings: 4 | Ready in about: 10 min

Ingredients:

2 lb baby spinach
1 lb kale leaves
½ lb Swiss chard
1 tbsp dried basil

Salt and black pepper to season
½ tbsp butter
½ cup water

Directions:

Turn on the Ninja Foodi, add the water and fit the reversible rack at the bottom of the pot. Put the spinach, swiss chard, and kale on the rack.

Close the lid, secure the pressure valve, and select Steam mode on High pressure for 3 minutes. Press Start/Stop.

Once the timer has ended, do a quick pressure release and open the lid.

Remove the trivet with the wilted greens onto a plate and discard the water in the pot.

Select Sear/Sauté mode on the pot and add the butter. Once it melts, add the spinach and kale back to the pot, and the dried basil. Season with salt and pepper and stir it. Close the crisping lid and cook for 4 minutes on Bake/Roast mode on 380 degrees F.

Dish the greens into serving plates and serve as a side dish.

Fall Celeriac Pumpkin Soup

Servings: 4 | Ready in about: 30 min

Ingredients:

1 celeriac, peeled and cubed
16 oz pumpkin puree
5 stalks celery, chopped
1 white onion, chopped
1 lb green beans, cut in 5 strips each
2 cups vegetable broth

3 cups spinach leaves
1 tbsp chopped basil leaves
¼ tsp dried thyme
⅛ tsp rubbed sage
Salt to taste

Directions:

Open the Ninja Foodi and pour in the celeriac, pumpkin puree, celery, onion, green beans, vegetable broth, basil leaves, thyme, sage, and a little salt.

Close the lid, secure the pressure valve, and select Steam mode on High pressure for 5 minutes. Press Start/Stop.

Once the timer has ended, do a quick pressure release and open the lid.

Add in the spinach and stir using a spoon. Close the crisping lid and cook for 3 minutes on Broil mode.

Use a soup spoon to fetch the soup into serving bowls.

Zucchini & Quinoa Stuffed Red Peppers

Servings: 4 | Ready in about: 40 min

Ingredients:

4 red bell peppers
2 large tomatoes, chopped
1 small onion, chopped
2 cloves garlic, minced
1 tbsp olive oil
1 cup quinoa, rinsed
2 cups chicken broth

1 small zucchini, chopped
1 ½ cup water
½ tsp smoked paprika
½ cup chopped mushrooms
Salt and black pepper to taste
1 cup grated Gouda cheese

Directions:

Select Sear/Sauté mode on High. Once it is ready, add the olive oil to heat and then add the onion and garlic. Sauté for 3 minutes to soften, stirring occasionally.

Include the tomatoes, cook for 3 minutes and then add the quinoa, zucchinis, and mushrooms. Season with paprika, salt, and black pepper and stir with a spoon. Cook for 5 to 7 minutes, then, turn the pot off.

Use a knife to cut the bell peppers in halves (lengthwise) and remove their seeds and stems.

Spoon the quinoa mixture into the bell peppers. Put the peppers in a greased baking dish and pour the broth over.

Wipe the pot clean with some paper towels, and pour the water into it. After, fit the steamer rack at the bottom of the pot.

Place the baking dish on top of the reversible rack, cover with aluminum foil, close the lid, secure the pressure valve, and select Pressure mode on High pressure for 15 minutes. Press Start/Stop.

Once the timer has ended, do a quick pressure release and open the lid. Remove the aluminum foil and sprinkle with the gouda cheese. Close the crisping lid, select Bake/Roast mode and cook for 10 minutes on 375 degrees F.

Arrange the stuffed peppers on a serving platter and serve right away or as a side to a meat dish.

Pine nuts and Steamed Asparagus

Servings: 4 | Ready in about: 15 min

Ingredients:

1 ½ lb asparagus, ends trimmed
Salt and pepper, to taste
1 cup water

1 tbsp butter
½ cup chopped Pine Nuts
1 tbsp olive oil to garnish

Directions:

Open the Ninja Foodi, pour the water in, and fit the reversible rack at the bottom.

Place the asparagus on the rack, close the crisping lid, select Air Crisp mode, and set the time to 8 minutes on 380 degrees F. Press Start/Stop.

At the 4-minute mark, carefully turn the asparagus over.

When ready, remove to a plate, sprinkle with salt and pepper, and set aside.

Select Sear/Sauté on your Ninja Foodi, set to Medium and melt the butter.

Add the pine nuts and cook for 2-3 minutes until golden. Scatter over the asparagus the pine nuts, and drizzle olive oil.

Bok Choy & Zoddle Soup

Servings: 6 | Ready in about: 35 min

Ingredients:

1 lb baby bok choy, stems removed
6 oz Shitake mushrooms, stems removed and sliced to a 2-inch thickness
3 carrots, peeled and sliced diagonally
2 zucchinis, spiralized
2 sweet onion, chopped
2-inch ginger, chopped
2 cloves garlic, peeled

2 tbsp sesame oil
2 tbsp soy sauce
2 tbsp chili paste
6 cups water
Salt to taste
Chopped green onion to garnish
Sesame seeds to garnish

Directions:

In a food processor, add the chili paste, ginger, onion, and garlic; and process them until they are pureed.

Turn on the Ninja foodi and select Sear/Sauté mode to High.

Pour in the sesame oil, once it has heated add the onion puree and cook for 3 minutes while stirring constantly to prevent burning. Add the water, mushrooms, soy sauce, and carrots.

Close the lid, secure the pressure valve, and select Pressure mode on High pressure for 5 minutes. Press Start/Stop.

Once the timer has ended, do a quick pressure release and open the lid.

Add the zucchini noodles and bok choy, and stir to ensure that they are well submerged in the liquid.

Adjust the taste with salt, cover the pot with the crisping lid, and let the vegetables cook for 10 minutes on Broil mode.

Use a soup spoon to dish the soup with veggies into soup bowls.

Sprinkle with green onions and sesame seeds.

Serve as a complete meal.

Mushroom Brown Rice Pilaf

Servings: 4 | Ready in about: 15 min

Ingredients:

2 cups brown rice, rinsed
4 cups vegetable broth
3 teaspoons olive oil
1 cup Portobello mushrooms, thinly sliced

¼ cup Romano cheese, grated
Salt to taste
2 sprigs parsley, to garnish

Directions:

Heat the oil on Sear/Sauté on Medium, and stir-fry the mushrooms for 3 minutes until golden. Season with salt, and add rice and broth.

Close the lid, secure the pressure valve, and select Pressure mode on High pressure for 5 minutes. Press Start/Stop to start cooking.

Once the timer has ended, do a quick pressure release and open the lid.

Spread the cheese over and close the crisping lid. Select Bake/Roast, adjust to 375°F and the timer to 2 minutes. Press Start/Stop to start cooking.

To serve, plate the pilaf and top with freshly chopped parsley.

Asian-Style Tofu Soup

Servings: 4 | Ready in about: 25 min

Ingredients:

16 oz firm Tofu, water- packed
7 cloves garlic, minced
2 tbsp Korean red pepper flakes (gochugaru)
1 tbsp sugar
1 tbsp olive oil
2 tbsp ginger paste

¼ cup soy sauce
3 cup sliced bok choy
6 ounces dry egg noodles
4 cups vegetable broth
1 cup sliced Shitake mushrooms
½ cup chopped cilantro

Directions:

Drain the liquid out of the tofu, pat the tofu dry with paper towels, and use a knife to cut them into 1-inch cubes.

Turn your Ninja Foodi on and select Sear/Sauté mode on Medium.

Pour the oil to heat, add the garlic and ginger, and sauté for 2 minutes.

Add the sugar, broth, and soy sauce. Stir and cook for 30 seconds. Include the tofu and bok choy, close the lid, secure the pressure valve, and select Pressure mode on High pressure for 10 minutes. Press Start/Stop.

Once the timer has ended, do a quick pressure release and open the lid. Add the zucchini noodles, give it a good stir using a spoon, and close the crisping lid. Let the soup cook for 4 minutes on Broil mode. Use a soup spoon to fetch the soup into soup bowls, top with cilantro and enjoy.

Cheesy Stuffed Mushrooms

Servings: 4 | Ready in about: 40 min

Ingredients:

10 large white mushrooms, stems removed
¼ cup roasted red bell peppers, chopped
1 red bell pepper, seeded and chopped
1 green onion, chopped
1 small onion, chopped

¼ cup grated Parmesan cheese
½ cup water
1 tbsp butter
½ tsp dried oregano
Salt and black pepper to taste

Directions:

Turn on the Ninja Foodi and select Sear/Sauté mode on Medium.

Put in the butter to melt and add the roasted and fresh peppers, green onion, onion, oregano, salt, and pepper. Use a spoon to mix and cook for 2 minutes.

Spoon the bell pepper mixture into the mushrooms and use a paper towel to wipe the pot and place the stuffed mushrooms in it, 5 at a time. Pour in water.

Close the lid, secure the pressure valve, and select pressure mode on High pressure for 5 minutes. Press Start/ Stop.

Once the timer has ended, do a quick pressure release and open the lid.

Sprinkle with parmesan cheese and close the crisping lid. Select Bake/Roast, adjust the temperature to 380°F and the time to 2 minutes and press

Start/Stop button.

Use a set of tongs to remove the stuffed mushrooms onto a plate and repeat the cooking process for the remaining mushrooms.

Serve hot with a side of steamed green veggies and a sauce.

Vegetarian Minestrone Soup

Servings: 4 | Ready in about: 40 min

Ingredients:

1 (15.5 oz) can Cannellini beans
1 Potato, peeled and diced
1 carrot, peeled and chopped
1 cup chopped butternut squash
2 small Red onions, cut in wedges
1 cup chopped celery
1 tbsp chopped fresh rosemary

8 sage leaves, chopped finely
1 bay leaf
4 cups vegetable broth
Salt and pepper, to taste
2 tsp olive oil
2 tbsp chopped fresh parsley

Directions:

Add the potato, carrot, squash, onion, celery, rosemary, sage leaves, bay leaf, vegetable broth, salt, pepper, and olive oil to the pot of your Ninja Foodi.

Close the lid, secure the pressure valve, and select Pressure mode on High pressure for 7 minutes. Press Start/ Stop.

Once the timer has ended, do a quick pressure release and open the lid. Add the cannellini beans and stir with a spoon. Close the crisping lid and cook for 5 minutes on Broil mode. Use a soup spoon to fetch the soup into soup bowls. Garnish with fresh parsley and serve with a side of crusted bread.

Green Cream Soup

Servings: 4 | Ready in about: 22 min

Ingredients:

½ lb kale leaves, chopped
½ lb spinach leaves, chopped
½ lb Swiss chard leaves, chopped
1 tbsp olive oil
1 onion, chopped
4 cloves garlic, minced

4 cups vegetable broth
1 ¼ cup heavy cream
Salt and pepper, to taste
1 ½ tbsp. white wine vinegar
Chopped Peanuts to garnish

Directions:

Turn on the Ninja Foodi and select Sear/Sauté mode on Medium.

Add the olive oil, once it has heated add the onion and garlic and sauté for 2-3 minutes until soft. Add greens and vegetable broth.

Close the lid, secure the pressure valve, and select Pressure mode on High pressure for 10 minutes. Press Start/Stop.

Once the timer has ended, do a quick pressure release.

Add the white wine vinegar, salt, and pepper. Use a stick blender to puree the ingredients in the pot. Close the crisping lid and cook for 3 minutes on Broil mode. Stir in the heavy cream.

Spoon the soup into bowls, sprinkle with peanuts, and serve.

Chipotle Chili

Servings: 4 | Ready in about: 35 min

Ingredients:

4 celery stalks, chopped
2 (15 oz) cans diced tomatoes
1 tbsp olive oil
3 carrots, chopped
2 cloves garlic, minced
2 tsp smoked paprika
2 green bell pepper, diced
½ cup water
1 tbsp cinnamon powder

1 tbsp cumin powder
1 sweet onion, chopped
2 cups tomato sauce
1.5 oz dark chocolate, chopped
1 small chipotle, minced
1 ½ cups raw walnuts, chopped + extra to garnish
Salt and pepper, to taste
Chopped cilantro to garnish

Directions:

Turn on the Ninja Foodi, open the lid and select Sear/Sauté mode on Medium.

Pour in the oil to heat and add the onion, celery, and carrots. Sauté for 4 minutes. Add the garlic, cumin, cinnamon, and paprika. Stir and let the sauce cook for 2 minutes.

Now, include the bell peppers, tomatoes, tomato sauce, chipotle, water, and walnuts Stir.

Close the lid, secure the pressure valve, and select Pressure mode on High pressure for 15 minutes. Press Start/Stop. Once the timer has ended, do a quick pressure release, and open the lid.

Pour the chopped chocolate in and stir it until it melts and is well incorporated into the chili. Adjust the taste with salt and pepper. Close the crisping lid and cook for 5 minutes on Broil mode.

Dish the chili into a serving bowl, garnish it with the remaining walnuts and cilantro. Serve with some noodles.

Vegan Carrot Gazpacho

Servings: 4 | Ready in about: 2 hr 30 min

INGREDIENTS

1 pound trimmed carrots
1 pinch salt
1 pound tomatoes, chopped
1 cucumber, peeled and chopped
1/4 cup extra-virgin olive oil

2 tbsp lemon juice
1 red onion, chopped
2 cloves garlic
2 tbsp white wine vinegar
salt and freshly ground black pepper to taste

DIRECTIONS

To the Foodi add carrots, salt and enough water. Seal the pressure lid, choose Pressure, set to High, and set the timer to 20 minutes. Press Start.

Once ready, do a quick release. Set the beets to a bowl and place in the refrigerator to cool. In a blender, add carrots, cucumber, red onion, pepper, garlic, olive oil, tomatoes, lemon juice, vinegar, and salt. Blend until very smooth. Place gazpacho to a serving bowl, chill while covered for 2 hours.

Pesto Quinoa Bowls with Veggies

Servings: 2 | Ready in about: 30 min

INGREDIENTS

1 cup quinoa, rinsed
2 cups water
salt and ground black pepper to taste
1 small beet, peeled and cubed
1 cup broccoli florets
1 carrot, peeled and chopped

½ pound Brussels sprouts
2 eggs
1 avocado, thinly sliced
¼ cup pesto sauce
lemon wedges, for serving

DIRECTIONS

In the pot, mix water, salt, quinoa and pepper.

Set the reversible rack to the pot over quinoa. To the reversible rack, add eggs, Brussels sprouts, broccoli, beet cubes, carrots, pepper and salt.

Seal the pressure lid, choose Pressure, set to High, and set the timer to 1 minute. Press Start. Release pressure naturally for 10 minutes, then release any remaining pressure quickly. Remove reversible rack from the pot and set the eggs to a bowl of ice water. Peel and halve the eggs. Use a fork to fluff quinoa.

Separate quinoa, broccoli, avocado, carrots, beet, Brussels sprouts, eggs, and a dollop of pesto into two bowls. Serve alongside a lemon wedge.

Indian Vegan Curry

Servings: 3 | Ready in about: 25 min

INGREDIENTS

1 tbsp butter
1 onion, chopped
2 cloves garlic, minced
1 tsp ginger, grated
1 tsp ground cumin
1 tsp red chilli powder
1 tsp salt

½ tsp ground turmeric
1 (15 ounces) can chickpeas, drained and rinsed
1 tomato, diced
⅓ cup water
5 cups collard greens, chopped
½ tsp garam masala
1 tsp lemon juice

DIRECTIONS

Melt butter on Sear/Sauté. Toss in the onion to coat. Close the pressure lid and cook for 2 minutes until soft. Mix in ginger, cumin powder, turmeric, red chili powder, garlic, and salt and cook for 30 seconds until crispy; stir in tomatoes. In the Foodi, mix in ⅓ water, tomato and chickpeas.

Seal the pressure lid, choose Pressure, set to High, and set the timer to 4 minutes. Press Start.

When ready, release the pressure quickly.

Into the chickpea mixture, stir in lemon juice, collard greens and garam masala until well coated. Cook for 2 to 3 minutes until collard greens wilt. Serve over rice or naan.

Green Minestrone

Servings: 4 | Ready in about: 30 min

INGREDIENTS

2 tbsp olive oil
1 head broccoli, cut into florets
4 celery stalks, sliced thinly
1 leek, sliced thinly
1 zucchini, chopped
1 cup green beans

2 cups vegetable broth
3 whole black peppercorns
salt to taste
water to cover
2 cups chopped kale

DIRECTIONS

Into the pressure cooker, add broccoli, leek, green beans, salt, peppercorns, zucchini, and celery. Mix in vegetable broth, oil, and water. Seal the pressure lid, choose Pressure, set to High, and set the timer to 4 minutes. Press Start.

Release pressure naturally for 5 minutes, then release the remaining pressure quickly. Add kale into the soup and stir; set to Keep Warm and cook until tender.

Creamy Mashed Potatoes with Spinach

Servings: 6 | Ready in about: 30 min

INGREDIENTS

3 pounds potatoes, peeled and quartered
1½ cups water
½ tsp salt
½ cup milk

⅓ cup butter
2 tbsp chopped fresh chives
fresh black pepper to taste
2 cups spinach, chopped

In the cooker, mix water, salt and potatoes. Seal the pressure lid, choose Pressure, set to High, and set the timer to 8 minutes. Press Start.

When ready, release the pressure quickly. Drain the potatoes, and reserve the liquid in a bowl. In a large bowl, mash the potatoes.

Mix with butter and milk; season with pepper and salt. With reserved cooking liquid, thin the potatoes to attain the desired consistency. Put the spinach in the remaining potato liquid and stir until wilted; season with salt and pepper. Drain and serve with potato mash. Garnish with black pepper and chives.

Herby-Garlic Potatoes

Servings: 4 | Ready in about: 30 min

INGREDIENTS

1½ pounds potatoes
3 tbsp butter
3 cloves garlic, thinly sliced
2 tbsp fresh rosemary, chopped

1/2 tsp fresh thyme, chopped
1/2 tsp fresh parsley, chopped
1/4 tsp ground black pepper
1/2 cup vegetable broth

DIRECTIONS

Use a small knife to pierce each potato to ensure there are no blowouts when placed under pressure.

Melt butter on Sear/Sauté. Add in potatoes, rosemary, parsley, pepper, thyme, and garlic, and cook for 10 minutes until potatoes are browned and the mixture is aromatic. In a bowl, mix miso paste and vegetable stock; stir into the mixture in the pressure cooker.

Seal the pressure lid, choose Pressure, set to High, and set the timer to 5 minutes. Press Start. Do a pressure quickly.

Punjabi Palak Paneer

Servings: 4 | Ready in about: 20 min

INGREDIENTS

¼ cup milk
2 tbsp butter
1 tsp cumin seeds
1 tsp coriander seeds
1 tomato, chopped
1 tsp minced fresh ginger
1 tsp minced fresh garlic

1 red onion, chopped
1 pound spinach, chopped
1 cup water
1 tsp salt, or to taste
2 cups paneer, cubed
1 tsp chilli powder

DIRECTIONS

Warm butter on Sear/Sauté, set to Medium High, and choose Start/Stop to preheat the pot. Press Start. Add in garlic, cumin seeds, coriander seeds, chilli powder, ginger, and garlic and fry for 1 minute until fragrant; add onion and cook for 2 more minutes until crispy. Add in salt, water and chopped spinach.

Seal the pressure lid, choose Pressure, set to High, and set the timer to 1 minute. Press Start.

When ready, release the pressure quickly. Add spinach mixture to a blender and blend to obtain a smooth paste. Mix paneer and tomato with spinach mixture.

Pilau Rice with Veggies

Servings: 4 | Ready in about: 30 min

INGREDIENTS

3 tbsp olive oil
1 tbsp ginger, minced
1 cup onion, chopped
1 cup green peas
1 cup carrot, chopped
1 cup mushroom, chopped
1 cup broccoli, chopped
1 tbsp chili powder

½ tbsp ground cumin
1 tsp garam masala
½ tsp turmeric powder
1 cup basmati rice, rinsed and drained
2 cups vegetable broth
1 tbsp lemon juice
2 tbsp chopped fresh cilantro

DIRECTIONS

Warm 1 tbsp olive oil on Sear/Sauté. Add in onion and ginger and cook for 3 minutes until soft. Stir in broccoli, green peas, mushrooms, and carrots; cook for 1 more minute. Add turmeric powder, chili powder, garam masala, and cumin for seasoning; cook for 1 minute until soft.

Add ¼ cup water into the pan to deglaze; scrape the bottom to get rid of any browned bits.

To the vegetables, add the remaining water and rice.

Seal the pressure lid, choose Pressure, set to High, and set the timer to 1 minute. Press Start. Release pressure naturally. Use a fork to fluff rice, sprinkle with lemon juice; divide onto plates and garnish with cilantro.

Carrot and Lentil Chili

Servings: 4 | Ready in about: 30 min

INGREDIENTS

1 tbsp olive oil
1 onion, chopped
1 cup celery, chopped
2 garlic cloves, sliced
1 onion, chopped
3 cups vegetable stock

1½ cups dried lentils, rinsed and stones removed
4 carrots, halved lengthwise
1 tbsp harissa, or more to taste
½ tsp sea salt
A handful of fresh parsley, chopped

DIRECTIONS

Warm olive oil on Sear/Sauté. Add in onion, garlic, and celery, and cook for 5 minutes until onion is soft. Mix in lentils, carrots, and vegetable stock. Seal the pressure lid, choose Pressure, set to High, and set the timer to 10 minutes. Press Start. Release pressure naturally. Mix lentils with salt and harissa and serve topped with parsley.

Steamed Artichokes with Lemon Aioli

Servings: 4 | Ready in about: 20 min

INGREDIENTS

4 artichokes, trimmed
1 lemon, halved
1 tsp lemon zest
1 tbsp lemon juice
3 cloves garlic, crushed

½ cup mayonnaise
1 cup water
Salt
1 small handful parsley, chopped

DIRECTIONS

On the artichokes cut ends, rub with lemon. Add water into the pot of pressure cooker. Set the reversible rack over the water,

Place the artichokes into the steamer basket with the points upwards; sprinkle each with salt.

Seal lid and cook on High pressure for 10 minutes. Press Start.

When ready, release the pressure quickly.

In a mixing bowl, combine mayonnaise, garlic, lemon juice, and lemon zest. Season to taste with salt.

Serve with warm steamed artichokes sprinkled with parsley.

Garlic Veggie Mash with Parmesan

Servings: 6 | Ready in about: 15 min

INGREDIENTS

3 pounds Yukon Gold potatoes, cut into 1-inch pieces
1 ½ cups cauliflower, broken into florets
1 carrot, chopped
1 cup Parmesan cheese, shredded
¼ cup butter, melted

¼ cup milk
1 tsp salt
1 garlic clove, minced
Fresh parsley for garnish

DIRECTIONS

Into your pot, add veggies, salt and cover with enough water.

Seal the pressure lid, choose Pressure, set to High, and set the timer to 10 minutes. Press Start.

When ready, release the pressure quickly.

Drain the vegetables and mash them with a potato masher; add garlic, butter and milk, and whisk until everything is well incorporated. Serve topped with parmesan cheese and chopped parsley.

Green Beans with Feta and Nuts

Servings: 6 | Ready in about: 15 min

INGREDIENTS

Juice from 1 lemon
1½ cups water
2 pounds green beans, trimmed
1 cup chopped toasted pine nuts

1 cup feta cheese, crumbled
6 tbsp olive oil
½ tsp salt
freshly ground black pepper to taste

DIRECTIONS

Add water to the pot. Set the reversible rack over the water.

Loosely heap green beans into the reversible rack.

Seal lid and cook on High Pressure for 5 minutes. Press Start. When the cooking cycle is complete,

When ready, release pressure quickly.

Drop green beans into a salad bowl; top with the olive oil, feta cheese, pepper, and pine nuts.

Mashed Parsnips and Cauliflower

Servings: 8 | Ready in about: 15 min

INGREDIENTS

1 ½ pounds parsnips, peeled and cubed
1 (1½ pounds) head cauliflower, cut into small florets
2 garlic cloves
¾ tsp salt
¼ tsp pepper

2 cups water
¼ cup sour cream
¼ cup grated Parmesan cheese
1 tbsp butter
2 tbsp minced chives

DIRECTIONS

In the pot, mix parsnips, garlic, water, salt, cauliflower, and pepper.

Seal the pressure lid, choose Pressure, set to High, and set the timer to 4 minutes. Press Start.

When ready, release the pressure quickly. Drain parsnips and cauliflower and return to pot; add Parmesan cheese, butter, and sour cream. Use a potato masher to mash until the desired consistency is attained.

Into the mashed parsnip, add 1 tbsp chives; place to a serving plate and garnish with remaining chives.

Tahini Sweet Potato Mash

Servings: 4 | Ready in about: 25 min

INGREDIENTS

1 cup water
2 pounds sweet potatoes, peeled and cubed
2 tbsp tahini
1 tbsp sugar

¼ tsp ground nutmeg
Chopped fresh chives, for garnish
sea salt to taste

DIRECTIONS

In the Foodi, add 1 cup cold water and set a steamer basket into the pot. Add sweet potato cubes into the steamer basket. Seal the pressure lid, choose Pressure, set to High, and set the timer to 8 minutes. Press Start. When ready, release the pressure quickly.

In a large mixing bowl, add cooked sweet potatoes and slightly mash.Using a hand mixer, whip in nutmeg, sugar, and tahini until the sweet potatoes attain the consistency you desire; add salt for seasoning. Top with chives and serve.

Aloo Gobi with Cilantro

Servings: 4 | Ready in about: 40 min

INGREDIENTS

1 tbsp vegetable oil
1 head cauliflower, cored and cut into florets
1 potato, peeled and diced
1 tbsp ghee
2 tsp cumin seeds
1 onion, minced
4 garlic cloves, minced
1 tomato, cored and chopped

1 jalapeño pepper, deseeded and minced
1 tbsp curry paste
1 tsp ground turmeric
½ tsp chili pepper
1 cup water
salt to taste
A handful of cilantro leaves, chopped

DIRECTIONS

Warm oil on Sear/Sauté. Add in potato and cauliflower and cook for 8 to 10 minutes until lightly browned; add salt for seasoning. Set the vegetables to a bowl.

Add ghee to the pot. Mix in cumin seeds and cook for 10 seconds until they start to pop; add onion and cook for 3 minutes until softened. Mix in garlic; cook for seconds. Add in tomato, curry paste, chili pepper, jalapeño pepper, curry paste, and turmeric; cook for 3 to 5 minutes until the tomato starts to break down.

Return potato and cauliflower to the pot. Add water over the vegetables, add more salt if need be, and stir.

Seal the pressure lid, choose Pressure, set to High, and set the timer to 4 minutes. Press Start. Release pressure naturally. Top with cilantro and serve.

Spicy Cauliflower Rice with Peas

Servings: 2 | Ready in about: 15 min

INGREDIENTS

1 head cauliflower, cut into florets
1 cup water
2 tbsp olive oil
salt to taste

1 tsp chili powder
¼ cup green peas
1 tbsp chopped fresh parsley

DIRECTIONS

Into the pressure cooker's pot, add water. Set the reversible rack over water. Add cauliflower into the steamer basket. Seal the pressure lid, choose Pressure, set to High, and set the timer to 1 minute. Press Start.

When ready, release the pressure quickly. Remove reversible rack. Drain water from the pot, pat dry, and return to pressure cooker base.

Set on Sear/Sauté. Warm oil. Add in cauliflower and stir to break into smaller pieces like rice; stir in chili powder, peas and salt. Place the cauliflower rice into plates and add parsley for garnishing.

Chipotle Vegetarian Chili

Servings: 12 | Ready in about: 45 min

INGREDIENTS

1 (28 ounces) can diced tomatoes
2 cups cashews, chopped
1 cup onion, chopped
1 cup red lentils
1 cup red quinoa
3 chipotle peppers, chopped
3 garlic cloves, minced

2 tbsp chili powder
1 tsp salt
4½ cups water
2 cups carrots, chopped
1 (15 ounces) can black beans, rinsed and drained
1/4 cup fresh parsley, chopped

DIRECTIONS

In the pot, mix tomatoes, onion, chipotle peppers, chili powder, lentils, walnuts, carrots, quinoa, garlic, and salt; stir in more water. Seal the pressure lid, choose Pressure, set to High, and set the timer to 30 minutes. Press Start.

When ready, release the pressure quickly. Into the chili, add black beans; simmer on Keep Warm until heated through. Add ¼ cup to 1 cup water if you want a thinner consistency. Top with a garnish of parsley.

Thai Vegetable Stew

Servings: 4 | Ready in about: 30 min

INGREDIENTS

1 tbsp coconut oil
1 cup onion, chopped
1 tbsp fresh ginger, minced
2 garlic cloves, minced
3 carrots, peeled and chopped
1 red bell pepper, sliced

1 orange bell pepper, sliced
1 (14 ounces) can coconut milk
1 cup bok choy, chopped
½ cup water
2 tbsp red curry paste

DIRECTIONS

Melt coconut oil on Sear/Sauté. Add in onion and cook for 3 to 4 minutes until soft; add garlic and ginger and cook for 30 more seconds until soft. Mix in orange bell pepper, red bell pepper and carrots; cook for 3 to 4 minutes until the peppers become soft and tender.

Add curry paste, bok choy, coconut milk, and water and stir well to obtain a consistent color of the sauce.

Seal lid and cook for 1 minute on High Pressure. Press Start.

When ready, release the pressure quickly. Serve hot!

Sweet Carrots with Crumbled Bacon

Servings: 8 | Ready in about: 30 min

INGREDIENTS

3 slices bacon, crumbled
4 pounds carrots, peeled and sliced
½ cup fresh orange juice
¼ cup olive oil

3 tbsp honey
1 tsp salt
2 tsp cornstarch
1 tbsp cold water

DIRECTIONS

Fry the bacon in your pressure cooker on Sear/Sauté until crisp, about 5 minutes. Set aside.

In a bowl, mix salt, olive oil, orange juice, and maple syrup; add the mixture and carrots to the pot and mix well to coat. Seal the pressure lid, choose Pressure, set to High, and set the timer to 6 minutes. Press Start.

When ready, release the pressure quickly. Transfer carrots to a serving dish. Press Sear/Sauté.

In a bowl, mix cold water and cornstarch until cornstarch dissolves completely; add to the liquid remaining in the pressure cooker. Simmer sauce as you stir for 2 minutes to obtain a thick and smooth consistency. Ladle sauce over the carrots and scatter over the crumbled bacon.

Honey-Glazed Acorn Squash

Servings: 4 | Ready in about: 30 min

INGREDIENTS

½ cup water
3 tbsp honey, divided
1 lb acorn squash, peeled and cut into chunks
2 tbsp butter

1 tbsp dark brown sugar
1 tbsp cinnamon
salt and ground black pepper to taste

DIRECTIONS

In a small bowl, mix 1 tbsp honey and water; pour into the pressure cooker's pot.

Add in squash. Seal the and cook on High pressure for 4 minutes. Press Start.

When ready, release the pressure quickly.

Transfer the squash to a serving dish. Turn Foodi to Sear/Sauté.

Mix brown sugar, cinnamon, the remaining 2 tbsp honey and the liquid in the pot; cook as you stir for 4 minutes to obtain a thick consistency and starts to turn caramelized and golden.

Spread honey glaze over squash; add pepper and salt for seasoning.

Artichoke with Garlic Mayo

Servings: 4 | Ready in about: 20 min

INGREDIENTS

2 large artichokes
2 cups water
2 garlic cloves, smashed

½ cup mayonnaise
Salt and black pepper to taste
Juice of 1 lime

DIRECTIONS

Using a serrated knife, trim about 1 inch from the artichokes' top. Into the pot, add water and set trivet over. Lay the artichokes on the trivet. Seal lid and cook for 14 minutes. Press Start.

When ready, release the pressure quickly. Mix the mayonnaise with garlic and lime juice; season with salt and pepper. Serve artichokes in a platter with garlic mayo on the side.

Asparagus with Feta

Servings: 4 | Ready in about: 15 min

INGREDIENTS

1 cup water
1 pound asparagus spears, ends trimmed
1 tbsp olive oil

salt and freshly ground black pepper to taste
1 lemon, cut into wedges
1 cup feta cheese, cubed

DIRECTIONS

Into the pot, add water and set trivet over the water. Place steamer basket on the trivet.

Place the asparagus into the steamer basket. Seal the pressure lid, choose Pressure, set to High, and set the timer to 1 minute. Press Start.

When ready, release the pressure quickly. Add olive oil in a bowl and toss in asparagus until well coated; season with pepper and salt. Serve alongside feta cheese and lemon wedges.

Parsley Mashed Cauliflower

Servings: 4 | Ready in about: 15 min

INGREDIENTS

2 cups water
1 head cauliflower
1 tbsp butter
¼ tsp celery salt

1/4 cup heavy cream
1 tbsp fresh parsley, finely chopped
⅛ tsp freshly ground black pepper

DIRECTIONS

Into the pot, add water and set trivet on top and lay cauliflower head onto the trivet.

Seal the pressure lid, choose Pressure, set to High, and set the timer to 8 minutes. Press Start.

When ready, release the pressure quickly.

Remove the trivet and drain liquid from the pot before returning to the base.

Take back the cauliflower to the pot alongside the pepper, heavy cream, salt and butter; use an immersion blender to blend until smooth. Top with parsley and serve.

Turkey Stuffed Potatoes

Servings: 4 | Ready in about: 30 min

INGREDIENTS

2 cups vegetable broth
1 tsp chili powder
1 tsp ground cumin
½ tsp onion powder
½ tsp garlic powder

1 pound turkey breasts
4 potatoes
2 tbsp fresh cilantro, chopped
1 Fresno chili pepper, chopped

DIRECTIONS

In the pot, combine chicken broth, cumin, garlic powder, onion powder, and chili powder; toss in turkey to coat. Place a reversible rack over the turkey. Use a fork to pierce the potatoes and set them into the reversible rack.

Seal the pressure lid, choose Pressure, set to High, and set the timer to 20 minutes. Press Start.

When ready, release the pressure quickly.

Remove reversible rack from the cooker. Place the potatoes on a plate.

Place turkey in a mixing bowl and use two forks to shred.

Half each potato lengthwise. Stuff with shredded turkey; top with cilantro, onion, and fresno pepper and serve.

Chorizo Mac and Cheese

Servings: 6 | Ready in about: 30 min

INGREDIENTS

1 pound macaroni
3 ounces chorizo, chopped
3 cups water
1 tbsp garlic powder

2 tbsp minced garlic
2 cups milk
2 cups Cheddar cheese, shredded
salt to taste

DIRECTIONS

Put chorizo in the pot of your Foodi, select Sear/Sauté and stir-fry until crisp, about 5 minutes. Press Start. Set aside. Wipe the pot with kitchen paper. Add in water, macaroni, and salt to taste.

Seal lid and cook on for 5 minutes High Pressure. Press Start.

When ready, release the pressure quickly. Stir in cheese and milk until the cheese melts. Divide the mac and cheese between serving bowls. Top with chorizo and serve.

Winter Minestrone with Pancetta

Servings: 6 | Ready in about: 40 min

INGREDIENTS

2 tbsp olive oil
2 ounces pancetta, chopped
1 onion, diced
1 parsnip, peeled and chopped
2 carrots, peeled and sliced into rounds
2 celery stalks,
2 garlic cloves, minced
1 tbsp dried basil
1 tbsp dried thyme

1 tbsp dried oregano
6 cups chicken broth
2 cups green beans, trimmed and chopped
1 (15 ounces) can diced tomatoes
1 (15 ounces) can chickpeas, rinsed and drained
1½ cups small shaped pasta
salt and ground black pepper to taste
½ cup grated Parmesan cheese

DIRECTIONS

Warm oil on Sear/Sauté. Add onion, carrots, garlic, pancetta, celery, and parsnip, and cook for 5 minutes until they become soft. Stir in basil, oregano, green beans, broth, tomatoes, pepper, salt, thyme, vegetable broth, chickpeas, and pasta.

Seal the pressure lid, choose Pressure, set to High, and set the timer to 6 minutes. Press Start. Release pressure naturally for 10 minutes then release the remaining pressure quickly. Ladle the soup into bowls and serve garnished with grated parmesan cheese.

Green Lasagna Soup

Servings: 4 | Ready in about: 30 min

INGREDIENTS

1 tsp olive oil
1 cup leeks, chopped
2 garlic cloves minced
1 cup tomato paste
1 cup tomatoes, chopped
1 carrot, chopped

1/2 pound broccoli, chopped
¼ cup dried green lentils
2 tsp Italian seasoning
salt to taste
2 cups vegetable broth
3 lasagna noodles

DIRECTIONS

Warm oil on Sear/Sauté. Add garlic and leeks and cook for 2 minutes until soft; add tomato paste, carrot, Italian seasoning, broccoli, tomatoes, lentils, and salt. Stir in vegetable broth and lasagna pieces.

Seal the pressure lid, choose Pressure, set to High, and set the timer to 3 minutes. Press Start. Release pressure naturally for 10 minutes, then release the remaining pressure quickly. Divide soup into serving bowls and serve.

Italian Sausage with Garlic Mash

Servings: 6 | Ready in about: 30 min

INGREDIENTS

1 ½ cups water
6 Italian sausages
1 tbsp olive oil
2 garlic cloves, smashed
4 large potatoes, peeled and cut into 1½-inch chunks

⅓ cup butter, melted
¼ cup milk, at room temperature, or more as needed
salt and ground black pepper to taste
1 tbsp chopped chives

DIRECTIONS

Select Sear/Sauté, set to Medium High, and choose Start/Stop to preheat the pot and heat olive oil. Cook for 8-10 minutes, turning periodically until browned. Set aside. Wipe the pot with paper towels. Add in water and set the reversible rack over water. Place potatoes onto the reversible rack.

Seal the pressure lid, choose Pressure, set to High, and set the timer to 12 minutes. Press Start.

When ready, release the pressure quickly.

Remove reversible rack from the pot. Drain water from the pot.

Return potatoes to pot. Add in salt, butter, pepper, garlic, and milk and use a hand masher to mash until no large lumps remain.

Using an immersion blender, blend potatoes on Low for 1 minute until fluffy and light. Avoid over-blending to ensure the potatoes do not become gluey!

Transfer the mash to a serving plate, top with sausages and scatter chopped chives over to serve.

Rosemary Sweet Potato Medallions

Servings: 4 | Ready in about: 25 min

INGREDIENTS

1 cup water
1 tbsp fresh rosemary
1 tsp garlic powder

4 sweet potatoes, scrubbed clean and dried
2 tbsp butter
salt to taste

DIRECTIONS

Into the pot, add water and place the reversible rack over the water. Use a fork to prick sweet potatoes all over and set onto the reversible rack. Seal the pressure lid, choose Pressure, set to High, and set the timer to 12 minutes. Press Start.

When ready, release the pressure quickly.

Transfer sweet potatoes to a cutting board and slice into 1/2-inch medallions and ensure they are peeled.

Melt butter in the pressure cooker on Sear/Sauté. Add in the medallions and cook each side for 2 to 3 minutes until browned. Apply salt and garlic powder to season. Serve topped with fresh rosemary.

Breakfast Burrito Bowls

Servings: 4 | Ready in about: 30 min

INGREDIENTS

2 tbsp olive oil
1 onion
2 garlic cloves, minced
1 tbsp chili powder
2 tsp ground cumin
2 tsp paprika
1 tsp salt
½ tsp black pepper
¼ tsp cayenne pepper

1 cup quinoa, rinsed
1 (14.5 ounces) can diced tomatoes
1 (14.5 ounces) can black beans, drained and rinsed
1 ½ cups vegetable stock
1 cup frozen corn kernels
2 tbsp chopped cilantro
1 tbsp roughly chopped fresh coriander
Cheddar cheese, grated for garnish
1 avocado, sliced

DIRECTIONS

Warm oil on Sear/Sauté. Add in onion and cook for 3 to 5 minutes until fragrant. Add garlic and cook for 2 more minutes until soft and golden brown. Add in chili powder, paprika, cayenne pepper, salt, cumin, and black pepper and cook for 1 minute until spices are soft.

Pour quinoa into onion and spice mixture and stir to coat quinoa completely in spices. Add diced tomatoes, black beans, vegetable stock, and corn; stir to combine.

Seal the pressure lid, choose Pressure, set to High, and set the timer to 7 minutes. Press Start.

When ready, release the pressure quickly. Open the lid and let sit for 6 minutes until flavors combine. Use a fork to fluff quinoa and season with pepper and salt if desired.

Into quinoa and beans mixture, stir in cilantro and divide among plates. Top with cheese and avocado slices.

Colorful Vegetable Medley

Servings: 4 | Ready in about: 15 min

INGREDIENTS

1 cup water
1 small head broccoli, broken into florets
16 asparagus, trimmed
1 small head cauliflower, broken into florets

5 ounces green beans
2 carrots, peeled and cut on bias into 1/4-inch rounds
salt to taste

DIRECTIONS

Into the pot, add water and set trivet on top of water and place steamer basket on top of the trivet. In an even layer, spread green beans, broccoli, cauliflower, asparagus, and carrots in the steamer basket.

Seal the pressure lid, choose Pressure, set to High, and set the timer to 3 minutes on High.

When ready, release the pressure quickly.

Remove steamer basket from cooker and add salt to vegetables for seasoning. Serve immediately.

Red Beans and Rice

Servings: 4 | Ready in about: 1 hr

INGREDIENTS

1 cup red beans, rinsed and stones removed
1/2 cup rice, rinsed
2 tbsp olive oil
1/2 tsp cayenne pepper
1 1/2 cup vegetable broth
water as needed

1 onion, diced
1 red bell pepper, diced
1 stalk celery, diced
1 tbsp fresh thyme leaves, or to taste
salt and freshly ground black pepper to taste

DIRECTIONS

Into the pot, add beans and water to cover about 1-inch. Seal the pressure lid, choose Pressure, set to High, and set the timer to 1 minute. Press Start.

When ready, release the pressure quickly. Drain the beans and set aside. Rinse and pat dry the inner pot.

Return inner pot to pressure cooker, add oil to the pot and press Sear/Sauté. Add onion to the oil and cook for 3 minutes until soft. Add celery and pepper and cook for 1 to 2 minutes until fragrant. Add garlic and cook for 30 seconds until soft; add rice.

Transfer the beans back into inner pot and top with broth. Stir black pepper, thyme, cayenne pepper, and salt into mixture. Seal the pressure lid, choose Pressure, set to High, and set the timer to 15 minutes. Press Start.

When ready, release pressure quickly. Add more thyme, black pepper and salt as desired.

Veggie Skewers

Servings: 4 | Ready in about: 20 min

INGREDIENTS:

2 tbsp corn flour
⅔ cup canned beans
⅓ cup grated carrots
2 boiled and mashed potatoes
¼ cup chopped fresh mint leaves
½ tsp garam masala powder

½ cup paneer
1 green chili
1-inch piece of fresh ginger
3 garlic cloves
Salt, to taste

DIRECTIONS:

Soak 12 skewers until ready to use.

Place the beans, carrots, garlic, ginger, chili, paneer, and mint, in a food processor and process until smooth; transfer to a bowl.

Add the mashed potatoes, corn flour, some salt, and garam masala powder to the bowl. Mix until fully incorporated. Divide the mixture into 12 equal pieces.

Shape each of the pieces around a skewer. Close the crisping lid and cook the skewers for 10 minutes on Air Crisp mode at 390 F.

Tasty Baby Porcupine Meatballs

Servings: 4 | Ready in about: 30 min

INGREDIENTS:

1 cup rice

1 lb of ground beef

1 onion, chopped

1 green bell pepper, finely chopped

1 tsp celery salt

2 tbsp Worcestershire sauce

1 garlic clove, minced

2 cups of tomato juice

1 tsp oregano

DIRECTIONS:

Combine the rice, ground beef, onion, celery, salt, green peppers, and garlic.

Shape into balls of 1 inch each.

Arrange the balls in the basket of the Ninja Foodi.

Close the crisping lid and cook for 15 minutes at 320°F.

After 8 minutes, shape the balls. Heat the tomato juice, cloves, oregano, and Worcestershire sauce in a saucepan over medium heat.

Pour in the meatballs, bring to a boil, reduce the heat and simmer for 10 minutes, stirring often. Serve warm.

Grilled Tofu Sandwich

Servings: 1 | Ready in about: 20 min

INGREDIENTS:

2 slices of bread

1-inch thick Tofu slice

¼ cup red cabbage, shredded

2 tsp olive oil divided

¼ tsp vinegar

Salt and pepper, to taste

DIRECTIONS:

Place the bread slices and toast for 3 minutes on Roast mode at 350 F; set aside.

Brush the tofu with 1 tsp of oil, and place in the basket of the Ninja Foodi. Bake for 5 minutes on each side on Roast mode at 350 F.

Combine the cabbage, remaining oil, and vinegar, and season with salt and pepper.

Place the tofu on top of one bread slice, place the cabbage over, and top with the other bread slice.

Spicy Pepper & Sweet Potato Skewers

Servings: 1 | Ready in about: 20 min

INGREDIENTS:

1 large sweet potato

1 beetroot

1 green bell pepper

1 tsp chili flakes

¼ tsp black pepper

½ tsp turmeric

¼ tsp garlic powder

¼ tsp paprika

1 tbsp olive oil

DIRECTIONS:

Soak 3 to 4 skewers until ready to use.

Peel the veggies and cut them into bite-sized chunks.

Place the chunks in a bowl along with the remaining ingredients. Mix until fully coated. Thread the veggies in this order: potato, pepper, beetroot.

Place in the Ninja Foodi, close the crisping lid and cook for 15 minutes on Air Crisp mode at 350 F; flip skewers halfway through.

Pasta with Roasted Veggies

Servings: 6 | Ready in about: 25 min

INGREDIENTS:

1 lb penne, cooked

1 zucchini, sliced

1 pepper, sliced

1 acorn squash, sliced

4 oz mushrooms, sliced

½ cup kalamata olives, pitted, halved

¼ cup olive oil

1 tsp Italian seasoning

1 cup grape tomatoes, halved

3 tbsp balsamic vinegar

2 tbsp chopped basil

Salt and pepper, to taste

DIRECTIONS:

Combine the pepper, zucchini, squash, mushrooms, and olive oil, in a large bowl.

Season with salt and pepper. Close the crisping lid and cook the veggies for 15 minutes on Air Crisp mode at 380 F.

In a large bowl, combine the penne, roasted vegetables, olives, tomatoes, Italian seasoning, and vinegar. Sprinkle basil and serve.

Paneer Cutlet

Servings: 1 | Ready in about: 15 min

INGREDIENTS:

2 cup grated paneer

1 cup grated cheese

½ tsp chai masala

1 tsp butter

½ tsp garlic powder

1 small onion, finely chopped

½ tsp oregano

½ tsp salt

DIRECTIONS:

Preheat the Ninja Foodi to 350 degrees F.

Oil the Ninja Foodi basket.

Mix all ingredients in a bowl, until well incorporated.

Make cutlets out of the mixture and place them on the greased baking dish.

Place the baking dish in the Ninja Foodi and cook the cutlets for 10 minutes.

Vegetable Tortilla Pizza

Servings: 1 | Ready in about: 15 min

INGREDIENTS:

1 ½ tbsp tomato paste

¼ cup grated cheddar cheese

¼ cup grated mozzarella cheese

1 tbsp cooked sweet corn

4 zucchini slices

4 eggplant slices

4 red onion Rings

½ green bell pepper, chopped

3 cherry tomatoes, quartered

1 tortilla

¼ tsp basil

¼ tsp oregano

DIRECTIONS:

Spread the tomato paste on the tortilla.

Arrange the zucchini and eggplant slices first, then green peppers, and onion rings.

Lay the cherry tomatoes and sprinkle the sweet corn over.

Sprinkle with oregano and basil. Top with cheddar and mozzarella.

Place in the Ninja Foodi close the crisping lid and cook for 10 minutes on Air Crisp mode at 350 F.

Poblano & Tomato Stuffed Squash

Servings: 3 | Ready in about: 50 min

INGREDIENTS:

½ butternut squash

6 grape tomatoes, halved

1 poblano pepper, cut into strips

¼ cup grated mozzarella, optional

2 tsp olive oil divided

Salt and pepper, to taste

DIRECTIONS:

Meanwhile, cut trim the ends and cut the squash lengthwise. You will only need one half for this recipe.

Scoop the flash out, so you make room for the filling.

Brush 1 tsp oil over the squash. Place in the Ninja Foodi and roast for 30 minutes.

Combine the other teaspoon of olive oil with the tomatoes and poblanos.

Season with salt and pepper, to taste. Place the peppers and tomatoes into the squash. Close the crisping lid and cook for 15 more minutes on Air Crisp mode at 350 F. If using mozzarella, add it on top of the squash, two minutes before the end.

Quinoa and Veggie Stuffed Peppers

Servings: 1 | Ready in about: 16 min

INGREDIENTS:

¼ cup cooked quinoa

1 bell pepper

½ tbsp diced onion

½ diced tomato, plus one tomato slice

¼ tsp smoked paprika

Salt and pepper, to taste

1 tsp olive oil

¼ tsp dried basil

DIRECTIONS:

Core and clean the bell pepper to prepare it for stuffing. Brush the pepper with half of the olive oil on the outside.

In a small bowl, combine all of the other ingredients, except the tomato slice and reserved half-teaspoon olive oil.

Stuff the pepper with the filling. Top with the tomato slice.

Brush the tomato slice with the remaining half-teaspoon of oil and sprinkle with basil. Close the crisping lid and cook for 10 minutes on Air Crisp mode at 350 F.

Avocado Rolls

Servings: 5 | Ready in about: 15 min | Servings: 5

INGREDIENTS:

3 avocados, pitted and peeled

10 egg roll wrappers

1 tomato, diced

¼ tsp pepper

½ tsp salt

DIRECTIONS:

Place all filling ingredients in a bowl. Mash with a fork until somewhat smooth. Divide the feeling between the egg wrappers. Wet your finger and brush along the edges so the wrappers can seal well.

Roll and seal the wrappers. Arrange them on the lined Ninja Foodi basket, and place into the Ninja Foodi.

Close the crisping lid and cook at 350 degrees F, for 5 minutes on Air Crisp mode. Serve with chili dipping.

Simple Air Fried Ravioli

Servings: 6 | Ready in about: 15 min

INGREDIENTS:

1 package cheese ravioli

2 cup Italian breadcrumbs

¼ cup Parmesan cheese

1 cup buttermilk

1 tsp olive oil

¼ tsp garlic powder

DIRECTIONS:

In a bowl, combine the crumbs, Parmesan cheese, garlic powder, and olive oil. Dip the ravioli in the buttermilk and then coat them with the breadcrumb mixture.

Line a baking sheet with parchment paper and arrange the ravioli on it. Place in the Ninja Foodi and cook for 5 minutes on Air Crisp mode at 390 F.

Serve the air-fried ravioli with marinara jar sauce.

Crispy Nachos

Servings: 2 | Ready in about: 20 min

INGREDIENTS:

1 cup sweet corn

1 cup all-purpose flour

1 tbsp butter

½ tsp chili powder

2-3 tbsp water

Salt to taste

DIRECTIONS:

Add a small amount of water to the sweet corn and grind until you obtain an excellent paste. In a large bowl, add the flour, the salt, the chili powder, the butter and mix very well. Add the corn and stir well.

Start to knead with your palm until you obtain a stiff dough. Meanwhile, dust a little bit of flour and spread the batter with a rolling pin.

Make it around ½ inch thick. Cut it in any shape you want and cook in the Ninja Foodi for 10 minutes on Air Crisp mode at 350 F. Serve with guacamole salsa.

Paneer Cheese Balls

Servings: 2 | Ready in about: 12 min

INGREDIENTS:

2 oz paneer cheese

2 tbsp flour

2 medium onions, chopped

1 tbsp corn flour

1 green chili, chopped

A 1-inch ginger piece, chopped

1 tsp red chili powder

a few leaves of coriander, chopped

Salt to taste

1 tbsp olive oil

DIRECTIONS:

Mix all ingredients, except the oil and the cheese.

Take a small part of the mixture, roll it up and slowly press to flatten it.

Stuff in 1 cube of cheese and seal the edges. Repeat with the rest of the mixture.

Close the crisping lid and fry the balls in the Ninja Foodi for 12 minutes on Air Crisp mode and at 370 F. Serve hot, with ketchup.

Potato Filled Bread Rolls

Servings: 4 | Ready in about: 25 min

INGREDIENTS:

8 slices of bread
5 large potatoes, boiled, mashed
½ tsp turmeric
2 green chilies, deseeded, chopped
1 medium onion, chopped

½ tsp mustard seeds
1 tbsp olive oil
2 sprigs curry leaf
Salt, to taste

DIRECTIONS:

Combine the olive oil, onion, curry leaves, and mustard seed, in the Ninja Foodi basket. Cook for 5 minutes.

Mix the onion mixture with the mashed potatoes, chilies, turmeric, and some salt. Divide the dough into 8 equal pieces.

Trim the sides of the bread, and wet it with some water.

Make sure to get rid of the excess water. Take one wet bread slice in your palm and place one of the potato pieces in the center.

Roll the bread over the filling, sealing the edges. Place the rolls onto a prepared baking dish, close the crisping lid and cook for 12 minutes on Air Crisp at 350 F.

Quick Crispy Kale Chips

Servings: 2 | Ready in about: 9 min

INGREDIENTS:

4 cups kale, stemmed and packed
2 tbsp of olive oil
1 tbsp of yeast flakes

1 tsp of vegan seasoning
Salt to taste

DIRECTIONS:

In a bowl, add the oil, the kale, the vegan seasoning, and the yeast and mix well.

Dump the coated kale in the Ninja Foodi's basket.

Set the heat to 370°F, close the crisping lid and fry for a total of 6 minutes on Air Crisp mode. Shake it from time to time.

Roasted Vegetable Salad

Servings: 1 | Ready in about: 25 min

INGREDIENTS:

1 potato, peeled and chopped
¼ onion, sliced
1 carrot, sliced diagonally
½ small beetroot, sliced
1 cup cherry tomatoes
Juice of 1 lemon
A handful of rocket salad
A handful of baby spinach

3 tbsp canned chickpeas
½ tsp cumin
½ tsp turmeric
¼ tsp sea salt
2 tbsp olive oil
Parmesan shavings

DIRECTIONS:

Combine the onion, potato, cherry tomatoes, carrot, beetroot, cumin, seas salt, turmeric, and 1 tbsp olive oil, in a bowl.

Place in the Ninja Foodi, close the crisping lid and cook for 20 minutes on Air Crisp mode at 370 F; let cool for 2 minutes.

Place the rocket, salad, spinach, lemon juice, and 1 tbsp olive oil, into a serving bowl. Mix to combine; stir in the roasted veggies.

Top with chickpeas and Parmesan shavings.

Quick Crispy Cheese Lings

Servings: 4 | Ready in about: 15 min

INGREDIENTS:

4 cups grated cheddar cheese
1 cup all-purpose flour
1 tbsp butter
1 tbsp baking powder

¼ tsp chili powder
¼ tsp salt, to taste
1-2 tbsp water

DIRECTIONS:

Mix the flour and the baking powder.

Add the chili powder, salt, butter, cheese and 1-2 tbsp of water to the mixture.

Make a stiff dough. Knead the dough for a while.

Sprinkle a tbsp or so of flour on the table.

Take a rolling pin and roll the dough into ½ -inch thickness.

Cut the dough in any shape you want. Close the crisping lid and fry the cheese lings for 6 minutes at 370° F on Air Crisp mode.

Prawn Toast

Servings: 2 | Ready in about: 12 min

INGREDIENTS:

6 large prawns, shells removed, chopped
1 large spring onion, finely sliced
3 white slices of bread

½ cup sweet corn
1 egg white, whisked
1 tbsp black sesame seeds

DIRECTIONS:

In a bowl, place the prawns, corn, spring onion and the black sesame seeds.

Add the whisked egg white, and mix the ingredients.

Spread the mixture over the bread slices.

Place the prawns in the Ninja Foodi's basket and sprinkle with oil.

Close the crisping lid and fry the prawns until golden, for 8-10 minutes at 370 F on Air Crisp mode. Serve with ketchup or chili sauce.

Pineapple Appetizer Ribs

Servings: 4 | Ready in about: 30 min

INGREDIENTS:

2 lb cut spareribs

7 oz salad dressing

5 oz canned pineapple juice

2 cups water

Garlic salt

Salt and black pepper

DIRECTIONS:

Sprinkle the ribs with salt and pepper and place them in a saucepan.

Pour water and cook the ribs for around 12 minutes on high heat.

Drain the ribs and arrange them in the Ninja Foodi.

Sprinkle with garlic salt. Close the crisping lid and cook for 15 minutes at 390 F on Air Crisp mode. Meanwhile, prepare the sauce by combining the salad dressing and the pineapple juice. Serve the ribs with this delicious dressing sauce!

Scottish Seafood Curry

Servings: 8 | Ready in about: 45 min

INGREDIENTS:

Seafood:

½ lb squid, trimmed and cut into 1-inch rings

½ lb langoustine tall meat

½ lb Sscallop meat

½ lb mussel meat

Curry:

4 tbsp olive oil

2 cups shellfish stock

2 curry leaves

2 tbsp Shallot puree

3 tbsp yellow curry paste

2 tbsp ginger paste

2 tbsp garlic paste

1 ½ tbsp chili powder

1 ½ tbsp chili paste

2 tbsp lemongrass paste

½ tsp turmeric powder

2 tsp shrimp powder

1 tsp shrimp paste

1 ½ cups coconut milk

1 cup milk

1 tbsp Grants Scotch Whiskey

2 tbsp fish curry powder

Salt to taste

Vegetables:

¼ cup diced tomatoes

¼ cup chopped onion

¼ cup chopped okra

¼ cup chopped eggplants

DIRECTIONS:

Add olive oil, shallot paste, yellow curry paste, ginger puree, garlic paste, lemongrass paste, chili paste, shrimp paste, and curry leaves.

Stir-fry for 10 minutes on Sear/Sauté mode, until well combined and aromatic.

Next, add turmeric powder, fish curry powder, and shrimp powder. Stir-fry for another minute. Pour in the shellfish stock and close the crisping lid. Cook on Broil mode for 15 minutes.

Open the lid, and add the scallops, squid, chopped onion, okra, tomatoes, and aubergine. Stir lightly.

Close the pressure lid, secure the pressure valve, and select Steam mode on High pressure for 5 minutes. Press Start/Stop to start cooking.

Once the timer has ended, do a quick pressure release, and open the lid.

Add milk, coconut milk, scotch whiskey, and salt. Stir carefully not to mash the aubergine.

Select Sear/Sauté and add mussel meat and langoustine. Stir carefully.

Simmer the sauce for 3 minutes, press Stop, and turn off the Ninja Foodi.

Dish the seafood with sauce and veggies into serving bowls.

Serve with a side of broccoli mash.

Buttery Herb Salmon with Barley Haricot Verts

Servings: 4 | Ready in about: 50 min

INGREDIENTS

1 cup pearl barley
2 cups water
4 salmon fillets
8 ounces green beans haricot verts, trimmed
1 tablespoon olive oil
1 teaspoon freshly ground black pepper, divided
1 teaspoon salt, divided

4 tablespoons melted butter
½ tablespoon brown sugar
½ tablespoon freshly squeezed lemon juice
½ teaspoon dried rosemary
2 garlic cloves, minced
½ teaspoon dried thyme

DIRECTIONS

Pour the barley and water in the pot and mix to combine. Place the reversible rack in the pot. Lay the salmon fillets on the rack.

Seal the pressure lid, choose Pressure, set to High and set the time to 2 minutes. Press Start.

In a bowl, toss the green beans with olive oil, ½ teaspoon of black pepper, and ½ teaspoon of salt. Then, in another bowl, mix the remaining black pepper and salt, the butter, brown sugar, lemon juice, rosemary, garlic, and rosemary.

When done cooking the rice and salmon, perform a quick pressure release. Gently pat the salmon dry with a paper towel, then coat with the buttery herb sauce.

Position the haricots vert around the salmon. Close the crisping lid; choose Broil and set the time to 7 minutes; press Start/Stop. When ready, remove the salmon from the rack, and serve with the barley and haricots vert.

Crispy Cod on Lentils

Servings: 4 | Ready in about: 65 min

INGREDIENTS

1 tablespoon olive oil
2 cups lentils, soaked
1 yellow bell pepper, diced
1 red bell pepper, diced
4 cups vegetable broth
1 cup panko breadcrumbs

4 tablespoons melted butter
¼ cup minced fresh cilantro
1 teaspoon lemon zest
1 lemon, juiced
1 teaspoon salt
4 cod fillets

DIRECTIONS

Choose Sear/Sauté on the pot and set to Medium High. Choose Start/Stop to preheat the pot.

Combine the oil, lentils, yellow and red bell peppers in the preheated pot and cook for 1 minute. Mix in the vegetable broth.

Seal the pressure lid, choose Pressure, set to High, and set the time to 6 minutes. Choose Start/Stop.

In a small bowl, combine the breadcrumbs, butter, cilantro, lemon zest, lemon juice, and salt. Spoon the breadcrumb mixture evenly on the cod fillet.

When cooking ended, perform a quick pressure release, and carefully open the pressure lid.

Fix the reversible rack in the pot, which will be over the lentils. Lay the cod fillets on the rack. Close the crisping lid. Choose Air Crisp, set the temperature to 350°F, and set the time to 12 minutes; press Start/Stop.

When ready, share the lentils into four serving plates, and top with salmon.

Potato Chowder with Peppery Prawns

Servings: 4 | Ready in about: 80 min

INGREDIENTS

4 slices serrano ham, chopped
4 tablespoons minced garlic, divided
1 onion, chopped
2 Yukon Gold potatoes, chopped
16 ounces frozen corn
2 cups vegetable broth
1 teaspoon dried rosemary

1 teaspoon salt, divided
1 teaspoon freshly ground black pepper, divided
16 prawns, peeled and deveined
2 tablespoons olive oil
½ teaspoon red chili flakes
¾ cup heavy cream

DIRECTIONS

Choose Sear/Sauté on the pot and set to Medium High. Choose Start/Stop to preheat the pot.

Add 1 tablespoon of the olive oil and cook the serrano ham, 2 tablespoons of garlic, and onion, stirring occasionally, for 5 minutes. Fetch out one-third of the serrano ham into a bowl for garnishing.

Add the potatoes, corn, vegetable broth, rosemary, half of the salt, and half of the black pepper to the pot.

Seal the pressure lid, hit Pressure and set to High. Set the time to 10 minutes, and press Start.

In a bowl, toss the prawns in the remaining garlic, salt, black pepper, the remaining olive oil, and the red chili flakes. When done cooking, do a quick pressure release and carefully open the pressure lid.

Stir in the heavy cream and fix the reversible rack in the pot over the chowder. Spread the prawn in the rack. Close the crisping lid. Choose Broil and set the time to 8 minutes. Choose Start/Stop. When the timer has ended, remove the rack from the pot.

Ladle the corn chowder into serving bowls and top with the prawns. Garnish with the reserved ham and serve immediately.

Traditional Mahi Mahi

Servings: 4 | Ready in about: 10 min

INGREDIENTS:

4 Mahi Mahi fillets, fresh
4 cloves garlic, minced
1 ¼ -inch ginger, grated
Salt and black pepper
2 tbsp chili powder

1 tbsp Sriracha sauce
1 ½ tbsp maple syrup
1 lime, juiced
1 cup water

DIRECTIONS:

Place mahi mahi on a plate and season with salt and pepper on both sides.

In a bowl, add garlic, ginger, chili powder, sriracha sauce, maple syrup, and lime juice. Use a spoon to mix it.

With a brush, apply the hot sauce mixture on the fillet.

Then, open the Ninja Foodi's lid, pour the water it and fit the rack at the bottom of the pot. Put the fillets on the trivet. Close the lid, secure the pressure valve, and select Steam mode on High pressure for 5 minutes. Press Start/Stop to start cooking.

Once the timer has ended, do a quick pressure release, and open the lid. Use a set of tongs to remove the mahi mahi onto serving plates. Serve with steamed or braised asparagus. For a crispier taste, cook them for 2 minutes on Air Crisp mode, at 300 degrees F.

Mushrooms and Shrimp Egg Wrappers

Servings: 4 AS AN APPETIZER | Ready in about: 70 min

INGREDIENTS

2 tablespoons coconut aminos
1 tablespoon dry white wine
2 teaspoons plain vinegar
3 cups shredded cabbage
3 green onions, chopped
1 large carrot, peeled and grated
1 teaspoon ginger puree
2 garlic cloves, minced
1 teaspoon sugar

2 teaspoons peanut oil
¼ teaspoon freshly ground black pepper
½ cup sautéed mushrooms, chopped
8 ounces shrimp, peeled and chopped
1 teaspoon arrowroot starch
1 tablespoon water
10 egg roll wrappers
Cooking spray

DIRECTIONS

Mix the coconut aminos, white wine, and vinegar in the inner pot of your Foodi. Stir in the cabbage, green onions, carrot, ginger, garlic, sugar, and peanut oil.

Seal the pressure lid, choose Pressure; adjust the pressure to High and the cook time to 2 minutes. Press Start to cook the vegetables.

After cooking, do a quick pressure release and carefully open the lid.

Stir in the black pepper, mushroom, and shrimp. Choose Sear/Sauté and adjust to Medium-High. Press Start to simmer the shrimp and mushrooms for about 5 minutes until almost all of the liquid has dried up.

Spoon the filling into a bowl and set aside to cool. Wipe out the inner pot with a paper towel and return the pot to the base.

Make the egg rolls

In a bowl, combine the arrowroot and water. Lay an egg roll wrapper on a clean flat surface with a corner side facing you. Dip your index finger in the starch mixture and lightly moisten the edges of the wrapper.

With a slotted spoon, fetch a ¼ cup of filling onto the wrapper, just below the center.

Fold the bottom corner of the wrapper over the filling, tuck under the filling, roll once and fold both sides in. Continue rolling up tightly and repeat the process with the remaining wrappers.

Close the crisping lid and Choose Air Crisp; adjust the temperature to 390°F and the time to 5 minutes; press Start. Lay 5 egg rolls in the Crisping Basket and oil with the cooking spray. Flip and oil the other sides. When the pot is ready, fix the basket in the inner pot.

Close the crisping lid and Choose Air Crisp; adjust the temperature to 390°F and the cook time to 15 minutes. Press Start.

After 6 minutes, open the lid and check the egg rolls, which should be golden brown and crisp on top. Otherwise, close the lid and cook for 2 minutes more. Flip the rolls with tongs and cook further for 5 to 6 minutes or until crisp on the other side too.

Repeat the frying process for the remaining egg rolls. When ready, use tongs to remove the egg rolls into a plate. Allow cooling for a few minutes before serving.

Sausage and Shrimp Paella

Servings: 4 | Ready in about: 70 min

INGREDIENTS

1 tablespoon melted butter
1 pound andouille sausage, sliced
1 white onion, chopped
4 garlic cloves, minced
½ cup dry white wine
2 cups Spanish rice
4 cups chicken stock

1½ teaspoons sweet paprika
1 teaspoon turmeric powder
½ teaspoon freshly ground black pepper
½ teaspoon salt
1 pound baby squid, cut into ¼-inch rings
1 pound jumbo shrimp, peeled and deveined
1 red bell pepper, diced

DIRECTIONS

Choose Sear/Sauté on the pot and set to Medium High. Choose Start/Stop to preheat the pot.

Melt the butter and add the sausage. Cook until browned on both sides, about 3 minutes while stirring frequently. Remove the sausage to a plate and set aside.

Sauté the onion and garlic in the same fat for 3 minutes until fragrant and pour in the wine. Use a wooden spoon to scrape the bottom of the pot of any brown bits and cook for 2 minutes or until the wine reduces by half.

Stir in the rice and water. Season with the paprika, turmeric, black pepper, and salt.

Seal the pressure lid, choose Pressure and set to High. Set the time to 5 minutes, then Choose Start/Stop. When done cooking, do a quick pressure release and carefully open the lid.

Choose Sear/Sauté, set to Medium High, and choose Start/Stop. Add the squid and shrimp to the pot and stir gently without mashing the rice.

Seal the pressure lid again and cook for 6 minutes, until the shrimp are pink and opaque.

Return the sausage to the pot and mix in the bell pepper. Warm through for 2 minutes.

Dish the paella and serve immediately.

Chorizo and Shrimp Boil

Servings: 4 | Ready in about: 30 min

INGREDIENTS

3 red potatoes
3 ears corn, cut into 1½-inch rounds
2 cups water
1 cup white wine
4 chorizo sausages, sliced

1 pound shrimp, peeled and deveined
2 tbsp of seafood seasoning
salt to taste
1 lemon, cut into wedges
¼ cup butter, melted

DIRECTIONS

To your Foodi add all ingredients except butter and lemon wedges. Do not stir.

Seal the pressure lid, choose Pressure, set to High, and set the timer to 2 minutes; press Start. When ready, release the pressure quickly.

Drain the mixture through a colander. Transfer to a serving platter. Serve with melted butter and lemon wedges.

Lemon Cod Goujons & Rosemary Chips

Servings: 4 | Ready in about: 100 min

INGREDIENTS

2 eggs

1 cup arrowroot starch

1 cup flour

½ tablespoon cayenne powder

1 tablespoon cumin powder

1 teaspoon black pepper, plus more for seasoning

1 teaspoon salt, plus more for seasoning

4 cod fillets, cut into strips

Zest and juice from   1 lemon

Cooking spray

2 potatoes, cut into chips

2 tablespoons olive oil

3 tbsp fresh rosemary, chopped

4 lemon wedges to serve

DIRECTIONS

Fix the Crisping Basket in the pot and close the crisping lid. Choose Air Crisp, set the temperature to 375°F, and the time to 5 minutes. Choose Start/Stop to preheat the pot.

In a bowl, whisk the eggs, lemon zest, and lemon juice. In another bowl, combine the arrowroot starch, flour, cayenne powder, cumin, black pepper, and salt.

Coat each cod strip in the egg mixture, and then dredge in the flour mixture, coating well on all sides.

Grease the preheated basket with cooking spray. Place the coated fish in the basket and oil with cooking spray.

Close the crisping lid. Choose Air Crisp, set the temperature to 375°F, and the time to 15 minutes; press Start/Stop. Toss the potatoes with oil and season with salt and pepper.

After 15 minutes, check the fish making sure the pieces are as crispy as desired. Remove the fish from the basket.

Pour the potatoes in the basket. Close the crisping lid; choose Air Crisp, set the temperature to 400°F, and the time to 24 minutes; press Start/Stop.

After 12 minutes, open the lid, remove the basket and shake the fries. Return the basket to the pot and close the lid to continue cooking until crispy. When ready, sprinkle with fresh rosemary. Serve the fish with the potatoes and lemon wedges.

Salmon with Dill Chutney

Servings: 2 | Ready in about: 15 min

INGREDIENTS

2 salmon fillets

Juice from ½ lemon

¼ tsp paprika

salt and freshly ground pepper to taste

2 cups water

For Chutney:

¼ cup fresh dill

Juice from ½ lemon

Sea salt to taste

¼ cup extra virgin olive oil

DIRECTIONS

In a food processor, blend all the chutney ingredients until creamy. Set aside.

To your Foodi, add the water and place a reversible rack.

Arrange salmon fillets skin-side down on the steamer basket. Drizzle lemon juice over salmon and apply a seasoning of paprika. Seal the pressure lid, choose Pressure, set to High, and set the timer to 3 minutes; press Start. When ready, release the pressure quickly.

Season the fillets with pepper and salt, transfer to a serving plate and top with the dill chutney.

Penne all'Arrabbiata with Seafood and Chorizo

Servings: 4 | Ready in about: 50 min

INGREDIENTS

1 tablespoon olive oil
1 onion, diced
16 ounces penne
1 (24-ounce) jar Arrabbiata sauce
3 cups fish broth
1 chorizo, sliced

½ teaspoon freshly ground black pepper
½ teaspoon salt
8 ounces shrimp, peeled and deveined
8 ounces scallops
12 clams, cleaned and debearded

DIRECTIONS

Choose Sear/Sauté on the pot and set to Medium High. Choose Start/Stop to preheat the pot.

Heat the oil and add the chorizo, onion, and garlic; sauté them for about 5 minutes. Stir in the penne, Arrabbiata sauce, and broth. Season with the black pepper and salt and mix. Seal the pressure lid, choose Pressure, set to High and set the time to 2 minutes; press Start. When the time is over, do a quick pressure release and carefully open the lid.

Choose Sear/Sauté and set to Medium High. Choose Start/Stop. Stir in the shrimp, scallops, and clams. Put the pressure lid together and set to the Vent position. Cover and cook for 5 minutes, until the clams have opened and the shrimp and scallops are opaque and cooked through. Discard any unopened clams. Spoon the seafood and chorizo pasta into serving bowls and serve warm.

Spaghetti with Arugula and Scallops

Servings: 4 | Ready in about: 50 min

INGREDIENTS

1¼ pounds scallops, peeled and deveined
1½ teaspoons salt, divided
1 tablespoon melted butter
2 large garlic cloves, minced, divided
¼ cup white wine
10 ounces spaghetti

2½ cups water
⅓ cup tomato puree
½ teaspoon red chili flakes or to taste
1 teaspoon grated lemon zest
1 tablespoon lemon juice
6 cups arugula

DIRECTIONS

Arrange the scallops in the Crisping Basket. Season with ½ teaspoon salt, melted butter, and 1 minced garlic clove. Toss to coat and put the basket in the inner pot.

Close the crisping lid; choose Air Crisp, adjust the temperature to 400°F and the cook time to 6 minutes. Press Start. After 3 minutes, open the lid and use tongs to turn the scallops. Close the lid and resume cooking. Remove onto a plate and set aside.

On the pot, choose Sear/Sauté and adjust to High. Press Start to preheat the pot. Pour in the white wine and simmer for 1 to 2 minutes until reduced by half.

Add the spaghetti, water, remaining salt, garlic, puréed tomato, and chili flakes. Stir to combine.

Lock the pressure lid into place and set to Seal. Choose Pressure; adjust the pressure to High and the cook time to 5 minutes. Press Start.

After cooking, perform a quick pressure release and carefully open the lid. Stir in the lemon zest, juice, and arugula until wilted and soft. Add the scallops and heat through for a few minutes. Serve immediately.

Mussel Chowder with Oyster Crackers

Servings: 4 | Ready in about: 75 min

INGREDIENTS

2 cups oyster crackers
2 tablespoons melted ghee
¼ cup finely grated Pecorino Romano cheese
½ teaspoon garlic powder
1 teaspoon salt, divided
2 thick pancetta slices, cut into thirds
2 celery stalks, chopped
1 medium onion, chopped
1 tablespoon flour

¼ cup white wine
1 cup clam juice
3 (6-ounce) cans chopped mussels, drained, liquid reserved
1 pound parsnips, peeled and cut into chunks
1 teaspoon dried rosemary
1 bay leaf
1½ cups heavy cream
2 tablespoons chopped fresh chervil

DIRECTIONS

To preheat the Foodi, close the crisping lid and Choose Air Crisp; adjust the temperature to 375°F and the time to 2 minutes; press Start.

In a bowl, pour in the oyster crackers. Drizzle with the melted ghee, add the cheese, garlic powder, and ½ teaspoon of salt. Toss to coat the crackers. Transfer to the crisping basket.

Once the pot is ready, open the pressure lid and fix the basket in the pot. Close the lid and Choose Air Crisp; adjust the temperature to 375°F and the cook time to 6 minutes; press Start.

After 3 minutes, carefully open the lid and mix the crackers with a spoon. Close the lid and resume cooking until crisp and lightly browned. Take out the basket and set aside to cool.

On the pot, choose Sear/Sauté and adjust to Medium. Press Start. Add the pancetta and cook for 5 minutes, turning once or twice, until crispy.

Remove the pancetta to a paper towel-lined plate to drain fat; set aside.

Sauté the celery and onion in the pancetta grease for 1 minute or until the vegetables start softening. Mix the flour into the vegetables to coat evenly and pour the wine over the veggies. Cook for about 1 minute or until reduced by about one-third.

Pour in the clam juice, the reserved mussel liquid, parsnips, remaining salt, rosemary, and bay leaf. Seal the pressure lid, choose Pressure; adjust the pressure to High and the cook time to 4 minutes. Press Start.

After cooking, perform a natural pressure release for 5 minutes. Stir in the mussels and heavy cream. Choose Sear/Sauté and adjust to Medium. Press Start to simmer to the chowder and heat the mussels. Carefully remove and discard the bay leaf after.

Spoon the soup into bowls and crumble the pancetta over the top. Garnish with the chervil and a handful of oyster crackers, serving the remaining crackers on the side.

Tuna Salad with Asparagus & Potatoes

Servings: 4 | Ready in about: 60 MINUTES

INGREDIENTS

1½ pounds potatoes, quartered
3 tablespoons olive oil
1 teaspoon salt, divided, plus more as needed
8 ounces asparagus, cut into three
2 tablespoons red wine vinegar, divided
¼ teaspoon freshly ground black pepper

½ cup pimento stuffed green olives
½ cup coarsely chopped roasted red peppers
2 tablespoons chopped fresh parsley
2 cans tuna, drained
1 cup water

DIRECTIONS

Pour the water into the inner pot and set the reversible rack. Place the potatoes on the rack.

Lock the pressure lid into place and set to Seal. Choose Pressure; adjust the pressure to High and the cook time to 4 minutes. Press Start/Stop.

After pressure cooking, perform a quick pressure release and carefully open the pressure lid. Take out the rack, empty the water in the pot, and return the pot to the base.

Arrange the potatoes and asparagus on the Crisping Basket. Drizzle the half of olive oil on them, and season with salt.

Place the basket in the pot. Close the crisping lid; choose Air Crisp, adjust the temperature to 375°F, and the cook time to 12 minutes. Press Start.

After 8 minutes, open the lid, and check the veggies. The asparagus will have started browning and crisping. Gently toss with the potatoes and close the lid. Continue cooking for the remaining 4 minutes.

Take out the basket, pour the asparagus and potatoes into a salad bowl. Sprinkle with 1 tablespoon of red wine vinegar and mix to coat.

In a bowl, pour the remaining oil, remaining vinegar, salt, and pepper. Whisk to combine.

To the potatoes and asparagus, add the roasted red peppers, olives, parsley, and tuna. Drizzle the dressing over the salad and mix to coat. Adjust the seasoning and serve immediately.

Crabmeat with Broccoli Risotto

Servings: 4 | Ready in about: 80 min

INGREDIENTS

1 pound broccoli, cut into florets and chopped into 1-inch pieces
1 tablespoon olive oil
1 teaspoon salt, divided
2 tablespoons ghee
1 small onion, chopped (about ½ cup)

1 cup short grain rice
⅓ cup white wine
2 cups vegetable stock
8 ounces lump crabmeat
⅓ cup grated Pecorino Romano cheese

DIRECTIONS

Preheat your Foodi by closing the crisping lid. Choose Air Crisp; adjust the temperature to 375°F and the time to 2 minutes. Press Start.

Add the broccoli in the crisping basket and drizzle with the olive oil. Season with ½ teaspoon of salt and toss.

Put the basket in the inner pot. Close the crisping lid; choose Air Crisp, adjust the temperature to 375°F and the cook time to 10 minutes. Press Start.

After 5 minutes, open the lid and stir the broccoli, then resume cooking. When done cooking, take out the basket and set aside.

Choose Sear/Sauté and adjust to Medium. Press Start and melt the ghee. Add and sauté the onion for 5 minutes until softened.

Stir in the rice and cook for 1 minute. Add the wine and cook for 2 to 3 minutes, stirring frequently, until the liquid has almost completely evaporated.

Pour in vegetable stock and the remaining salt. Stir to combine. Seal the pressure lid, choose Pressure, adjust the pressure to High, and the cook time to 8 minutes. Press Start.

After cooking, perform a quick pressure release and carefully open the pressure lid. Gently stir in the crabmeat, and cheese. Taste and adjust the seasoning. Serve immediately.

Seafood Gumbo

Servings: 4 | Ready in about: 90 min

INGREDIENTS

1 pound jumbo shrimp
8 ounces lump crabmeat
1½ teaspoons salt divided
¼ cup olive oil, plus 2 teaspoons
⅓ cup all-purpose flour
1½ teaspoons Cajun Seasoning
1 medium onion, chopped
1 small red bell pepper, chopped (about ⅔ cup)

2 celery stalks, chopped
2 garlic cloves, minced
1 small banana pepper, seeded and minced
3 cups chicken broth
1 cup jasmine rice
¾ cup water
2 green onions, finely sliced

DIRECTIONS

Lay the shrimp in the Crisping Basket. Season with ½ teaspoon of salt and 2 teaspoons of olive oil. Toss to coat and fix the basket in the inner pot.

Close the crisping lid and Choose Air Crisp; adjust the temperature to 400°F and the cook time to 6 minutes. Press Start.

After 3 minutes, open the lid and toss the shrimp. Close the lid and resume cooking. When ready, the shrimp should be opaque and pink. Remove the basket and set aside.

Choose Sear/Sauté and adjust to High. Press Start. Heat the remaining ¼ cup of olive oil. Whisk in the flour with a wooden spoon and cook the roux that forms for 3 to 5 minutes, stirring constantly, until the roux has the color of peanut butter. Turn the pot off.

Stir in the Cajun, onion, bell pepper, celery, garlic, and banana pepper for about 5 minutes until the mixture slightly cools. Add the chicken broth and crabmeat, stir.

Put the rice into a heatproof bowl. Add the water and the remaining salt. Cover the bowl with foil. Put the reversible rack in the lower position of the pot and set the bowl in the rack.

Seal the pressure lid, choose Pressure; adjust the pressure to High and the cook time to 6 minutes; press Start.

After cooking, perform a natural pressure for 8 minutes. Take out the rack and bowl and set aside. Stir the shrimp into the gumbo to heat it up for 3 minutes.

Fluff the rice with a fork and divide into the center of four bowls. Spoon the gumbo around the rice and garnish with the green onions.

Haddock with Sanfaina

Servings: 4 | Ready in about: 40 min

INGREDIENTS

4 haddock fillets
¼ teaspoon salt
3 tablespoons olive oil
½ small onion, sliced
1 small jalapeño pepper, seeded and minced
2 large garlic cloves, minced
1 eggplant, cubed

1 bell pepper, chopped
1 (14.5-ounce) can diced tomatoes, drained
1 bay leaf
½ teaspoon dried basil
⅓ cup sliced green olives
¼ cup chopped fresh chervil, divided
3 tablespoons capers, divided

DIRECTIONS

Season the fish on both sides with salt, place in the refrigerator, and make the sauce. Press Sear/Sauté and set to Medium. Press Start.

Melt the butter until no longer foaming. Add onion, eggplant, bell pepper, jalapeño, and garlic; sauté for 5 minutes.

Stir in the tomatoes, bay leaf, basil, olives, half of the chervil, and half of the capers. Remove the fish from the refrigerator and lay on the vegetables in the pot.

Seal the pressure lid, choose Pressure; adjust the pressure to Low and the cook time to 3 minutes; press Start.

After cooking, do a quick pressure release and carefully open the lid. Remove and discard the bay leaf.

Transfer the fish to a serving platter and spoon the sauce over. Sprinkle with the remaining chervil and capers. Serve.

Cajun Salmon with Creamy Grits

Servings: 4 | Ready in about: 100 min

INGREDIENTS

¾ cup corn grits
1½ cups coconut milk
1½ cups vegetable stock
3 tablespoons butter, divided
2 teaspoons salt

3 tablespoons Cajun
1 tablespoon packed brown sugar
4 salmon fillets, skin removed
Cooking spray

DIRECTIONS

Pour the grits into a heatproof bowl. Add the coconut milk, stock, 1 tablespoon of butter, and ½ teaspoon of salt. Stir and cover the bowl with foil.

Pour the water into the inner pot. Put the reversible rack in the pot and place the bowl on top.

Seal the pressure lid, choose Pressure; adjust the pressure to High and the cook time to 15 minutes. Press Start to begin cooking.

In a bowl combine the Cajun, brown sugar, and remaining salt.

Oil the fillets on one side with cooking spray and place one or two at a time with sprayed-side down into the spice mixture. Oil the other sides and turn over to coat that side in the seasoning. Repeat the process with the remaining fillets.

Once the grits are ready, perform a natural pressure release for 10 minutes. Remove the rack and bowl from the pot. Add the remaining butter to the grits and stir to combine well. Cover again with aluminum foil and return the bowl to the pot (without the rack).

Fix the rack in the upper position of the pot and put the salmon fillets on the rack.

Close the crisping lid and Choose Bake/Roast; adjust the temperature to 400°F and the cook time to 12 minutes. Press Start. After 6 minutes, open the lid and use tongs to turn the fillets over. Close the lid and continue cooking.

When the salmon is ready, take out the rack. Remove the bowl of grits and take off the foil. Stir and serve immediately with the salmon.

Autumn Succotash with Basil-Crusted Fish

Servings: 4 | Ready in about: 65 min

INGREDIENTS

1 tablespoon olive oil
½ small onion, chopped
1 garlic clove, minced
1 medium red chili, seeded and chopped
1 cup frozen corn
1 cup frozen mixed beans
1 cup butternut squash, cubed
1 bay leaf
¼ teaspoon cayenne pepper
¼ cup chicken stock

½ teaspoon Worcestershire sauce
1 teaspoon salt, divided
4 firm white fish fillets, at least 1 inch thick
¼ cup mayonnaise
1 tablespoon Dijon-style mustard
1 ½ cups breadcrumbs
1 large tomato, seeded and chopped
¼ cup chopped fresh basil
Cooking spray

DIRECTIONS

Press Sear/Sauté and adjust to Medium. Press Start to preheat the pot. Heat the oil and sauté the onion, garlic, and red chili pepper in the oil for 4 minutes or until the vegetables are soft.

Stir in the corn, squash, mixed beans, bay leaf, cayenne, chicken stock, Worcestershire sauce, and ½ teaspoon salt.

Seal the pressure lid, choose Pressure; adjust the pressure to High and the cook time to 5 minutes. Press Start.

Season the fish fillets with the remaining salt. In a small bowl, mix the mayonnaise and mustard. Pour the breadcrumbs and basil into another bowl. Use a brush to spread the mayonnaise mixture on all sides of the fish and dredge each piece in the basil breadcrumbs to be properly coated.

Once the succotash is ready, perform a quick pressure release and carefully open the pressure lid. Stir in the tomato and remove the bay leaf.

Set the reversible rack in the upper position of the pot, line with aluminum foil, and carefully lay the fish in the rack. Oil the top of the fish with cooking spray.

Close the crisping lid and Choose Bake/Roast; adjust the temperature to 375°F and the cook time to 8 minutes. Press Start. After 4 minutes, open the lid. Use tongs to turn them over and oil the other side with cooking spray. Close the lid and continue cooking.

Serve the fillets with the succotash.

Farfalle Tuna Casserole with Cheese

Servings: 4 | Ready in about: 60 min

INGREDIENTS

1 tablespoon olive oil
1 medium onion, chopped
1 large carrot, chopped
6 ounces farfalle
1 (12-ounce) can full cream milk, divided
1 cup vegetable broth
1 teaspoon salt

2 cups shredded Monterey Jack cheese
2 teaspoons corn starch
2 (5- to 6-ounce) cans tuna, drained
1 cup chopped green beans
2½ cups panko bread crumbs
3 tablespoons butter, melted

DIRECTIONS

On the Foodi, Choose Sear/Sauté and adjust to Medium. Press Start to preheat the pot. Heat the oil until shimmering and sauté the onion and carrots for 3 minutes, stirring, until softened.

Add the farfalle, ¾ cup of milk, broth, and salt to the pot. Stir to combine and submerge the farfalle in the liquid with a spoon.

Seal the pressure lid, choose pressure; adjust the pressure to Low and the cook time to 5 minutes; press Start. After cooking, do a quick pressure release and carefully open the pressure lid.

Choose Sear/Sauté and adjust to Less for low heat. Press Start. Pour the remaining milk on the farfalle.

In a medium bowl, mix the cheese and cornstarch evenly and add the cheese mixture by large handfuls to the sauce while stirring until the cheese melts and the sauce thickens. Add the tuna and green beans, gently stir. Heat for 2 minutes.

In another bowl, mix the crumbs and melted butter well. Spread the crumbs over the casserole.

Close the crisping lid and press Broil. Adjust the cook time to 5 minutes; press Start. When ready, the topping should be crisp and brown. If not, broil for 2 more minutes. Serve immediately.

Mackerel en Papillote with Vegetables

Servings: 6 | Ready in about: 25 min + 2 h for marinating

INGREDIENTS:

3 large whole mackerel, cut into 2 pieces
1 pound asparagus, trimmed
1 carrot, cut into sticks
1 celery stalk, cut into sticks
½ cup butter, at room temperature
6 medium tomatoes, quartered
1 large brown onion, sliced thinly

1 Orange Bell pepper, seeded and cut into sticks
Salt and black pepper to taste
2 ½ tbsp Pernod
3 cloves garlic, minced
2 lemons, cut into wedges
1 ½ cups water

DIRECTIONS:

Cut out 6 pieces of parchment paper a little longer and wider than a piece of fish with kitchen scissors. Then, cut out 6 pieces of foil slightly longer than the parchment papers.

Lay the foil wraps on a flat surface and place each parchment paper on each aluminium foil.

In a bowl, add tomatoes, onions, garlic, bell pepper, pernod, butter, asparagus, carrot, celery, salt, and pepper. Use a spoon to mix them.

Place each fish piece on the layer of parchment and foil wraps. Spoon the vegetable mixture on each fish. Then, wrap the fish and place the fish packets in the refrigerator to marinate for 2 hours. Remove the fish to a flat surface.

Open the Ninja Foodi, pour the water in, and fit the reversible rack at the bottom of the pot. Put the packets on the trivet. Seal the lid and select Steam mode on High pressure for 3 minutes. Press Start/Stop to start cooking.

Once the timer has ended, do a quick pressure release, and open the lid.

Remove the trivet with the fish packets onto a flat surface. Carefully open the foil and using a spatula. Return the packets to the pot, on top of the rack.

Close the crisping lid and cook on Air Crisp for 3 minutes at 300 F.

Then, remove to serving plates. Serve with lemon wedges.

Smoked Salmon Pilaf with Walnuts

Servings: 4 | Ready in about: 60 min

INGREDIENTS

½ cup walnut pieces

1 tablespoon ghee

4 green onions, chopped (white part separated from the green part)

1 cup basmati rice

1 cup frozen corn, thawed

2 cups water

1 teaspoon salt

1 smoked salmon fillet, flaked

2 teaspoons prepared horseradish

1 medium tomato, seeded and diced

DIRECTIONS

Pour the walnuts into a heatproof bowl. Put the Crisping basket in the inner pot and the bowl in the basket.

Close the crisping lid and Choose Air Crisp; adjust the temperature to 375°F and the time to 5 minutes. Press Start to begin toasting the walnuts. After the cooking time is over, carefully take the bowl and basket out of the pot and set aside.

On the Foodi, choose Sear/Sauté and adjust to Medium to preheat the inner pot. Add the ghee to melt and sauté the white part of the green onions for about a minute, or until starting to soften. Stir in the rice and corn, stirring occasionally for 2 to 3 minutes, or until starting to be fragrant. Add the water and salt.

Seal the pressure lid, choose Pressure; adjust the pressure to High and the cook time to 3 minutes; press Start.

After cooking, perform a natural pressure release for 5 minutes, then a quick pressure and carefully open the lid.

Fluff the rice gently with a fork. Stir in the flaked salmon, green parts of the green onions, and the horseradish. Add the tomato and allow sitting a few minutes to warm through. Spoon the pilaf into serving bowls and top with the walnuts. Serve.

Italian-Style Flounder

Servings: 4 | Ready in about: 70 min

INGREDIENTS

3 slices prosciutto, chopped

½ small red onion, chopped

½ teaspoon salt, divided

2 (6-ounce) bags baby kale

½ cup whipping cream

4 flounder fillets

3 tablespoons unsalted butter, melted and divided

¼ teaspoon fresh ground black pepper

2 tablespoons chopped fresh parsley

1 cup panko breadcrumbs

DIRECTIONS

On the Foodi, choose Sear/Sauté and adjust to Medium. Press Start to preheat the inner pot.

Add the prosciutto and cook until crispy, about 6 minutes. Stir in the red onions and cook for about 2 minutes or until the onions start to soften. Sprinkle with half of the salt.

Fetch the kale into the pot and cook, stirring frequently until wilted and most of the liquid has evaporated, about 4-5 minutes. Mix in the whipping cream.

Lay the flounder fillets over the kale in a single layer. Brush 1 tablespoon of the melted butter over the fillets and sprinkle with the remaining salt and black pepper.

Close the crisping lid and choose Bake/Roast. Adjust the temperature to 300°F and the cook time to 3 minutes. Press Start.

Combine the remaining butter, the parsley and breadcrumbs in a bowl.

When done cooking, open the crisping lid. Spoon the breadcrumbs mixture on the fillets.

Close the crisping lid and Choose Bake/Roast. Adjust the temperature to 400°F and the cook time to 6 minutes. Press Start.

After about 4 minutes, open the lid and check the fish. The breadcrumbs should be golden brown and crisp. If not, close the lid and continue to cook for an additional two minutes.

Monk Fish with Greens

Servings: 4 | Ready in about: 22 min

INGREDIENTS:

2 tbsp olive oil
4 (8 oz) monk fish fillets, cut in 2 pieces each
½ cup chopped green beans
2 cloves garlic, sliced
1 cup kale leaves

½ lb baby bok choy, stems removed and chopped largely
1 lemon, zested and juiced
Lemon wedges to serve
Salt and white pepper to taste

DIRECTIONS:

Pour in the coconut oil, garlic, red chili, and green beans. Stir fry for 5 minutes on Sear/Sauté mode.

Add the kale leaves, and cook them to wilt, about 3 minutes.

Meanwhile, place the fish on a plate and season with salt, white pepper, and lemon zest. After, remove the green beans and kale into a plate and set aside.

Back to the pot, add the olive oil and fish. Brown the fillets on each side for about 2 minutes and then add the bok choy in.

Pour the lemon juice over the fish and gently stir. Cook for 2 minutes and then press Start/Stop to stop cooking. Spoon the fish with bok choy over the green beans and kale. Serve with a side of lemon wedges and there, you have a complete meal.

Paprika & Garlic Salmon

Servings: 4 | Ready in about: 10 min

INGREDIENTS:

4 (5 oz) salmon fillets
1 cup water
Salt and black pepper to taste
2 tsp cumin powder
1 ½ tsp paprika
2 tbsp chopped parsley

2 tbsp olive oil
2 tbsp hot water
1 tbsp maple syrup
2 cloves garlic, minced
1 lime, juiced

DIRECTIONS:

In a bowl, add cumin, paprika, parsley, olive oil, hot water, maple syrup, garlic, and lime juice. Mix with a whisk. Set aside.

Open the Ninja Foodi and pour the water in. Then, fit the rack. Season the salmon with pepper and salt; and place them on the rack. Close the lid, secure the pressure valve, and select Steam mode on High pressure for 3 minutes. Press Start/Stop. Once the timer has ended, do a quick pressure release, and open the pot.

Close the crisping lid and cook on Air Crisp mode for 3 minutes at 300 F. Use a set of tongs to transfer the salmon to a serving plate and drizzle the lime sauce all over it. Serve with steamed swiss chard.

Alaskan Cod with Fennel & Beans

Servings: 4 | Ready in about: 25 min

INGREDIENTS:

2 (18 oz) Alaskan cod, cut into 4 pieces each
4 tbsp olive oil
2 cloves garlic, minced
2 small onions, chopped
½ cup olive brine
3 cups chicken broth
Salt and black pepper to taste

½ cup tomato puree
1 head fennel, quartered
1 cup Pinto beans, soaked, drained and rinsed
1 cup green olives, pitted and crushed
½ cup basil leaves
Lemon slices to garnish

DIRECTIONS:

Heat the olive oil and add the garlic and onion. Stir-fry on Sear/Sauté mode until the onion softens.

Pour in chicken broth and tomato puree. Let simmer for about 3 minutes.

Add fennel, olives, beans, salt, and pepper. Seal the lid and select Steam mode on High pressure for 10 minutes. Press Start/Stop to start cooking.

Once the timer has stopped, do a quick pressure release, and open the lid.

Transfer the beans to a plate with a slotted spoon. Adjust broth's taste with salt and pepper and add the cod pieces to the cooker.

Close the lid again, secure the pressure valve, and select Steam mode on Low pressure for 3 minutes. Press Start/Stop.

Once the timer has ended, do a quick pressure release, and open the lid.

Remove the cod into soup plates, top with the beans and basil leaves, and spoon the broth over them.

Serve with a side of crusted bread.

White Wine Black Mussels

Servings: 4 | Ready in about: 45 min

INGREDIENTS:

1 ½ lb black mussels, cleaned and de-bearded
3 tbsp olive oil
3 large chilies, seeded and chopped
3 cloves garlic, peeled and crushed
1 white onion, chopped finely
10 tomatoes, skin removed and chopped

4 tbsp tomato paste
1 cup dry white wine
3 cups vegetable broth
⅓ cup fresh basil leaves
1 cup fresh parsley leaves

DIRECTIONS:

Heat the olive oil on Sear/Sauté mode, and stir-fry the onion, until soft. Add the chilies and garlic, and cook for 2 minutes, stirring frequently.

Stir in the tomatoes and tomato paste, and cook for 2 more minutes. Then, pour in the wine and vegetable broth. Let simmer for 5 minutes.

Add the mussels, close the lid, secure the pressure valve, and press Steam mode on High pressure for 3 minutes. Press Start/Stop to start cooking. Once the timer has ended, do a natural pressure release for 15 minutes, then a quick pressure release, and open the lid.

Remove and discard any unopened mussels. Then, add half of the basil and parsley, and stir. Close the crisping lid and cook on Broil mode for 5 minutes.

Dish the mussels with sauce in serving bowls and garnish it with the remaining basil and parsley. Serve with a side of crusted bread.

Parsley Oyster Stew

Servings: 4 | Ready in about: 12 min

INGREDIENTS:

2 cups heavy cream
2 cups chopped celery
2 cups bone broth
3 (10 oz) jars shucked oysters in liqueur
3 Shallots, minced

3 tbsp olive oil
Salt and white pepper to taste
3 cloves garlic, minced
3 tbsp chopped parsley

DIRECTIONS:

Add oil, garlic, shallot, and celery. Stir-fry them for 2 minutes on Sear/Sauté mode, and add the heavy cream, broth, and oysters. Stir once or twice.

Close the lid, secure the pressure valve, and select Steam mode on High pressure for 3 minutes. Press Start/Stop.

Once the timer has stopped, do a quick pressure release, and open the lid.

Season with salt and white pepper. Close the crisping lid and cook for 5 minutes on Broil mode. Stir and dish the oyster stew into serving bowls.

Garnish with parsley and top with some croutons.

Creamy Crab Soup

Servings: 4 | Ready in about: 45 min

INGREDIENTS:

2 lb Crabmeat Lumps
6 tbsp butter
6 tbsp flour
Salt to taste
1 white onion, chopped
3 tsp minced garlic
2 celery stalk, diced
1 ½ cup chicken broth

¾ cup heavy cream
½ cup Half and Half cream
2 tsp Hot sauce
3 tsp Worcestershire sauce
3 tsp old bay Seasoning
¾ cup Muscadet
Lemon juice to serve
Chopped dill to serve

DIRECTIONS:

Melt the butter on Sear/Sauté mode, and mix in the all-purpose flour, in a fast motion to make a rue. Add celery, onion, and garlic.

Stir and cook until soft and crispy, for 3 minutes.

While stirring, gradually add the half and half cream, heavy cream, and broth.

Let simmer for 2 minutes. Add Worcestershire sauce, old bay seasoning, Muscadet, and hot sauce. Stir and let simmer for 15 minutes. Add the crabmeat and mix it well into the sauce.

Close the crisping lid and cook on Broil mode for 10 minutes to soften the meat. Dish into serving bowls, garnish with dill and drizzle squirts of lemon juice over. Serve with a side of garlic crusted bread.

Paella Señorito

Servings: 5 | Ready in about: 25 min

INGREDIENTS

¼ cup olive oil
1 onion, chopped
1 red bell pepper, diced
2 garlic cloves, minced
1 tsp paprika
1 tsp turmeric
salt and ground white pepper to taste

1 cup bomba rice
¼ cup frozen green peas
2 cups fish broth
1 pound frozen shrimp, peeled and deveined
chopped fresh parsley
1 lemon, cut into wedges

DIRECTIONS

Warm oil on Sear/Sauté. Add in bell pepper and onions and cook for 5 minutes until fragrant. Mix in garlic and cook for one more minute until soft.

Add paprika, ground white pepper, salt and turmeric to the vegetables and cook for 1 minute.

Stir in fish broth and rice. Add shrimp in the rice mixture.

Seal the pressure lid, choose Pressure, set to High, and set the timer to 5 minutes; press Start. When ready, release the pressure quickly. Stir in green peas and let sit for 5 minutes until green peas are heated through. Serve warm garnished with parsley and lemon wedges.

Steamed Mediterranean Cod

Servings: 4 | Ready in about: 20 min

INGREDIENTS

1 pound cherry tomatoes, halved
1 bunch fresh thyme sprigs
4 fillets cod
1 tsp olive oil
1 clove garlic, pressed
3 pinches salt

2 cups water
1 cup white rice
1 cup Kalamata olives
2 tbsp pickled capers
1 tbsp olive oil, divided
1 pinch ground black pepper

DIRECTIONS

Line a parchment paper to the steamer basket of your Foodi. Place about half the tomatoes in a single layer on the paper. Sprinkle with thyme, reserving some for garnish.

Arrange cod fillets on the top of tomatoes. Sprinkle with a little bit of olive oil.

Spread the garlic, pepper, salt, and remaining tomatoes over the fish. In the pot, mix rice and water. Lay a trivet over the rice and water. Lower steamer basket onto the trivet.

Seal the pressure lid, choose Pressure, set to High, and set the timer to 7 minutes. Press Start. When ready, release the pressure quickly.

Remove the steamer basket and trivet from the pot. Use a fork to fluff rice.

Plate the fish fillets and apply a garnish of olives, reserved thyme, pepper, remaining olive oil, and capers. Serve with rice.

Seared Scallops with Butter-Caper Sauce

Servings: 6 | Ready in about: 18 min

INGREDIENTS:

2 lb sea scallops, foot removed
10 tbsp butter, unsalted
4 tbsp capers, drained

4 tbsp olive oil
1 cup dry white wine
3 tsp lemon zest

DIRECTIONS:

Melt the butter to caramel brown on Sear/Sauté. Use a soup spook to fetch the butter out into a bowl.

Next, heat the oil in the pot, once heated add the scallops and sear them on both sides to golden brown which is about 5 minutes.

Remove to a plate and set aside.

Pour the white wine in the pot to deglaze the bottom while using a spoon to scrape the bottom of the pot of any scallop bits.

Add the capers, butter, and lemon zest. Use a spoon to stir the mixture once gently. After 40 seconds, spoon the sauce with capers over the scallops.

Serve with a side of braised asparagus.

Steamed Sea Bass with Turnips

Servings: 4 | Ready in about: 15 min

INGREDIENTS

1½ cups water
1 lemon, sliced
4 sea bass fillets
4 sprigs thyme
1 white onion, sliced into thin rings

2 turnips, sliced
2 pinches salt
1 pinch ground black pepper
2 tsp olive oil

DIRECTIONS

Add water to the Foodi. Set a reversible rack into the pot.

Line a parchment paper to the bottom of steamer basket. Place lemon slices in a single layer on the reversible rack.

Arrange fillets on the top of the lemons, cover with onion and thyme sprigs and top with turnip slices.

Drizzle pepper, salt, and olive oil over the mixture. Put steamer basket onto the reversible rack. Seal lid and cook on Low for 8 minutes; press Start.

When ready, release pressure quickly. Serve over the delicate onion rings and thinly sliced turnips.

White Wine Mussels

Servings: 5 | Ready in about: 15 min

INGREDIENTS

1 cup white wine
½ cup water
1 tsp garlic powder

2 pounds mussels, cleaned and debearded
Juice from 1 lemon

DIRECTIONS

In the Foodi, mix garlic powder, water and wine. Put the mussels into the steamer basket, rounded-side should be placed facing upwards to fit as many as possible.

Insert reversible rack in the Foodi and lower steamer basket onto the reversible rack. Seal lid and cook on Low pressure for 1 minute. When ready, release the pressure quickly.

Remove unopened mussels. Coat the mussels with the wine mixture. Serve with a side of French fries or slices of toasted bread.

Delicious Coconut Shrimp

Servings: 2 | Ready in about: 30 min

INGREDIENTS:

8 large shrimp
½ cup breadcrumbs
8 oz coconut milk
½ cup shredded coconut
¼ tsp salt
¼ tsp pepper

½ cup orange jam
1 tsp mustard
1 tbsp honey
½ tsp cayenne pepper
¼ tsp hot sauce

DIRECTIONS:

Combine the breadcrumbs, cayenne pepper, shredded coconut, salt, and pepper in a small bowl.

Dip the shrimp in the coconut milk, first, and then in the coconut crumbs.

Arrange in the lined Ninja Foodi basket, close the crisping lid and cook for 20 minutes on Air Crisp mode at 350 F. Meanwhile whisk the jam, honey, hot sauce, and mustard. Serve the shrimp with the sauce.

Fish Finger Sandwich

Servings: 4 | Ready in about: 20 min

INGREDIENTS:

4 cod fillets
2 tbsp flour
10 capers
4 bread rolls

2 oz breadcrumbs
4 tbsp pesto sauce
4 lettuce leaves
Salt and pepper, to taste

DIRECTIONS:

Season the fillets with some salt and pepper, and coat them with the flour, and then dip in the breadcrumbs. You should get at the layer of breadcrumbs, that's why we don't use eggs for this recipe. Arrange the fillets onto a baking mat.

Close the crisping lid and cook for about 10 to 15 minutes on Air Crisp mode at 370 F. Cut the bread rolls in half.

Place a lettuce leaf on top of the bottom halves; place the fillets over.

Spread a tbsp of pesto sauce on top of each fillet; top with the remaining halves.

Parmesan Tilapia

Servings: 4 | Ready in about: 15 min

INGREDIENTS:

¾ cup grated Parmesan cheese
1 tbsp olive oil
2 tsp paprika
1 tbsp chopped parsley

¼ tsp garlic powder
¼ tsp salt
4 tilapia fillets

DIRECTIONS:

Mix parsley, Parmesan, garlic, salt, and paprika, in a shallow bowl.

Brush the olive oil over the fillets, and then coat them with the Parmesan mixture.

Place the tilapia onto a lined baking sheet, and then into the Ninja Foodi.

Close the crisping lid and cook for about 4 to 5 minutes on all sides on Air Crisp mode at 350 F.

Crab Cakes

Servings: 4 | Ready in about: 55 min

INGREDIENTS:

½ cup cooked crab meat
¼ cup chopped red onion
1 tbsp chopped basil
¼ cup chopped celery
¼ cup chopped red pepper
3 tbsp mayonnaise

Zest of ½ lemon
¼ cup breadcrumbs
2 tbsp chopped parsley
Old Bay seasoning, as desired
Cooking spray

DIRECTIONS:

Place all ingredients in a large bowl and mix well until thoroughly incorporated.

Make 4 large crab cakes from the mixture and place on a lined sheet.

Refrigerate for 30 minutes, to set.

Spay the air basket with cooking spray and arrange the crab cakes in it.

Close the crisping lid and cook for 7 minutes on each side on Air Crisp at 390 F.

Quick and Easy Air Fried Salmon

Servings: 1 | Ready in about: 13 min

INGREDIENTS:

1 salmon fillet

1 tbsp soy sauce

¼ tsp garlic powder

Salt and pepper

DIRECTIONS:

Combine the soy sauce with the garlic powder, salt, and pepper.

Brush the mixture over the salmon.

Place the salmon onto a sheet of parchment paper and inside the Ninja Foodi.

Close the crisping lid and cook for 10 minutes on Air Crisp at 350 F, until crispy on the outside and tender on the inside.

Cajun Salmon with Lemon

Servings: 1 | Ready in about: 10 min

INGREDIENTS:

1 salmon fillet

¼ tsp brown sugar

Juice of ½ lemon

1 tbsp Cajun seasoning

2 lemon wedges

1 tbsp chopped parsley, for garnishing

DIRECTIONS:

Meanwhile, combine the sugar and lemon and coat the salmon with this mixture thoroughly. Coat the salmon with the Cajun seasoning as well.

Place a parchment paper into the Ninja Foodi, close the crisping lid and cook the salmon for 7 minutes on Air Crisp mode at 350 F.

If you use a thicker fillet, cook no more than 6 minutes. Serve with lemon wedges and chopped parsley.

Tuna Patties

Servings: 2 | Ready in about: 50 min

INGREDIENTS:

5 oz of canned tuna

1 tsp lime juice

1 tsp paprika

¼ cup flour

½ cup milk

1 small onion, diced

2 eggs

1 tsp chili powder, optional

½ tsp salt

DIRECTIONS:

Place all ingredients in a bowl, and mix to combine.

Make two large patties, or a few smaller ones, out of the mixture.

Place them on a lined sheet and refrigerate for 30 minutes.

Close the crisping lid and cook the patties for about 6 minutes on each side on Roast mode at 350 F.

Cod Cornflakes Nuggets

Servings: 4 | Ready in about: 25 min

INGREDIENTS:

1 ¼ lb cod fillets, cut into chunks
½ cup flour
1 egg
1 tbsp water

1 cup cornflakes
1 tbsp olive oil
Salt and pepper, to taste

DIRECTIONS:

Add the oil and cornflakes in a food processor, and process until crumbed.

Season the fish chunks with salt and pepper.

Beat the egg along with 1 tbsp water. Dredge the chunks in flour first, then dip in the egg, and coat with cornflakes.

Arrange on a lined sheet. Close the crisping lid and cook at 350 F for 15 minutes on Air Crisp mode.

Pistachio Crusted Salmon

Servings: 1 | Ready in about: 15 min

INGREDIENTS:

1 salmon fillet
1 tsp mustard
3 tbsp pistachios
Pinch of sea salt
Pinch of garlic powder

Pinch of black pepper
1 tsp lemon juice
1 tsp grated Parmesan cheese
1 tsp olive oil

DIRECTIONS:

Whisk the mustard and lemon juice together. Season the salmon with salt, pepper, and garlic powder. Brush the olive oil on all sides.

Brush the mustard-lemon mixture on top of the salmon.

Chop the pistachios finely, and combine them with the Parmesan cheese.

Sprinkle them on top of the salmon. Place the salmon in the Ninja Foodi basket with the skin side down. Close the crisping lid and cook for 10 minutes on Air Crisp mode at 350 F.

Lemon Chicken Tenders with Broccoli

Servings: 2 | Ready in about: 70 min

INGREDIENTS

1 cup basmati rice
1 cup plus 2 tbsp water
1 head broccoli, cut into florets
2 tbsp melted butter, divided
¼ tsp salt
¼ tsp freshly ground black pepper
Cooking spray

4 boneless, skinless chicken tenders
¼ cup barbecue sauce
¼ cup lemon marmalade
½ tbsp soy sauce
1 tbsp sesame seeds, for garnish
2 tbsp sliced green onions, for garnish

DIRECTIONS

Pour the rice and water in the pot and stir to combine. Seal the pressure lid, choose Pressure, set to High, and the timer to 2 minutes. Press Start/Stop to boil the rice.

Meanwhile, in a medium bowl, toss the broccoli with 1 tablespoon of melted butter, and season with the salt and black pepper.

When done cooking, perform a quick pressure release, and carefully open the lid.

Place the reversible rack in the higher position inside the pot, which will be over the rice. Then, spray the rack with cooking spray. Lay the chicken tenders on the rack and brush with the remaining 1 tablespoon of melted butter. Arrange the broccoli around the chicken tenders.

Close the crisping lid. Choose Air Crisp, set the temperature to 400°F, and set the time to 10 minutes. Press Start/Stop to begin.

In a bowl, mix the barbecue sauce, lemon marmalade, and soy sauce until well combined.

When done crisping, coat the chicken with the lemon sauce. Use tongs to turn the chicken over and apply the lemon sauce in the other side. Close the crisping lid, select Broil and set the time to 5 minutes; press Start/Stop.

After cooking is complete, check for your desired crispiness and remove the rack from the pot.

Spoon the rice into serving plates with the chicken and broccoli. Garnish with the sesame seeds and green onions and serve.

Garlic Herb Roasted Chicken

Servings: 4 | Ready in about: 70 min

INGREDIENTS

1 (3½-pound) whole chicken
½ cup white wine
Juice of 1 lemon
2 limes, juiced
3 tbsp olive oil

¼ cup coconut aminos
2 tbsp Italian herb mix
1½ tbsp ground cumin
6 cloves garlic, grated
1 tbsp salt

DIRECTIONS

Remove the neck from inside the chicken's cavity, trim off the excess fat and any remaining feathers. Rinse the chicken thoroughly with water and tie the legs with butcher's twine.

Pour the wine and lemon juice into the pot. Place the chicken in the crisping basket and fix the basket in the higher position of the pot.

Put the pressure lid together and lock in the Seal position. Choose Pressure and set to High. Set the time to 20 minutes, then Choose Start/Stop to begin cooking the chicken.

When the timer is done, perform a quick pressure release, and carefully open the pressure lid.

In a bowl, combine the lime juice, the olive oil, coconut aminos, Italian herb mix, cumin, garlic and salt; mix until thoroughly combined. Brush the mixture over the chicken.

Close the crisping lid. Choose Air Crisp, set the temperature to 400°F, and set the time to 15 minutes. Choose Start/Stop to begin. If you prefer a crispier chicken, cook further for 5 to 10 minutes.

After about 10 minutes, lift the crisping lid and sprinkle the chicken with the fresh rosemary. Close the crisping lid and continue cooking.

Carefully open the lid and transfer the chicken to a plate.

Let the chicken rest for 10 minutes before cutting and serving.

Sweet Sesame Chicken Wings

Servings: 4 | Ready in about: 65 min

INGREDIENTS

24 chicken wings
2 tbsp sesame oil
2 tbsp hot garlic sauce

2 tbsp honey
2 garlic cloves, minced
1 tbsp toasted sesame seeds

DIRECTIONS

Pour 1 cup of water into the Foodi's inner pot and place the reversible rack in the lower position of the pot. Place the chicken wings on the rack.

Seal the pressure lid, choose Pressure; adjust the pressure to High and the cook time to 10 minutes. Press Start to begin cooking the chicken.

While the wings cook, prepare the glaze. In a large bowl, whisk the sesame oil, hot garlic sauce, honey, and garlic.

After cooking, perform a quick pressure release, and carefully open the lid.

Remove the rack from the pot and empty the water in the pot. Return the pot to the base.

Close the crisping lid and Choose Air Crisp; adjust the temperature to 375°F and the time to 3 minutes to preheat the inner pot. Press Start.

Toss the wings in the sauce to properly coat. Put the wings in the Crisping Basket, leaving any excess sauce in the bowl.

Place the basket in the Foodi and close the crisping lid. Choose Air Crisp and adjust the cook time to 15 minutes. Press Start to commence crisping.

After 8 minutes, open the lid and use tongs to turn the wings. Close the lid to resume browning until the wings are crisp and the glaze set.

Before serving, drizzle with any remaining sauce and sprinkle with the sesame seeds.

Crispy Chicken Thighs with Thyme Carrot Roast

Servings: 4 | Ready in about: 50 min

INGREDIENTS

1 ½ cups chicken broth
1 cup basmati rice
4 bone-in, skin-on chicken thighs
2 carrots, chopped

2 tbsp melted butter
2 tsp chicken seasoning
1 tsp salt, divided
2 tsp chopped fresh thyme

DIRECTIONS

Pour the chicken broth and rice in the pot.

Then, put the reversible rack in the pot. Arrange the chicken thighs on the rack, skin side up, and arrange the carrots around the chicken.

Put the pressure lid together and lock in the Seal position. Choose Pressure, set to High, and the time to 2 minutes. Choose Start/Stop to begin cooking the chicken.

When done cooking, perform a quick pressure release, and carefully open the lid.

Brush the carrots and chicken with the melted butter. Season the chicken with the chicken seasoning and half of the salt. Also, season the carrots with the thyme and remaining salt.

Close the crisping lid; choose Broil and set the time to 10 minutes. Choose Start/Stop to begin crisping. When done cooking, check for your desired crispiness, and the turn the Foodi off.

Spoon the rice into serving plates, and serve the chicken and carrots over the rice.

Quick Chicken Fried Rice

Servings: 4 | Ready in about: 60 min

INGREDIENTS

1 tbsp ghee
1 onion, diced
4 garlic cloves, minced
1 pound boneless, skinless chicken breasts, diced
⅛ tsp salt

⅛ tsp freshly ground black pepper
2 cups chicken broth
¼ cup coconut aminos
1 cup long grain rice
1 (16-ounce) bag frozen mixed vegetables

DIRECTIONS

Press Sear/Sauté on the pot and set to Medium High. Choose Start/Stop to preheat the pot.

Melt the ghee and sauté the onion for 3 minutes. Add and sauté the garlic until fragrant, about 1 minute. Put the chicken in the pot and season with the salt and black pepper. Cook for 5 minutes to brown the chicken.

Pour the chicken broth, coconut aminos, and rice into the pot.

Put the pressure lid together and lock the pressure release valve in the Seal position. Choose Pressure, set to High, and set the time to 3 minutes. Choose Start/Stop to begin cooking.

When the timer is done, perform a quick pressure and carefully open the lid.

Pour the frozen vegetables into the pot. Choose Sear/Sauté and set to Medium High. Choose Start/Stop to begin heating the vegetables through. Cook for 5 minutes while stirring occasionally.

When ready, dish the fried rice with chicken and serve.

Chicken with Crunchy Coconut Dumplings

Servings: 6 | Ready in about: 70 min

INGREDIENTS

1 tbsp ghee
1 white onion, chopped
2 carrots, diced
2 celery stalks, diced
1 pound skinless, boneless chicken breasts, cubed

2 cups chicken stock
1 tsp fresh rosemary
½ tsp salt
½ cup heavy cream
1 package refrigerated biscuits, at room temperature

DIRECTIONS

Choose Sear/Sauté on the pot and set to Medium High. Choose Start/Stop to preheat the pot.

Melt the ghee and sauté the onion until softened, about 3 minutes.

Pour the carrots, celery, chicken, and stock into the pot. Season with the rosemary and salt.

Put the pressure lid together and lock in the Seal position. Choose Pressure, set to High, and set the time to 2 minutes. Choose Start/Stop to begin

When done cooking, perform a quick pressure release, and carefully open the lid.

Stir the heavy cream into the soup. Place the reversible rack in the higher position inside the pot, which will be over the soup and arrange the biscuits in a single layer in the rack.

Close the crisping lid. Choose Broil and set the time to 15 minutes. Choose Start/Stop to begin crisping. When ready, allow the biscuit and soup to rest for a few minutes and then serve.

Creamy Turkey Enchilada Casserole

Servings: 6 | Ready in about: 70 min

INGREDIENTS

1 tbsp butter
1 yellow onion, diced
2 garlic cloves, minced
1 pound boneless, skinless turkey breasts
2 cups enchilada sauce
¼ tsp salt

¼ tsp freshly ground black pepper
1 (15-ounce) can pinto beans, drained and rinsed
8 tortillas, each cut into 8 pieces
1 (16-ounce) bag frozen corn
2 cups shredded Monterey Jack cheese, divided

DIRECTIONS

Choose Sear/Sauté on the pot and set to Medium High. Choose Start/Stop to preheat the pot.

Melt the butter and cook the onion for 3 minutes, stirring occasionally. Stir in the garlic and cook until fragrant, about 1 minute more.

Put the turkey and enchilada sauce in the pot, and season with salt and black pepper. Stir to combine. Seal the pressure lid, choose Pressure, set to High, and set the time to 15 minutes. Choose Start/Stop.

When done cooking, perform a quick pressure release and carefully open the lid.

Shred the turkey with two long forks while being careful not to burn your hands. Mix in the pinto beans, tortilla pieces, corn, and half of the cheese to the pot. Sprinkle the remaining cheese evenly on top of the casserole.

Close the crisping lid. Choose Broil and set the time to 5 minutes. Press Start/Stop to begin broiling. When ready, allow the casserole to sit for 5 minutes before serving.

Chicken Cassoulet with Frijoles

Servings: 4 | Ready in about: 60 min

INGREDIENTS

4 small chicken thighs, bone-in skin-on
1½ tsp salt
¼ tsp black pepper
2 pancetta slices, cut into thirds
1 medium carrot, diced
½ small onion, diced

½ cup dry red wine
1 cup Pinto Beans Frijoles, soaked
3 cups chicken stock
1 cup panko breadcrumbs
Olive oil, as needed

DIRECTIONS

Season the chicken on both sides with salt and black pepper and set aside on a wire rack.

On your Foodi, choose Sear/Sauté and adjust to Medium. Press Start to preheat the inner pot.

Add the pancetta slices in a single layer and cook for 3 to 4 minutes or until browned on one side. Turn and brown the other side. Remove the pancetta to a paper towel-lined plate.

Put the chicken thighs in the pot, and fry for about 6-7 minutes or until is golden brown on both sides. Use tongs to pick the chicken into a plate.

Carefully pour out all the fat in the pot leaving about 1 tablespoon to coat the bottom of the pot. Reserve the remaining fat in a small bowl.

Sauté the carrots and onion in the pot for 3 minutes with frequent stirring, until the onion begins to brown. Stir in the wine while scraping off the brown bits at the bottom. Allow boiling until the wine reduces by one-third and stir in the beans and chicken stock.

Seal the pressure lid, choose pressure; adjust the pressure to High and the cook time to 25 minutes. Press Start to commence cooking.

When done cooking, perform a quick pressure release and carefully open the lid. Return the chicken to the pot and cook for 10 minutes.

Combine the breadcrumbs with the reserved fat until evenly mixed.

When done cooking, perform a natural pressure release for 5 minutes, then a quick pressure release to let out any remaining steam, and carefully open the lid.

Crumble the pancetta over the cassoulet. Spoon the breadcrumbs mixture on top of the beans while avoiding the chicken as much as possible.

Close the crisping lid; choose Broil, adjust the cook time to 7 minutes, and press Start/Stop. When the cassoulet is ready, allow resting for a few minutes before serving.

Chicken with Cilantro Rice

Servings: 4 | Ready in about: 70 min

INGREDIENTS

2 tbsp ghee divided
1 red onion, diced
1 yellow bell pepper, diced
1 tbsp cayenne powder
1 tsp ground cumin
1 tsp Italian herb mix
½ tsp salt

1 cup basmati rice
¾ cup chicken broth
½ cup tomato sauce
1 pound bone-in, skin-on chicken thighs
Chopped fresh cilantro, for garnish
Lime wedges, for serving

DIRECTIONS

Choose Sear/Sauté on the pot and set to Medium High. Choose Start/Stop to preheat the pot.

Melt half of the ghee in the pot, and cook the onion for 3 minutes, stirring occasionally, until softened. Include the yellow bell pepper, cayenne pepper, cumin, herb mix, and salt, and cook for 2 minutes more with frequent stirring.

Pour the rice, broth, and tomato sauce into the pot. Place the reversible rack in the higher position of the pot, which is over the rice. Put the chicken on the rack.

Seal the pressure lid, choose pressure, set to High, and set the time to 30 minutes. Choose Start/Stop to begin cooking the rice. When the time is over, perform a quick pressure release and carefully open the lid.

Brush the chicken thighs with the remaining 1 tablespoon of ghee. Close the crisping lid. Choose Broil and set the time to 5 minutes. Press Start/Stop.

When ready, check for your desired crispiness and remove the rack from the pot. Plate the chicken, garnish with cilantro, and serve with lime wedges.

Black Refried Beans and Chicken Fajitas

Servings: 4 | Ready in about: 40 min

INGREDIENTS

1 large (27-ounce) can black beans
1 garlic clove, crushed
1 bacon slice, halved widthwise
¼ cup water
4 tbsp olive oil, divided
1 pound chicken breasts, sliced
1 yellow bell pepper, sliced
1 red bell pepper, sliced

1 small onion, cut into 8 wedges
1 jalapeño pepper, sliced
1 tsp salt
1 tbsp Mexican seasoning mix
Corn tortillas to serve
Avocado slices to serve
Salsa to serve

DIRECTIONS

Pour the beans with liquid into the Foodi's inner pot. Stir in the garlic, bacon, water, and 2 tablespoons of olive oil. Seal the pressure lid, choose Pressure; adjust to High and the cook time to 5 minutes. Press Start.

In a large bowl, mix the chicken, yellow and red bell peppers, jalapeño, and onion. Drizzle with the remaining oil, sprinkle with the salt and Mexican seasoning and toss to coat. Set aside.

When the beans are ready, do a quick pressure release, and carefully open the lid. Pour out the beans with liquid into a large bowl and cover with aluminum foil to keep warm; set aside.

Place the Crisping Basket into the inner pot. Close the crisping lid and select Air Crisp. Adjust the temperature to 375°F and the time to 4 minutes. Press Start to preheat.

Uncover the beans. Remove and discard the bacon pieces and garlic clove. Fetch out about ¼ cup of the liquid and reserve it. Then, use a potato masher to break the beans into the remaining liquid until smooth while adding more liquid if needed. Cover the bowl again with aluminum foil.

When the pot has preheated, open the lid and add the vegetables and chicken to the basket. Close the crisping lid. Choose Air Crisp; adjust the temperature to 375°F and the cook time to 10 minutes. Press Start to begin browning.

After 5 minutes, open the lid and use tongs to turn the vegetables and chicken. Continue cooking until the vegetables are slightly browned and the chicken tender. Wrap the chicken and beans in warm tortillas and garnish with the avocado and salsa to serve.

Chicken Potato Pot Pie

Servings: 6 | Ready in about: 70 min

INGREDIENTS

4 tbsp butter
1 onion, diced
2 garlic cloves, minced
2 pounds boneless chicken breasts, cubed
2 potatoes, diced
1 cup chicken broth

½ tsp salt
½ tsp freshly ground black pepper
8 oz frozen sweetcorn
½ cup whipping cream
1 piecrust, at room temperature

DIRECTIONS

Choose Sear/Sauté on the pot and set to Medium High. Choose Start/Stop to preheat the inner pot. Melt the ghee and sauté garlic and onion until softened, about 3 minutes.

Add the chicken, potatoes, and broth to the pot. Season with the salt and black pepper.

Put the pressure lid together and lock in the Seal position. Choose Pressure, set to High, and the time to 10 minutes; press Start/Stop. When done cooking, do a quick pressure release.

Select Sear/Sauté and set to Medium High. Choose Start/Stop keep the pot in a simmering mode. Pour the frozen sweetcorn and whipping cream into the pot. Stir until the sauce thickens, about 3 minutes.

Place the piecrust on top of vegetables and cream mixture, folding over the edges if necessary. Cut out a small dent in the center of the pie to allow steam to escape when baking.

Close the crisping lid. Choose Broil and set the time to 10 minutes; press Start/Stop.

When ready, remove the inner pot from the Foodi and place on a heat-resistant surface. Let the potpie rest for 10 to 15 minutes before serving.

Herbed Chicken and Biscuit Chili

Servings: 6 | Ready in about: 90 min

INGREDIENTS

1 tbsp olive oil
1 onion, chopped
2 garlic cloves, minced
1½ pounds ground chicken
1 tbsp ground cilantro

1 tbsp dried oregano
4 cups chicken broth
⅛ tsp salt
⅛ tsp black pepper
1 package refrigerated biscuits, at room temperature

DIRECTIONS

Choose Sear/Sauté on the Foodi and set to Medium-High; press Start/Stop to preheat the pot.

Pour the oil, chicken, onion, and garlic into the inner pot and sauté until the onion is softened, about 3 minutes. Add the cilantro, oregano, broth, salt, and black pepper to the pot.

Put the pressure lid together and lock in the Seal position. Choose Pressure and set to High. Set the time to 10 minutes, then Choose Start/Stop to begin cooking.

When the time is over, perform a quick pressure release, and carefully open the lid.

Spread the biscuits in a single layer over the chili. Close the crisping lid. Choose Broil and set the time to 15 minutes. Choose Start/Stop to commence browning.

When ready, remove the pot from the Foodi and place on a heat-resistant surface. Let the chili and biscuits rest for 10 to 15 minutes before serving.

Hot Crispy Chicken with Carrots and Potatoes

Servings: 4 | Ready in about: 35 min

INGREDIENTS

4 bone-in skin-on chicken thighs
½ tsp salt
2 tbsp melted butter
2 tsp Worcestershire sauce
2 tsp turmeric powder
1 tsp dried oregano
½ tsp dry mustard

½ tsp garlic powder
¼ tsp sweet paprika
2 dashes hot sauce
¼ cup chicken stock
1 tbsp olive oil
1 pound potatoes, quartered
2 carrots, sliced into rounds

DIRECTIONS

Season the chicken on both sides with salt. In a small bowl, mix the melted butter, Worcestershire sauce, turmeric, oregano, dry mustard, garlic powder, sweet paprika, and hot sauce to be properly combined and stir in the chicken stock.

On your Foodi, choose Sear/Sauté and adjust to Medium-High. Press Start to preheat the inner pot. Heat olive oil and add the chicken thighs and fry for 4 to 5 minutes or until browned. Turn and briefly sear the other side, about 1 minute. Remove from the pot.

Add the potatoes and carrots to the pot and stir to coat with the fat. Pour in about half of the spicy sauce and mix to coat. Put the chicken thighs on top and drizzle with the remaining sauce.

Seal the pressure lid, choose pressure; adjust the pressure to High and the cook time to 3 minutes; press Start. After cooking, do a quick pressure release, and carefully open the lid.

Transfer the chicken to the reversible rack. Use a spoon to gently move the potatoes and carrots aside and fetch some of the sauce over the chicken. Mix the potatoes and carrots back into the sauce and carefully set the rack in the pot.

Close the crisping lid and Choose Bake/Roast; adjust the temperature to 375°F and the cook time to 16 minutes. Press Start to begin crisping the chicken.

When done cooking, open the lid and transfer the potatoes, carrots and chicken to a serving platter, drizzling with any remaining sauce.

Herby Chicken Breasts

Servings: 4 | Ready in about: 15 min

INGREDIENTS

4 boneless, skinless chicken breasts
½ tsp salt
1 cup water
1/4 cup dry white wine

½ tsp rosemary
½ tsp mint
½ tsp marjoram
½ tsp sage

DIRECTIONS

Sprinkle salt over the chicken and set in the pot of the Foodi. Mix in mint, rosemary, marjoram, and sage. Pour wine and water around the chicken.

Seal the pressure lid, choose Pressure, set to High, and set the timer to 6 minutes. Press Start. Release the pressure naturally for 10 minutes.

Herby Dumplings and Italian Season Chicken

Servings: 4 | Ready in about: 40 min

INGREDIENTS

For the Dumplings
1 large egg
¾ cup heavy cream

6 ounces self-rising flour
1 tsp dried mixed herbs

For the Chicken
3 tbsp butter
3 tbsp flour
1 tsp Italian seasoning mix
3 cups chicken stock
1¼ lb skinless, boneless chicken thighs, cubed

1 bay leaf
2 large celery stalks, chopped
3 large carrots, cut into coins
⅔ cup peas, frozen
1 cup frozen pearl onions

DIRECTIONS

To make the dumplings, whisk the egg and cream in a medium bowl until evenly combined and stir in the flour and mixed herbs until a stiff but soft dough forms. Refrigerate the dough while you make the chicken.

Select Sear/Sauté and adjust to Medium and press Start to preheat the pot for 5 minutes.

Melt the butter, stir in the flour and Italian seasoning. Cook for 3 to 4 minutes, stirring occasionally, until the roux is golden brown. Pour in stock, whisking until combined.

Cook until the sauce has slightly thickened. Add the chicken, bay leaf, celery, and carrots to the inner pot. Seal the pressure lid, choose Pressure; adjust the pressure to High and the cook time to 6 minutes; press Start.

Once ready, perform a quick pressure release and carefully open the lid. Remove and discard the bay leaf. Stir in the peas and onion.

Take out the dumpling from the fridge and drop in small spoonfuls into the chicken and vegetables. Seal the pressure lid, choose Pressure; adjust the pressure to High and the cook time to 2 minutes; press Start.

After cooking, perform a quick pressure release and carefully open the lid. The dumplings will have cooked through and be pale in color.

Close the crisping lid and Choose Broil. Adjust the cook time to 7 minutes; press Start. When done cooking, the dumplings should be golden brown on top. Ladle into bowls and serve.

Tandoori Chicken Thighs

Servings: 4 | Ready in about: 45 min

INGREDIENTS

1½ pounds chicken thighs, boneless skinless
2½ tsp salt
1 cup plain Greek yogurt
1½ tsp garlic puree
1 tbsp ginger puree
1 tsp sweet paprika
½ tsp chili pepper
½ tsp garam masala
½ tsp ground cumin

1 tsp turmeric powder
⅛ tsp freshly ground black pepper
1 cup long grain white rice, rinsed and drained
¾ cup coconut milk
¼ cup water
½ cup cooked lima beans
Cooking spray
1 tbsp chopped fresh parsley

DIRECTIONS

Season the chicken on both sides with salt and place the meat in a plastic zipper bag. Set aside and make the marinade.

In a medium bowl, mix the yogurt, salt, garlic, ginger, paprika, chili pepper, garam masala, cumin, turmeric, and black pepper. Pour the marinade over the chicken. Zip the bag and rub the marinade on the chicken to coat properly. Set aside.

Pour the rice into the Foodi's inner pot and mix in the coconut milk, water, and some salt to taste. Seal the pressure lid, choose Pressure; adjust the pressure to High and the cook time to 3 minutes. Press Start to commence cooking the rice.

After cooking, perform a natural pressure release for 6 minutes and then a quick pressure release to let out the remaining pressure. Carefully open the lid.

Stir in the lima beans and cover the rice with aluminum foil to prevent the rice from drying out.

Oil the reversible rack with cooking spray. Place in the pot and slide the legs of the rack under the foil. Remove the chicken from the marinade, hold for a while to allow the excess liquid drip back into the bag. Arrange the chicken on the greased rack in a single layer.

Close the crisping lid and choose Broil. Adjust the cook time to 16 minutes. Press Start/Stop.

After 8 minutes, open the lid and flip the chicken and close the lid. Cook until the second side is crisp and browned on the edges. Serve the chicken with rice and garnish with the parsley.

Saucy Shredded Chicken

Servings: 4 | Ready in about: 35 min

INGREDIENTS:

4 chicken breasts, skinless
¼ cup Sriracha sauce
2 tbsp butter
1 tsp grated ginger
2 cloves garlic, minced
½ tsp Cayenne pepper

½ tsp red chili flakes
½ cup honey
½ cup chicken broth
Salt and black pepper to taste
Chopped scallion to garnish

DIRECTIONS:

In a bowl, pour the chicken broth. Mix in honey, ginger, sriracha sauce, red pepper flakes, cayenne pepper, and garlic. Set aside.

Put the chicken on a plate and season with salt and pepper. Set aside too. Select Sear/Sauté mode on High on your Ninja Foodi.

Melt the butter, and add the chicken in 2 batches to brown on both sides for about 3 minutes. Add the chicken back, and pour the pepper sauce over.

Close the pressure lid, secure the pressure valve, and select Pressure mode on High for 20 minutes. Press Start/Stop.

When ready, do a natural pressure release for 5 minutes and open the lid. Remove the chicken onto a cutting board and shred using two forks.

Return the shredded chicken to the pot, close the crisping lid and Select Air Crisp mode. Adjust the time to 4 minutes at 385 degrees F.

When ready, transfer the chicken to a serving bowl, pour the sauce over, and garnish with the scallions.

Serve with a side of sauteéd mushrooms.

Wine Braised Chicken with Mushrooms and Brussel Sprouts

Servings: 4 | Ready in about: 40 min

INGREDIENTS

4 chicken thighs, bone-in skin-on
1 tsp salt or to taste, divided
1 tbsp olive oil
½ small onion, sliced
½ cup dry white wine
⅓ cup chicken stock

1 cup frozen halved Brussel sprouts, thawed
1 bay leaf
¼ tsp dried rosemary
Freshly ground black pepper
1 cup sautéed Mushrooms
¼ cup heavy cream

DIRECTIONS

Season the chicken on both sides with half of the salt. On your pot, Choose Sear/Sauté and adjust to Medium-High. Press Start to preheat the inner pot.

Heat olive oil and add the chicken thighs. Fry for 4 to 5 minutes or until browned. Turn and lightly sear the other side, about 1 minute. Use tongs to remove the chicken into a plate and spoon out any thick coating of oil in the pot.

Sauté the onion in the pot and season with the remaining salt. Cook for about 2 minutes to soften and just beginning to brown for 2 minutes. Stir in the white wine and bring to a boil for 2 to 3 minutes or until reduced by about half.

Mix in the chicken stock, brussel sprouts, bay leaf, rosemary, and several grinds of black pepper. Arrange the chicken thighs on top with skin-side up.

Seal the pressure lid, choose Pressure; adjust the pressure to High and the cook time to 5 minutes. Press Start to begin cooking.

When the timer is over, perform a quick pressure release and carefully open the lid. Remove the bay leaf.

Remove the chicken onto the reversible rack, and stir the mushrooms into the sauce. Carefully set the rack in the upper position of the pot.

Close the crisping lid and Choose Bake/Roast; adjust the temperature to 375°F and the cook time to 12 minutes. Press Start to commence browning.

When ready, open the lid and transfer the chicken to a platter. Stir the heavy cream into the sauce and adjust the taste with salt and pepper.

Spoon the sauce and vegetables around the chicken and serve.

Mexican Green Chili Chicken

Servings: 4 | Ready in about: 40 min

INGREDIENTS

1 tbsp olive oil
12 ounces, baby plum tomatoes, halved
¾ cup chicken stock
½ tsp salt
½ tsp ground cumin
1 tsp Mexican seasoning mix
1½ pounds boneless skinless chicken breasts
2 jalapeño peppers, seeded and chopped

2 large serrano pepper seeded and cut into chunks
2 large garlic cloves, minced
1 small onion, sliced
¼ cup minced fresh cilantro
Cooking spray
Tortilla chips
½ cup shredded Cheddar Cheese
½ lime, juiced

DIRECTIONS

Choose Sear/Sauté on your Foodi and adjust to High. Press Start to preheat the inner pot.

Heat the olive oil add the plum tomatoesl; cook without turning, for 3 to 4 minutes.

Add the chicken stock while scraping the bottom of the pot to dissolve any browned bits. Stir in the cumin, Mexican seasoning, and salt. Add the chicken, jalapeños, serrano pepper, garlic, onion, and half the cilantro.

Seal the pressure lid, choose pressure; adjust the pressure to High and the cook time to 10 minutes. Press Start.

Meanwhile, grease the reversible rack with cooking spray and fix the rack in the upper position of the pot. Cut out a circle of aluminum foil to fit the rack and place on the rack.

Lay on a single layer of tortilla chips, sprinkle with half of the Cheddar cheese and repeat with another layer of chips and cheese. Set aside.

After cooking, perform a natural pressure release for 5 minutes. Take out the chicken from the pot and set aside. Then, with an immersion blender, purée the vegetables into the sauce.

Shred the chicken with two forks and return the pieces to the sauce. Add the remaining cilantro and the lime juice. Taste and adjust the seasoning and carefully transfer the rack of chips to the pot.

Close the crisping lid and Choose Air Crisp; adjust the temperature to 375°F and the time to 5 minutes; press Start. When done cooking, open the lid. Carefully take out the rack and pour the chips into a platter. Serve the chili in bowls with the chips on the side.

Lemon and Paprika Chicken Thighs

Servings: 4 | Ready in about: 26 min

INGREDIENTS:

4 chicken thighs
1 ½ tbsp olive oil
½ tsp garlic powder
Salt and black pepper to taste
½ tsp red pepper flakes
½ tsp smoked paprika
1 small onion, chopped

2 cloves garlic, sliced
½ cup chicken broth
1 tsp Italian Seasoning
1 lemon, zested and juiced
1 ½ tbsp heavy cream
Lemon slices to garnish
Chopped parsley to garnish

DIRECTIONS:

Preheat the Ninja Foodi by selecting Sear/Sauté mode on Medium. Warm the olive oil and add the chicken thighs; cook to brown on each side for about 3 minutes. Remove the browned chicken onto a plate.

Melt the butter in the pot, then, add garlic, onions, and lemon juice. Deglaze the bottom of the pot and cook for 1 minute. Add the Italian seasoning, chicken broth, lemon zest, and the chicken.

Close the pressure lid, secure the pressure valve, select Pressure on High for 10 minutes. Press Start/Stop.

When ready, do a quick pressure release. Open the lid. Stir in the heavy cream. Close the crisping lid and select Broil mode. Set the time to 5 minutes. Serve with the steamed kale and spinach mix. Garnish with the lemons slices and parsley.

BBQ Chicken & Kale Quesadillas

Servings: 4 | Ready in about: 40 min

INGREDIENTS

¼ cup butter, divided
1 (10-to 12-ounce) bag fresh baby kale
1 jalapeño pepper, minced
¼ cup minced onion
3 ounces cottage cheese, at room temperature
2 tsp Mexican seasoning mix

1 cup shredded cooked chicken
6 ounces shredded Cheddar cheese
Cooking spray
4 medium flour tortillas
⅓ cup grated Pecorino Romano cheese

DIRECTIONS

On your Foodi, choose Sear/Sauté and adjust to Medium. Press Start to preheat the inner pot.

Drop in 1 tablespoon of butter and melt until foaming. Add the kale and cook for 1 to 2 minutes or until wilted while stirring occasionally.

Mix in the jalapeño and onion, continue cooking for 3 to 4 minutes, stirring occasionally, until the vegetables have softened and most of the liquid from the kale has evaporated.

Mix in the cottage cheese to melt and add the Mexican seasoning and the chicken. Stir to combine. Spoon the filling into a large bowl and stir in the shredded cheddar cheese. Set aside.

Use a paper towel to wipe out the inner pot and return the pot to the base. Oil the reversible rack with cooking spray and fix in the upper position of the pot.

Close the crisping lid and Choose Air Crisp; adjust the temperature to 375°F and the time to 5 minutes. Press Start to preheat.

To assemble the quesadillas, place a tortilla on a clean flat surface. Brush the top with olive oil and sprinkle 1 teaspoon of Pecorino Romano cheese on top. Press the cheese down with the palm of your hand to stick to the tortilla.

Spread about a ⅓ cup of filling over half the tortilla, leaving a ¼-inch border. Fold the other half over the filling and press gently. Repeat the process with the remaining tortillas, filling, and Pecorino Romano cheese.

Carefully transfer two quesadillas to the prepared rack. Close the crisping lid and Choose Air Crisp; adjust the temperature to 375°F and the cook time to 6 minutes. Press Start.

After 3 minutes, or when they are browned on top, use a spatula to flip the quesadillas. Continue cooking until browned on both sides.

Once ready, carefully remove the rack from the pot and use the spatula to transfer the quesadillas to the bottom of the pot to keep warm while you work on the other quesadillas.

Return the empty rack to the upper position of the pot and place the two remaining uncooked quesadillas on the rack. Repeat the cooking process. Serve the quesadillas with guacamole.

Chicken Florentine

Servings: 4 | Ready in about: 30 min

INGREDIENTS:

4 chicken thighs, cut into 1-inch pieces
1 tbsp olive oil
1 ½ cups chicken broth
Salt to taste
1 cup chopped sun dried tomatoes with herbs

2 tbsp Italian Seasoning
2 cups baby spinach
¼ tsp red pepper flakes
6 oz softened cream cheese, cut into small cubes
1 cup shredded Pecorino cheese

DIRECTIONS:

Pour the chicken broth into the pressure cooker, and add the Italian seasoning, chicken, tomatoes, salt, and red pepper flakes. Stir them with a spoon. Close the lid, secure the pressure valve, and select Pressure mode on High for 12 minutes. Press Start/Stop.

Once the timer has ended, do a quick pressure release, and open the lid. Add and stir in the spinach, parmesan cheese, and cream cheese until the cheese melts and is fully incorporated. Close the crisping lid and cook on Broil mode for 5 minutes. Dish the chicken over a bed of zoodles or a side of steamed asparagus.

Chicken Caesar Salad with Salted Croutons

Servings: 4 | Ready in about: 45 min

INGREDIENTS

2 chicken breasts, skinless boneless
¾ tsp salt plus more for sprinkling the croutons
1 garlic clove, minced
1 tbsp unsalted butter
1½ tbsp olive oil
½ small Italian bread loaf, cubed

⅓ cup Caesar dressing, divided
1 romaine lettuce heart, torn into bite-size pieces
1 oz coarsely grated Parmigiano Reggiano cheese
Grated Parmigiano Reggiano cheese, for serving
Freshly ground black pepper

DIRECTIONS

Season the chicken with salt on both sides. Pour 1 cup of water into the inner pot. Put the reversible rack in the pot and place the chicken on the rack.

Seal the pressure lid, choose Pressure; adjust the pressure to Low and the cook time to 5 minutes. Press Start.

Once done cooking, perform a natural pressure release for 8 minutes, and then a quick pressure release to let out any remaining pressure. Carefully open the lid. Set aside.

In a heatproof bowl, combine garlic, butter, and olive oil. Put the bowl in the Crisping Basket and place the basket in the pot.

Close the crisping lid and Choose Air Crisp; adjust the temperature to 375°F and the cook time to 2 minutes. Press Start to preheat the pot and melt the butter.

When done preheating, take out the basket from the pot and the bowl from the basket.

Pour the bread cubes into the bowl and toss to be well-coated in the butter and oil. Transfer the bread to the Crisping Basket and the basket into the pot.

Close the crisping lid and Choose Air Crisp; adjust the temperature to 375°F and the cook time to 10 minutes; press Start.

After 5 minutes, open the lid and toss the bread. Close the lid and continue cooking until the croutons are golden brown. Remove the basket from the pot and lightly season the croutons with salt. Allow cooling.

Cut the chicken into bite-size chunks. In a small bowl, toss the chicken with 3 tablespoons of Caesar dressing and set aside. Place the lettuce on a salad bowl, pour the remaining dressing over nad toss to coat well. Mix with chesse and black pepper.

Share the salad into four bowls, top with chicken, then croutons, and sprinkle with extra cheese.

Chicken Shawarma Wrap

Servings: 4 | Ready in about: 35 min

INGREDIENTS

1 ½ pounds boneless skinless chicken breasts
1 tsp salt
2 tbsp olive oil, divided
2 tbsp yogurt
2 tbsp freshly squeezed lemon juice
3 garlic cloves, minced
1 tsp ground cumin

¼ tsp cinnamon powder
1 tsp smoked paprika
¼ tsp turmeric
¼ tsp freshly ground black pepper
¼ tsp cayenne pepper
4 flat breads, halved
Cooking spray

For the Sauce

½ cup yogurt
½ tsp salt
1 tsp olive oil

1 small garlic clove, minced
2 tbsp Italian herb mix
1 tbsp chopped fresh cilantro

To Assemble

2 large tomatoes, sliced

½ medium cucumber, sliced

DIRECTIONS

Season the chicken with salt on both sides, put in a plastic zipper bag, and set aside while you make the marinade.

In a bowl, evenly mix the olive oil, yogurt, lemon juice, garlic, cumin, cinnamon, paprika, turmeric, black pepper, and cayenne pepper. Pour the marinade over the chicken, zip up the bag, and massage the bag to coat the chicken well with the marinade. Refrigerate the chicken for 1 hour or more to marinate. Cover the flatbread with foil and place at the bottom of the pot. Grease the reversible rack with cooking spray and fix in the upper position of the pot.

Close the crisping lid and choose Air Crisp; adjust the temperature to 390°F and the time to 4 minutes. Press Start to preheat the pot.

Take the chicken out of the refrigerator and remove from the bag while holding each piece to allow excess liquid drip into the bag. Lay the chicken on the rack in a single layer.

Close the crisping lid and choose Air Crisp. Adjust the temperature to 390°F and the cook time to 16 minutes. Press Start to begin cooking.

After 8 minutes, open the lid and flip the chicken and close the lid. Cook to crisp and brown the other side for 8 minutes. When the breasts are ready, transfer to a cutting board, and cut into thin slices. Take out the bread from the pot and set aside.

Meanwhile, prepare the sauce: pour the yogurt into a small bowl; add the salt, olive oil, garlic, and Italian herb mix. Whisk the ingredients to combine and stir in the parsley.

Spread 1 to 2 tablespoons of yogurt sauce into half a side of flatbread. Spoon in some chicken and add the tomato and cucumber slices. Repeat the process for the remaining bread. Wrap the bread over the filling, repeat the assembling process for the remaining bread and serve.

Coq au Vin

Servings: 4 | Ready in about: 60 min

INGREDIENTS

4 chicken leg quarters, skin on
1½ tsp salt
1 tbsp olive oil
4 serrano ham slices, cut into thirds
¼ cup brown onion slices
1¼ cups dry red wine

⅓ cup chicken stock
1½ tsp tomato puree
½ tsp brown sugar
Black pepper to taste
½ cup sautéed mushrooms
¾ cup shallots, sliced

DIRECTIONS

Season the chicken on both sides with 1 teaspoon of salt and set aside on a wire rack. On the Foodi, choose Sear/ Sauté and adjust to Medium. Press Start to preheat the inner pot.

Heat the olive oil and place the ham in the pot in a single layer and cook for 3 to 4 minutes or until browned. Remove the ham to a plate and set aside.

Add the chicken quarters to the pot. Cook for 5 minutes or until the skin is golden brown. Turn the chicken over and cook further for 2 minutes; remove to a plate.

Carefully pour out almost all the fat leaving about a tablespoon to cover the bottom of the pot. Then, stir in the sliced onion and cook until the onion begins to brown.

Add ½ cup of red wine, stir, and scrape the bottom of the pan to let off any browned bits. Then, boil the mixture until the wine reduces by about 1/3, about 2 minutes.

Pour the remaining red wine, chicken stock, tomato puree, brown sugar, and a few grinds of black pepper into the pot. Boil the sauce for 1 minute, stirring to make sure the tomato paste is properly mixed. Add the chicken pieces with skin- side up, to the pot.

Put the pressure lid in place and lock to seal. Choose Pressure; adjust the pressure to High and the cook time to 12 minutes. Press Start to continue cooking.

After cooking, perform a natural pressure release for 10 minutes. Remove the chicken from the pot. Pour the sauce into a bowl and allow sitting until the fat rises to the top and starts firming up. Use a spoon to fetch off the fat on top of the sauce.

Pour the sauce back into the pot and stir in the mushrooms and pearl onions. Place the chicken on the sauce with skin side up. Close the crisping lid and select Broil. Adjust the cook time to 7 minutes; press Start.

When done cooking, open the lid and transfer the chicken to a serving platter. Spoon the sauce with mushrooms and pearl onions all around the chicken and crumble the reserved ham on top.

Cajun Roasted Chicken with Potato Mash

Servings: 4 | Ready in about: 70 min

INGREDIENTS

2 bone-in chicken breasts
2½ tsp salt
4 tsp Cajun seasoning
¾ cup chicken stock

3 medium Yukon Gold potatoes, scrubbed
3 tbsp melted butter
2 tbsp warm heavy cream

DIRECTIONS

Pat the chicken dry with a paper towel and carefully slide your hands underneath the skin to slightly separate the meat from the skin. Then in a small bowl, combine the salt and Cajun seasoning, and rub half of the mixture under the skin and cavity of the chicken.

Pour the chicken stock into the inner pot of the Foodi. Fix the reversible rack in a lower position of the pot and lay the chicken, on the side in the center of the rack. Also, arrange the potatoes around the chicken.

Seal the pressure lid, choose pressure; adjust the pressure to High and the cook time to 13 minutes. Press Start to begin cooking the chicken. Mix the remaining spice mixture with 2 tablespoons of the melted butter, and set aside.

When done pressure cooking, perform a natural pressure release for 10 minutes. Remove the potatoes and chicken onto a cutting board. Pour the cooking juices into a bowl and return the rack with chicken only to the pot. Baste the outer side of the chicken with half of the spice- butter mixture.

Close the crisping lid and choose Air Crisp; adjust the temperature to 360°F and the cook time to 16 minutes. Press Start. After 8 minutes, open the lid and flip the chicken over. Baste this side with the remaining butter mixture and close the lid to continue cooking.

With a potato masher, smoothly puree the potatoes, and add the remaining salt, melted butter, heavy cream, and 2 tablespoons of the reserved cooking juice; stir to combine. Taste and adjust the seasoning with salt and pepper and cover the bowl with aluminum foil to keep warm.

After cooking, transfer the chicken to a cutting board, leaving the rack in the pot.

Pour the remaining cooking sauce into the pot, choose Sear/Sauté and adjust to Medium-High. Place the bowl of potatoes on the rack to keep warm as the sauce reduces. Press Start and boil the sauce for 2 to 3 minutes or until reduced by about half.

Meanwhile, slice the chicken and lay the pieces on a platter. Remove the mashed potato from the pot and remove the rack. Spoon the sauce over the chicken slices and serve with the creamy potatoes.

Chicken Chili with Cannellini Beans

Servings: 4 | Ready in about: 40 min

INGREDIENTS:

3 chicken breasts, cubed
3 cups chicken broth
1 tbsp butter
1 white onion, chopped
Salt and black pepper

2 (14.5 ounces) cans Cannellini beans, drained
1 tsp cumin powder
1 tsp dried oregano
½ cup heavy whipping cream
1 cup sour cream

DIRECTIONS:

Select Sear/Sauté mode and set to Medium. Melt the butter, and add onion and chicken.

Stir and let cook the chicken for 6 minutes. Stir in the cannellini beans, cumin powder, oregano, salt, and pepper.

Pour in the broth, stir, close the pressure lid, and secure the pressure valve.Select Pressure mode on High for 10 minutes. Press Start/Stop.

Once the timer has ended, let the pot sit uncovered for 10 minutes, then do a quick pressure release. Stir in the whipping and sour cream.

Close the crisping lid and select Broil mode. Cook for 2 minutes.

Serve warm with a mix of steamed bell peppers and broccoli.

Traditional Chicken Cordon Bleu

Servings: 4 | Ready in about: 35 min

INGREDIENTS

2 large boneless skinless chicken breasts
¾ tsp salt
12 ounces broccoli, cut into florets
3 tbsp melted butter
Cooking spray

4 tsp Dijon mustard
4 thin ham slices
4 thin slices Emmental cheese
⅔ cup panko bread crumbs
¼ cup grated Pecorino Romano cheese

DIRECTIONS

Put the chicken breasts on a cutting board and slice through the breasts to form two thinner pieces from each breast to make 4 pieces in total. Season the chicken on both sides with ½ teaspoon of salt. Pour a cup of water into the inner pot. Put the reversible rack in the lower position of the pot and lay the broccoli florets on the rack. After, put the chicken on the broccoli.

Seal the pressure lid, choose Pressure; adjust the pressure to High and the cook time to 1 minute. Press Start to begin cooking the broccoli and chicken.

After cooking, perform a quick pressure release and carefully open the pressure lid. Take out the rack and set aside. Pour the water out of the pot and put the pot back on the base.

Place the chicken on the cutting board and the broccoli into the pot. Put 1 tablespoon of melted butter on the broccoli florets and sprinkle with the remaining salt. Stir to coat the broccoli with the butter.

Grease the reversible rack with cooking spray and fix in the upper position of the pot. Close the crisping lid and Choose Air Crisp; adjust the temperature to 360°F and the time to 4 minutes. Press Start to preheat.

Smear 1 teaspoon of mustard on each chicken piece. Lay each ham slice on each chicken and each Emmental cheese slice on each ham.

In a small bowl, combine the breadcrumbs, remaining butter, and the Pecorino Romano cheese. Sprinkle the breadcrumb mixture equally over the chicken.

Open the crisping lid and carefully transfer the chicken pieces to the rack. Close the crisping lid and choose Air Crisp; adjust the temperature to 360°F and the cook time to 10 minutes; press Start.

When done cooking, the crumbs should be crisp and have obtained a deep golden brown. Transfer the chicken pieces to a platter and serve with the broccoli.

Pesto Chicken with Roasted Red Pepper Sauce

Servings: 4 | Ready in about: 23 min

INGREDIENTS:

4 chicken breasts, skinless and boneless
½ cup heavy cream
½ cup chicken broth
⅓ tsp minced garlic
Salt and black pepper to taste

⅓ tsp Italian Seasoning
¼ cup roasted red peppers, chopped
1 tbsp basil pesto
1 tbsp cornstarch

DIRECTIONS:

In the inner pot of the Ninja Foodi, add the chicken at the bottom. Pour the chicken broth and add Italian seasoning, garlic, salt, and pepper.

Close the pressure lid, secure the pressure valve, and select Pressure mode on High for 15 minutes. Press Start/Stop.

Once the timer has ended, do a natural pressure release for 5 minutes and open the lid.

Use a spoon to remove the chicken onto a plate. Scoop out any fat or unwanted chunks from the sauce.

In a small bowl, add the cream, cornstarch, red peppers, and pesto. Mix them with a spoon. Pour the creamy mixture into the pot and close the crisping lid.

Select Broil mode and cook for 4 minutes. Serve the chicken with sauce over on a bed of cooked quinoa.

Mexican Chicken & Wild Rice Bowls

Servings: 4 | Ready in about: 30 min

INGREDIENTS:

4 chicken breasts
2 cups chicken broth
2 ¼ packets Taco Seasoning
1 cup wild rice, rinsed
1 green bell pepper, seeded and diced

1 red bell pepper, seeded and diced
1 cup salsa
Salt and black pepper to taste
1 cup sour cream

To Serve:

Grated cheese, of your choice
Chopped cilantro

Avocado slices

DIRECTIONS:

Pour the chicken broth into the inner pot, add the chicken. Pour the taco seasoning over. Add the salsa and stir lightly with a spoon.

Close the pressure lid, secure the pressure valve, and select Pressure on High for 15 minutes. Press Start/Stop.

Once the timer has ended, do a quick pressure release, and open the lid.

Add the wild rice and peppers, and use a spoon to push them into the sauce. Close the pressure lid, secure the pressure valve, and select Pressure mode on High for 8 minutes. Press Start/Stop.

Once the timer has ended, do a quick pressure release, and open the lid. Gently stir the mixture, adjust the taste with salt and pepper.

Stir in sour cream, close the crisping lid and select Broil mode; cook for 2 minutes. Spoon the chicken dish into serving bowls. Top it with avocado slices, sprinkle with chopped cilantro and some cheese. Serve.

White Wine Chicken

Servings: 4 | Ready in about: 9 hrs

INGREDIENTS:

3 chicken legs, cut into drumsticks and thighs
2 bacon slices, chopped
1 ½ cups dry white wine
Salt and black pepper to taste+
½ bunch thyme, divided
8 oz Shiitake mushrooms, stems removed and cut into
4 pieces

3 Shallots, peeled
3 tbsp butter, divided
3 skinny carrots, cut into 4 crosswise pieces each
2 cloves garlic, crushed
1 tbsp flour
3 tbsp chopped parsley for garnishing

DIRECTIONS:

Put the chicken on a clean flat surface and season on both sides with salt and pepper. In a plastic zipper bag, pour the wine.

Add half of the thyme and chicken. Zip the bag and shake to coat the chicken well with the wine. Place it in the refrigerator for 6 to 8 hours.

After 8 hours, turn on the Ninja Foodi on High and fry the bacon on Sear/Sauté mode for about 8 minutes. Remove the bacon without the fat onto a plate using a slotted spoon. Set aside.

Pour the mushroom into the pot, season with salt and cook for 5 minutes. Then, remove at the side of the bacon.

Remove the chicken from the refrigerator onto a clean flat surface. Take out and discard the thyme but reserve the marinade. Pat the chicken dry with paper towels.

Melt half of the butter in the pot on Sauté. Place the chicken in the butter in batches and fry until dark golden brown on each side, about 12 minutes.

Add bacon, mushrooms, shallots, garlic, carrots, and a bit of salt. Cook the ingredients for 4 minutes and top with the wine and remaining thyme.

Close the pressure lid, secure the pressure valve, and select Pressure mode on High for 15 minutes. Press Start/ Stop.

Meanwhile, add the flour and the remaining butter in a bowl, and smash them together with a fork. Set aside. Once the timer has ended, do a natural pressure release for 10 minutes.

Discard the thyme. Add the flour mixture to the sauce in the pot, stir until well incorporated. Adjust the seasoning with salt and black pepper.

Close the crisping lid and select Broil mode. Cook for 4 minutes. Press Start. Garnish with parsley and serve with steamed asparagus.

Chicken with Tomato Salsa

Servings: 4 | Ready in about: 30 min

INGREDIENTS:

4 chicken thighs, skinless but with bone
4 tbsp olive oil
1 cup crushed tomatoes
1 large red bell pepper, seeded and diced
1 large green bell pepper, seeded and diced
1 Red onion, diced

Salt and black pepper to taste
1 tbsp chopped basil
½ cup chicken broth
1 bay leaf
½ tsp dried oregano

DIRECTIONS:

Place the chicken on a clean flat surface and season with salt and pepper. Select Sear/Sauté mode on High, and heat the oil.

Once heated add the chicken to brown on both sides for 6 minutes. Then, add the onions and peppers. Cook for 5 minutes until nice and soft.

Add bay leaf, salt, broth, pepper, and oregano. Stir using a spoon. Close the pressure lid, secure the pressure valve, and select Pressure mode on High for 15 minutes. Press Start/Stop.

Once the timer has ended, do a natural pressure release for 5 minutes.

Discard the bay leaf. Stir in tomatoes, close the crisping lid, select Broil mode and cook for 25 minutes.

Dish the chicken with the sauce into a serving bowl and garnish with the chopped basil. Serve over a bed of steamed squash spaghetti.

Cheesy Buffalo Chicken

Servings: 4 | Ready in about: 37 min

INGREDIENTS:

4 chicken breasts, boneless and skinless
½ cup Hot sauce
2 large white onion, finely chopped
2 cups finely chopped celery
1 tbsp olive oil
1 tsp dried thyme

3 cups chicken broth
1 tsp garlic powder
½ cup crumbled Blue cheese + extra for serving
4 oz cream cheese, cubed in small pieces
Salt and pepper, to taste

DIRECTIONS:

Put the chicken on a clean flat surface and season with pepper and salt. Set aside. Select Sear/Sauté mode on High.

Heat in olive oil, add onion and celery. Sauté them, constant stirring, until they are nice and soft, for about 5 minutes.

Then, add garlic powder and thyme. Stir and cook for about a minute, and add the chicken, hot sauce, and chicken broth. Season with salt and pepper. Close the pressure lid, secure the pressure valve, and select Pressure mode on High for 15 minutes. Press Start/Stop.

Meanwhile, put the blue cheese and cream cheese in a bowl, and use a fork to smash them together. Set the resulting mixture aside.

Once the timer has ended, do a natural pressure release for 5 minutes. Take out the chicken on to a flat surface with a slotted spoon and use two forks to shred them. Return shredded chicken to the pot, close the crisping lid, select Broil mode and cook for 5 minutes.

Add the cheese to the pot and stir until is slightly incorporated into the sauce.

Dish the buffalo chicken soup into bowls. Sprinkle the remaining cheese over the soup and serve with sliced baguette.

Chicken Noodle Soup with Crispy Bacon

Servings: 8 | Ready in about: 33 min

INGREDIENTS:

5 oz dry egg noodles
4 chicken breasts, skinless and boneless
1 large white onion, chopped
8 bacon slices, chopped
4 cloves garlic, minced
Salt and black pepper to taste

2 medium carrots, sliced
2 cups sliced celery
½ cup chopped parsley
1 ½ tsp dried thyme
8 cups chicken broth

DIRECTIONS:

Turn on the Ninja Foodi, and select Sear/Sauté mode on High. Press Start. Add the chopped bacon and fry for 5 minutes until nicely brown and crispy.

Remove to a paper towel to soak up excess oil and set aside.

Add the onion and garlic to the pot and cook for 3 minutes until tender. Add the chicken breasts, noodles, carrots, celery, chicken broth, thyme, salt, and pepper. Close the pressure lid, secure the valve to seal, and select Pressure mode on High pressure. Adjust the time to 5 minutes and press Start/Stop.

Once the timer has ended, do a quick pressure release, and open the lid. Use a wooden spoon to remove the chicken onto a plate. Shred the chicken with two forks and add it back to the soup.

Stir in the bacon. Adjust the seasoning as desired. Close the crisping lid and cook on Broil mode for 5 minutes. Adjust the seasoning. Ladle the soup into serving bowls and serve with a side of bread.

Chicken & Green Bean Coconut Curry

Servings: 8 | Ready in about: 32 min

INGREDIENTS:

4 chicken breasts
4 tbsp red curry paste
½ cup chicken broth
2 cups coconut milk
4 tbsp sugar

Salt and black pepper to taste
2 red bell pepper, seeded and cut in 2-inch sliced
2 yellow bell pepper, seeded and cut in 2-inch slices
2 cup green beans, cut in half
2 tbsp lime juice

DIRECTIONS:

Add the chicken, red curry paste, salt, pepper, coconut milk, broth, and sugar, in the Ninja Foodi inner pot.

Close the pressure lid, secure the pressure valve, and select Pressure mode on High for 15 minutes. Press Start/Stop.

Once the timer has ended, do a quick pressure release, and open the lid.

Remove the chicken onto a cutting board and close the crisping lid. Select Broil mode. Add the bell peppers, green beans, and lime juice.

Stir the sauce with a spoon and cook for 4 minutes. Slice the chicken with a knife, pour the sauce and vegetables over and serve warm.

Chicken & Veggie Tacos with Guacamole

Servings: 4 | Ready in about: 30 min

INGREDIENTS:

2 lb chicken breasts, skinless and cut in 1-inch slices
½ cup chicken broth
1 yellow onion, sliced
1 green bell pepper, seeded and sliced
1 yellow bell pepper, seeded and sliced
1 red bell pepper, seeded and sliced

2 tbsp cumin powder
2 tbsp chili powder
Salt to taste
½ Lime
Cooking spray
Fresh cilantro, to garnish

Assembling:
Tacos, Guacamole, sour cream, Salsa, cheese

DIRECTIONS:

Grease the inner pot with cooking spray and line the bottom with the peppers and onion. Lay the chicken on the bed of peppers.

Sprinkle with salt, chili powder, and cumin powder. Squeeze some lime juice and pour in chicken broth. Close the lid, secure the pressure valve, and select Pressure mode on High pressure for 15 minutes. Press Start/Stop.

Once the timer has ended, do a quick pressure release, and open the lid. Close the crisping lid and cook for 5 minutes on Bake/Roast mode at 370 F. Dish the chicken with the vegetables and juice onto a large serving platter.

Add sour cream, cheese, guacamole, salsa, and tacos in one layer on the side of the chicken.

Chicken Meatballs Primavera

Servings: 4 | Ready in about: 30 min

INGREDIENTS:

1 lb ground chicken
1 egg, cracked into a bowl
6 tsp flour
Salt and black pepper to taste
2 tbsp chopped basil + extra to garnish
1 tbsp olive oil + ½ tbsp olive oil

1 ½ tsp Italian Seasoning
1 red bell pepper, seeded and sliced
2 cups chopped green beans
½ lb chopped asparagus
1 cup chopped tomatoes
1 cup chicken broth

DIRECTIONS:

In a mixing bowl, add the chicken, egg, flour, salt, pepper, 2 tablespoons of basil, 1 tablespoon of olive oil, and Italian seasoning. Mix them well with hands and make 16 large balls out of the mixture. Set the meatballs aside.

Select Sear/Sauté mode. Heat half teaspoon of olive oil, and add peppers, green beans, and asparagus. Cook for 3 minutes, stirring frequently.

After 3 minutes, use a spoon the veggies onto a plate and set aside.

Pour the remaining oil in the pot to heat and then fry the meatballs in it in batches. Fry them for 2 minutes on each side to brown them lightly.

After, put all the meatballs back into the pot as well as the vegetables. Also, pour the chicken broth over it.

Close the lid, secure the pressure valve, and select Pressure mode on High pressure for 10 minutes. Press Start/ Stop. Do a quick pressure release. Close the crisping lid and select Air Crisp. Cook for 5 minutes at 400 degrees F, until nice and crispy.

Dish the meatballs with sauce into a serving bowl and garnish it with basil. Serve with over cooked pasta.

Mediterranean Stuffed Chicken Breasts

Servings: 4 | Ready in about: 30 min

INGREDIENTS:

4 chicken breasts, skinless
Salt and black pepper to taste
1 cup baby spinach, frozen
½ cup crumbled Feta cheese
½ tsp dried oregano

½ tsp garlic powder
2 tbsp olive oil
2 tsp dried parsley
1 cup water

DIRECTIONS:

Wrap the chicken in plastic and put on a cutting board. Use a rolling pin to pound flat to a quarter inch thickness. Remove the plastic wrap.

In a bowl, mix spinach, salt, and feta cheese and scoop the mixture onto the chicken breasts. Wrap the chicken to secure the spinach filling in it.

Use toothpicks to secure the wrap firmly from opening. Gently season the chicken pieces with oregano, parsley, garlic powder, and pepper.

Select Sear/Sauté mode on Foodi Ninja. Heat the oil, add the chicken, and sear to golden brown on each side. Work in 2 batches. Remove the chicken onto a plate and set aside.

Pour the water into the pot and use a spoon to scrape the bottom of the pot to let loose any chicken pieces or seasoning that is stuck to the bottom of the pot. Fit the reversiblerack into the pot with care as the pot will still be hot.

Transfer the chicken onto the rack. Seal the lid and select Pressure mode on High pressure for 10 minutes. Press Start/Stop.

Once the timer has ended, do a quick pressure release. Close the crisping lid and cook on Bake/Roast mode for 5 minutes at 370 F. Plate the chicken and serve with a side of sautéed asparagus, and some slices of tomatoes.

Sticky Orange Chicken

Servings: 4 | Ready in about: 30 min

INGREDIENTS

2 chicken breasts, cubed
½ cup honey
½ cup orange juice
⅓ cup soy sauce
⅓ cup chicken stock
⅓ cup hoisin sauce

1 garlic clove, minced
2 tsp cornstarch
2 tsp water
1 cup diced orange
3 cups hot cooked quinoa

DIRECTIONS

Arrange the chicken to the bottom of the Foodi's pot.

In a bowl, mix honey, soy sauce, garlic, hoisin sauce, chicken stock, and orange juice, until the honey is dissolved; pour the mixture over the chicken. Seal the pressure lid, choose Pressure, set to High, and set the timer to 7 minutes. Press Start. When ready, release the pressure quickly. Take the chicken from the pot and set to a bowl. Press Sear/Sauté.

In a small bowl, mix water with cornstarch; pour into the liquid within the pot and cook for 3 minutes until thick. Stir diced orange and chicken into the sauce until well coated. Serve with quinoa.

Spinach & Mushroom Chicken Stew

Servings: 4 | Ready in about: 56 min

INGREDIENTS:

4 chicken breasts, diced
1 ¼ lb white Button mushrooms, halved
3 tbsp olive oil
1 large onion, sliced
5 cloves garlic, minced
Salt and black pepper to taste
1 ¼ tsp cornstarch

½ cup spinach, chopped
1 bay leaf
1 ½ cups chicken stock
1 tsp Dijon mustard
1 ½ cup sour cream
3 tbsp chopped parsley

DIRECTIONS:

Select Sear/Sauté mode and set to medium High to preheat.

Once the pot is ready, heat the olive oil then include the onion and sauté for 3 minutes until soft. Add the mushrooms, chicken, garlic, bay leaf, salt, pepper, Dijon mustard, and chicken broth. Stir well.

Close the lid, secure the pressure valve, and press Pressure mode on High pressure for 15 minutes. Press Start/Stop.

Once the timer has ended, do a natural pressure release for 5 minutes and carefully open the lid. Stir the stew, remove the bay leaf, and scoop some of the liquid into a bowl. Add the cornstarch to the liquid and mix them until completely lump free.

Pour the liquid into the sauce, stir it, and let the sauce thicken to your desired consistency. Top it with the sour cream, close the crisping lid and select Broil mode. Cook for 2 minutes.

Garnish with the chopped parsley and serve with steamed green peas.

BBQ Chicken Drumettes

Servings: 4 | Ready in about: 30 min

INGREDIENTS:

2 lb chicken drumettes, bone in and skin in
½ cup chicken broth
½ tsp dry mustard
½ tsp sweet paprika
½ tbsp. cumin powder
½ tsp onion powder

¼ tsp Cayenne powder
Salt and pepper, to taste
1 stick butter, sliced in 5 pieces
BBQ sauce to taste
Cooking spray

DIRECTIONS:

Pour the chicken broth into the inner pot of Ninja Foodi P and insert the reversiblerack. In a zipper bag, pour in dry mustard, cumin powder, onion powder, cayenne powder, salt, and pepper.

Add the chicken, close the bag and shake to coat the chicken well with the spices. You can toss the chicken in the spices in batches too.

Then, remove the chicken from the bag and place on the rack. Spread the butter slices on the drumsticks. Close the lid, secure the pressure valve, and select Pressure mode on High pressure for 10 minutes. Press Start/Stop.

Once the timer has ended, do a quick pressure release, and open the lid.

Remove the chicken onto a clean flat surface like a cutting board and brush them with the barbecue sauce using the brush. Return to the rack and close the crisping lid. Cook for 10 minutes at 400 F on Air Crisp mode.

Sage Chicken Thighs

Servings: 4 | Ready in about: 35 min

INGREDIENTS:

2 lb chicken thighs, bone in and skin on
2 tbsp olive oil
Salt and pepper, to taste
1 ½ cups diced tomatoes
¾ cup yellow onion

2 tsp minced garlic
½ cup balsamic vinegar
3 tsp chopped fresh sage
1 cup chicken broth
2 tbsp chopped parsley

DIRECTIONS:

With paper towels, pat dry the chicken and season with salt and pepper.

Select Sear/Sauté mode. Warm the olive and add the chicken with skin side down. Cook to golden brown on each side, for about 9 minutes. Remove onto a clean plate.

Then, add onions and tomatoes to the pot and sauté for 3 minutes, stirring occasionally with a spoon. Add in garlic and cook for 30 seconds, until fragrant.

Pour the chicken broth, and add some salt, sage, and balsamic vinegar. Stir them using a spoon. Add the chicken back to the pot.

Close the lid, secure the pressure valve, and select Pressure mode on High pressure for 15 minutes. Press Start/Stop to start cooking. When ready, do a quick pressure release.

Close the crisping lid and cook on Air Crisp mode for 5 minutes at 400 F.

Garnish with parsley and serve with roasted tomatoes, carrots, and potatoes.

Whole Chicken with Lemon & Onion Stuffing

Servings: 6 | Ready in about: 55 min

INGREDIENTS:

4 lb whole chicken
1 tbsp herbes de Provence Seasoning
1 tbsp olive oil
Salt and black pepper to season
2 cloves garlic, peeled

1 tsp garlic powder
1 yellow onion, peeled and quartered
1 lemon, quartered
1 ¼ cups chicken broth

DIRECTIONS:

Put the chicken on a clean flat surface and pat dry using paper towels.

Sprinkle the top and cavity of the chicken with salt, black pepper, Herbes de Provence, and garlic powder.

Stuff the onion, lemon quarters, and garlic cloves into the cavity. In the Ninja Foodi, fit the reversiblerack. Pour the broth in and place the chicken on the rack. Seal the lid, and select Pressure mode on High for 25 minutes.

Press Start/Stop to start cooking.

Once ready, do a natural pressure release for about 10 minutes, then a quick pressure release to let the remaining steam out, and press Stop.

Close the crisping lid and broil the chicken for 5 minutes on Broil mode, to ensure that it attains a golden brown color on each side.

Dish the chicken on a bed of steamed mixed veggies. Right here, the choice is yours to whip up some good veggies together as your appetite tells you.

Za'atar Chicken with Lemony Couscous

Servings: 4 | Ready in about: 40 min

INGREDIENTS

4 chicken thighs
2 tbsp za'atar mix
1 tbsp ground sumac
sea salt and freshly ground black pepper to taste
2 tbsp butter
2 ½ cups chicken stock, divided

1 onion, thinly sliced
1 garlic clove, minced
1½ cups couscous
Juice from 1 lemon
Fresh parsley, chopped

DIRECTIONS

Season the chicken with salt, sumac, za'atar, and pepper.

Melt butter on Sear/Sautéand sear the chicken in batches for 5 minutes per batch until lightly browned; set aside.

In the Foodi, add ¼ cup chicken stock to deglaze the pan, scrape the bottom to get rid of any browned bits of food.

Add garlic and onion to the stock; cook for 3 minutes until soft.

Add the remaining chicken stock into the pan; add lemon juice and couscous. Add in chicken.

Seal the pressure lid, choose Pressure, set to High, and set the timer to 5 minutes. Press Start. Naturally release the pressure for 5 minutes.

Transfer the couscous and chicken to a serving plate; add parsley to garnish.

Lettuce Carnitas Wraps

Servings: 6 | Ready in about: 50 min

INGREDIENTS

2 tbsp canola oil
2 pounds chicken thighs, boneless, skinless
1 cup pineapple juice
⅓ cup water
¼ cup soy sauce
2 tbsp maple syrup

1 tbsp rice vinegar
1 tsp chili-garlic sauce
3 tbsp cornstarch
salt and freshly ground black pepper to taste
12 large lettuce leaves
2 cups canned pinto beans, rinsed and drained

DIRECTIONS

Warm oil on Sear/Sauté. In batches, sear chicken in the oil for 5 minutes until browned. Set aside in a bowl.

Into your pot, mix chili-garlic sauce, pineapple juice, soy sauce, vinegar, maple syrup, and water; stir in chicken to coat.

Seal the pressure lid, choose Pressure, set to High, and set the timer to 7 minutes. Press Start. Release pressure naturally for 10 minutes. Shred the chicken with two forks. Take ¼ cup liquid from the pot to a bowl; stir in cornstarch to dissolve.

Mix the cornstarch mixture with the mixture in the pot and return the chicken.

Select Sear/Sauté and cook for 5 minutes until the sauce thickens; add pepper and salt for seasoning.

Transfer beans into lettuce leaves; apply a topping of chicken carnitas and serve.

Lemon Turkey Risotto

Servings: 4 | Ready in about: 40 min

INGREDIENTS

2 boneless turkey breasts, cut into strips
2 lemons, zested and juiced
1 tbsp dried oregano
2 garlic cloves, minced
½ tsp sea salt
1½ tbsp olive oil

1 onion, diced
2 cups chicken broth
1 cup Arborio rice, rinsed
salt and freshly ground black pepper to taste
¼ cup chopped fresh parsley, or to taste
8 lemon slices

DIRECTIONS

In a ziplock back, mix turkey, oregano, sea salt, garlic, juice and zest of two lemons. Marinate for 10 minutes.

Warm oil on Sear/Sauté. Add onion and cook for 3 minutes until fragrant; add rice and chicken broth and season with pepper and salt.

Empty the ziplock having the chicken and marinade into the pot.

Seal the pressure lid, choose Pressure, set to High, and set the timer to 12 minutes. Press Start. When ready, release the pressure quickly.

Divide the rice and turkey between 4 serving bowls; garnish with lemon slices and parsley.

Thyme Chicken with Veggies

Servings: 4 | Ready in about: 40 min

INGREDIENTS

4 skin-on, bone-in chicken legs
2 tbsp olive oil
salt and freshly ground black pepper to taste
4 cloves garlic, minced
1 tsp fresh chopped thyme
½ cup dry white wine
1¼ cups chicken stock

1 cup carrots, thinly sliced
1 cup parsnip, thinly sliced
3 tomatoes, thinly sliced
1 tbsp honey
4 slices lemon
Fresh thyme, chopped for garnish

DIRECTIONS

Season the chicken with pepper and salt. Warm oil on Sear/Sauté.

Arrange chicken legs into the hot oil; cook for 3 to 5 minutes each side until browned. Place in a bowl and set aside. Cook thyme and garlic in the chicken fat for 1 minute until soft and lightly golden.

Add wine into the pot to deglaze, scrape the pot's bottom to get rid of any brown bits of food. Simmer the wine for 2 to 3 minutes until slightly reduced in volume.

Add stock, carrots, parsnips, tomatoes, pepper and salt into the pot.

Lay reversible rack onto veggies. Into the Foodi's steamer basket, arrange chicken legs. Set the steamer basket onto the reversible rack.

Drizzle the chicken with honey then top with lemon slices.

Seal the pressure lid, choose Pressure, set to High, and set the timer to 12 minutes. Press Start. Release pressure naturally for 10 minutes. Place the chicken onto a bowl. Drain the veggies and place them around the chicken. Garnish with fresh thyme leaves before serving.

Juicy Orange Chicken

Servings: 6 | Ready in about: 50 min

INGREDIENTS

2 tbsp olive oil
6 chicken breasts, boneless, skinless, cubed
⅓ cup chicken stock
¼ cup soy sauce
2 tbsp brown sugar
1 tbsp lemon juice

1 tbsp garlic powder
1 tsp chili sauce
1 cup orange juice
salt and black pepper to taste
2 cups cooked gnocchi

DIRECTIONS

Warm oil on Sear/Sauté. In batches, sear chicken in the oil for 5 minutes until browned. Set aside in a bowl.

In your pot, mix orange juice, water, sugar, chili sauce, garlic powder, vinegar, and soy sauce; stir in chicken to coat. Seal the pressure lid, choose Pressure, set to High, and set the timer to 7 minutes; press Start. When ready, release the pressure quickly.

Take ¼ cup liquid from the pot to a bowl; stir in cornstarch to dissolve; mix into sauce in the pot until the color is consistent. Press Sear/Sauté. Cook sauce for 5 minutes until thickened; season with pepper and salt. Serve the chicken with gnocchi.

Beef Congee (Chinese Rice Porridge)

Servings: 6 | Ready in about: 1 hr

INGREDIENTS

1 cup jasmine rice
2 cloves garlic, minced
1 (1 inch) piece fresh ginger, minced
6 cups beef stock
1 cup kale, roughly chopped

1 cups water
2 pounds ground beef
salt and ground black pepper to taste
Fresh cilantro, chopped

DIRECTIONS

Run cold water and rinse rice. Add garlic, rice, and ginger into the Foodi. Pour water and stock into the pot and spread the beef on top of rice.

Seal the pressure lid, choose Pressure, set to High, and set the timer to 30 minutes. Press Start. Once ready, release pressure naturally for 10 minutes. Stir in kale to obtain the desired consistency. Add pepper and salt for seasoning. Divide into serving plates and top with cilantro.

Creamy Chicken and Quinoa Soup

Servings: 6 | Ready in about: 30 min

INGREDIENTS

2 tbsp butter
1 cup red onion, chopped
1 cup carrots, chopped
1 cup celery, chopped
2 large boneless, skinless chicken breasts, cubed
4 cups chicken broth

6 ounces quinoa, rinsed
1 tbsp fresh parsley, chopped
Salt and freshly ground black pepper to taste
4 ounces mascarpone cheese, at room temperature
1 cup milk
1 cup heavy cream

DIRECTIONS

Melt butter on Sear/Sauté. Add carrot, onion, and celery and cook for 5 minutes until tender.

Add chicken broth to the pot; mix in parsley, quinoa and chicken. Add pepper and salt for seasoning.

Seal the pressure lid, choose Pressure, set to High, and set the timer to 5 minutes. Press Start. When ready, release the pressure quickly. Press Sear/Sauté. Add mascarpone cheese to the soup and stir well to melt completely; mix in heavy cream and milk. Simmer the soup for 3 to 4 minutes until thickened and creamy.

Creamy Chicken Pasta with Pesto Sauce

Servings: 8 | Ready in about: 30 min

INGREDIENTS

3½ cups water
4 chicken breast, boneless, skinless, cubed
8 oz macaroni pasta
1 tbsp butter
1 tbsp salt, divided
2 cups fresh collard greens, trimmed
1 cup cherry tomatoes, halved

½ cup basil pesto sauce
¼ cup cream cheese, at room temperature
1 garlic clove, minced
1 tsp freshly ground black pepper to taste
1/4 cup Asiago cheese, grated
Freshly chopped basil for garnish

DIRECTIONS

To the inner steel pot of the Foodi, add water, chicken, 2 tsp salt, butter, and macaroni, and stir well to mix and be submerged in water.

Seal the pressure lid, choose Pressure, set to High, and set the timer to 2 minutes. Press Start. When ready, release the pressure quickly. Press Start/Stop, open the lid, get rid of ¼ cup water from the pot.

Set on Sear/Sauté. Into the pot, mix in collard greens, pesto sauce, garlic, remaining 1 tsp salt, cream cheese, tomatoes, and black pepper. Cook, for 1 to 2 minutes as you stir, until sauce is creamy.

Place the pasta into serving plates; top with asiago cheese and basil before serving.

Chicken and Sweet Potato Corn Chowder

Servings: 8 | Ready in about: 40 min

INGREDIENTS

4 boneless, skinless chicken breast, diced
3 garlic cloves, minced
1 cup chicken stock
19 ounces corn kernels, frozen
1 sweet potato, peeled and cubed
4 ounces canned diced green chiles, drained

2 tsp chili powder
1 tsp ground cumin
2 cups cheddar cheese, shredded
2 cups creme fraiche
Salt and black pepper to taste
Cilantro leaves, chopped

DIRECTIONS

Mix chicken, corn, chili powder, cumin, chicken stock, sweet potato, green chiles, and garlic in the pot of the Foodi. Seal the pressure lid, choose Pressure, set to High, and set the timer to 10 minutes. Press Start.

When ready, release the pressure quickly. Set the chicken to a cutting board and use two forks to shred it. Return to pot and stir well into the liquid. Stir in cheese and creme fraiche; season with pepper and salt. Cook for 2 to 3 minutes until cheese is melted.

Place chowder into plates and top with cilantro.

Cajun Shredded Chicken and Wild Rice

Servings: 6 | Ready in about: 45 min

INGREDIENTS

6 chicken thighs, skinless
1 tsp salt
½ tsp ground red pepper
½ tsp onion powder
½ tsp ground white pepper
1 tsp Cajun seasoning
1/8 tsp smoked paprika

2 tbsp olive oil
1 cup pumpkin, peeled and cubed
2 celery stalks, diced
2 onions, diced
2 garlic cloves, crushed
3 cups chicken broth, divided
1 ½ cups wild rice

DIRECTIONS

Season the chicken with salt, onion powder, Cajun seasoning, ground white pepper, ground red pepper, and smoked paprika. Warm oil on Sear/Sauté. Stir in celery and pumpkin and cook for 5 minutes until tender; set the vegetables on a plate. In batches, sear chicken in oil for 3 minutes each side until golden brown; set on a plate.

In the Foodi, add 1/4 cup chicken stock to deglaze the pan, scrape away any browned bits from the bottom; add garlic and onion and cook for 2 minutes until fragrant.

Take back the celery and pumpkin to Foodi; add the wild rice and remaining chicken stock. Place the chicken over the rice mixture.

Seal the pressure lid, choose Pressure, set to High, and set the timer to 10 minutes. Press Start. When ready, release the pressure quickly. Place rice and chicken pieces in serving plates and serve.

Hawaiian-Style Chicken Sliders with Pineapple Salad

Servings: 12 | Ready in about: 2 hr

INGREDIENTS

Mango Slaw:
¼ cup apple cider vinegar
¼ cup olive oil
1 small pineapple, chopped
4 cups arugula
¼ cup chopped fresh cilantro
4 green onions, sliced
Hawaiian-Style Chicken:
1 cup brown sugar
½ cup chicken broth

½ cup soy sauce
½ cup honey
¼ cup orange juice
2 garlic cloves, minced
2 tbsp grated fresh ginger
1 tsp freshly ground black pepper
6 skinless, boneless chicken breasts, halved
2 tbsp cornstarch
2 tbsp water
12 Hawaiian bread rolls

DIRECTIONS

In a bowl, mix oil and vinegar; add pineapple, green onions, cilantro, and arugula and toss well to coat. Refrigerate for 1 hour while the bowl is covered.

In the Foodi, mix in brown sugar, soy sauce, garlic, black pepper, ginger, honey, chicken broth, and orange juice.

Press Sear/Sauté. Allow the liquid to a simmer. Cook until the honey and brown sugar dissolves. Arrange chicken into the sauce and toss to coat.

Seal the pressure lid, choose Pressure, set to High, and set the timer to 16 minutes. Press Start. When ready, release the pressure quickly.

Transfer chicken to a cutting board; use 2 forks to shred it.

Preheat your oven's broiler. In a small bowl, mix water and cornstarch; stir into the sauce in the cooker.

Set cooker to Sear/Sauté. Cook sauce for 2 to 3 minutes until it begins to thicken. Stir in the shredded chicken. Halve the loaf of Hawaiian rolls.

Set the halves, cut-side up, onto a Cook & Crisp Basket in the pot.

Close the crisping lid. Select Bake/Roast, set the temperature to 400°F, and set the time to 3 minutes. Press Start.

When cooking is complete, remove, transfer the shredded chicken to the bottom half of the rolls and apply a topping of salad. Replace the top half of the rolls and cut into individual sliders before serving.

Asian Turkey Lettuce Cups

Servings: 4 | Ready in about: 45 min

INGREDIENTS

¾ cup olive oil
4 cloves garlic, minced
3 tbsp maple syrup
2 tbsp pineapple juice
1 cup coconut milk
3 tbsp rice wine vinegar

3 tbsp soy sauce
1 tbsp Thai-style chili paste
1 pound boneless, skinless turkey breasts, cut into strips
1 romaine lettuce, leaves separated
⅓ cup chopped peanuts
¼ cup chopped fresh cilantro leaves

DIRECTIONS

In the Foodi's pressure, mix peanut butter, garlic, rice wine vinegar, soy sauce, pineapple juice, honey, coconut milk, and chili paste until smooth; add turkey strips and ensure they are submerged in the sauce.

Seal the pressure lid, choose Pressure, set to High, and set the timer to 12 minutes. Press Start. When ready, release the pressure quickly.

Place the turkey at the center of each lettuce leaf; top with cilantro and chopped peanuts.

Honey-Garlic Chicken

Servings: 4 | Ready in about: 30 min

INGREDIENTS

4 boneless, skinless chicken breast, cut into chunks
1 onion, diced
4 garlic cloves, smashed
½ cup honey
3 tbsp soy sauce
2 tbsp lime juice

2 tsp sesame oil
1 tsp rice vinegar
Salt and black pepper to taste
1 tbsp cornstarch
1 tbsp water

DIRECTIONS

Mix garlic, onion and chicken in your Foodi.

In a bowl, combine honey, sesame oil, lime juice, soy sauce, and rice vinegar; pour over the chicken mixture.

Seal the pressure lid, choose Pressure, set to High, and set the timer to 15 minutes. Press Start. When ready, release the pressure quickly.

Mix water and cornstarch until well dissolved; stir into the sauce. Press Sear/Sauté.

Simmer the sauce and cook for 2 to 3 minutes as you stir until thickened.

Pulled Chicken and Peach Salsa

Servings: 4 | Ready in about: 40 min

INGREDIENTS

15 ounces canned peach chunks
4 boneless, skinless chicken thighs
14 ounces canned diced tomatoes
2 cloves garlic, minced

½ tsp cumin
½ tsp salt
Cheddar shredded cheese
Fresh chopped mint leaves

DIRECTIONS

Strain canned peach chunks. Reserve the juice and set aside. In your Foodi, add chicken, tomatoes, cumin, garlic, peach juice (about 1 cup), and salt.

Seal the pressure lid, choose Pressure, set to High, and set the timer to 15 minutes. Press Start. When ready, do a quick pressure release.

Shred chicken with the use of two forks. Transfer to a serving plate. Add peach chunks to the cooking juices and mix until well combined. Pour the peach salsa over the chicken, top with chopped mint leaves and shredded cheese. Serve immediately.

Chicken with Beans and Bacon

Servings: 4 | Ready in about: 45 min

INGREDIENTS

1 tbsp olive oil
4 slices bacon, crumbled
4 boneless, skinless chicken thighs
1 onion, diced
4 garlic cloves, minced
1 tbsp tomato paste
1 tbsp oregano
1 tbsp ground cumin
1 tsp chili powder
½ tsp cayenne pepper

1 (14.5 ounces) can whole tomatoes
1 cup chicken broth
1 tsp salt
1 cup cooked corn
1 red bell pepper, chopped
15 ounces red kidney beans, drained and rinsed
1 cup shredded Monterey Jack cheese
1 cup sliced red onion
¼ cup chopped cilantro

DIRECTIONS

Warm oil on Sear/Sauté. Sear the chicken for 3 minutes for each side until browned. Set the chicken on a plate. In the same oil, fry bacon until crispy, about 5 minutes and set aside.

Add in onions and cook for 2 to 3 minutes until fragrant. Stir in garlic, oregano, cayenne pepper, cumin, tomato paste, bell pepper, and chili powder and cook for 30 more seconds. Pour the chicken broth, salt, and tomatoes and bring to a boil. Press Start/Stop.

Take back the chicken and bacon to the pot and ensure it is submerged in the braising liquid.

Seal the pressure lid, choose Pressure, set to High, and set the timer to 15 minutes. Press Start. When ready, release the pressure quickly.

Pour the kidney beans in the cooker, press Sear/Sauté and bring the liquid to a boil; cook for 10 minutes. Serve topped with shredded cheese and chopped cilantro.

Chicken Cacciatore

Servings: 4 | Ready in about: 40 min

INGREDIENTS

2 tsp olive oil
1 pound chicken drumsticks, boneless, skinless
2 tsp salt
1½ tsp freshly ground black pepper
1carrot, chopped
1 red bell pepper, chopped
1 yellow bell pepper, chopped
1 onion, chopped
4 garlic cloves, thinly sliced

2 tsp dried oregano
1 tsp dried basil
1 tsp dried parsley
1 pinch red pepper flakes
1 (28 ounces) can diced tomatoes
½ cup dry red wine
¾ cup chicken stock
1 cup black olives, pitted and sliced
2 bay leaves

DIRECTIONS

Warm oil on Sear/Sauté. Add pepper and salt to the chicken drumsticks. In batches, sear the chicken for 5-6 minutes until golden-brown. Set aside on a plate. Drain the cooker and remain with 1 tbsp of fat.

In the hot oil, sauté onion, garlic, and bell peppers for 4 minutes until softened; add red pepper flakes, basil, parsley, and oregano, and cook for 30 more seconds. Season with salt and pepper.

Stir in tomatoes, olives, chicken stock, red wine and bay leaves.

Return chicken to the pot. Seal the pressure lid, choose Pressure, set to High, and set the timer to 15 minutes. Press Start. When ready, release the pressure quickly.

Divide chicken between four serving bowls; top with tomato mixture before serving.

Vietnamese Pork Soup

Servings: 4 | Ready in about: 40 min

INGREDIENTS

2 tbsp olive oil
2 yellow onions, halved
1 large piece fresh ginger, halved lengthwise
2 tsp fennel seeds
1 tsp red pepper flakes
½ tsp coriander seeds
10 black peppercorns

2-star anise
8 cups water
1 pound pork tenderloin, cut into thin strips
2 tsp salt
8 ounces rice noodles
1 lime, cut into wedges
A handful of fresh cilantro leaves

DIRECTIONS

Set your Foodi to Sear/Sauté, set to Medium High, and choose Start/Stop to preheat the pot. Warm oil on Normal.

Add ginger and onions and cook for 4 minutes; add in red pepper flakes, fennel seeds, star anise, peppercorns, and coriander seeds; cook for 1 minute as you stir. Add water, salt and pork into the pot.

Seal the pressure lid, choose Pressure, set to High, and set the timer to 60 minutes. Press Start. Release the pressure naturally for 10 minutes.

As the pho continues to cook, soak rice noodles in hot water for 8 minutes until softened and pliable; stop the cooking process by draining and rinsing with cold water. Separate the noodles into four soup plates.

Remove the pork from the cooker and ladle among bowls. Strain the broth to get rid of solids. Pour it over the pork and noodles; season with red pepper flakes. Garnish with lime wedges and cilantro leaves.

Tandoori Chicken with Cilantro Sauce

Servings: 4 | Ready in about: 9 hr

INGREDIENTS

4 chicken thighs, skinless
½ cup Greek yogurt
1 tbsp olive oil
1 tbsp lemon juice
1 tbsp red chili powder
2 tsp salt

1 tsp garam masala
½ tsp ground turmeric
½ tbsp grated fresh ginger
½ tbsp minced garlic
1 cup water
Cooking spray

Cilantro Sauce:

A handful of fresh cilantro leaves
1 tsp cumin seeds
½ jalapeno pepper
2-3 garlic cloves

2 tsp honey
2 tsp lemon juice
¾ cup olive oil
salt to taste

DIRECTIONS

In a large bowl, mix yogurt, lemon juice, garam masala, garlic, turmeric, red chili powder, vegetable oil, salt, and ginger. Use a paper towel to pat thighs. Place the thighs into a resealable plastic bag; add in yogurt mixture and seal. Massage bag to ensure the marinade coats the chicken completely and place in the refrigerator for 12 hours. Take the chicken out of the refrigerator and set aside for 30 minutes before cooking.

Add water into the Foodi. Apply a cooking spray to your steamer and set in the pot over the water. Remove chicken from marinade and arrange on the trivet.

Seal the pressure lid, choose Pressure, set to High, and set the timer to 15 minutes. Press Start.

When ready, release the pressure quickly. In a blender, blend cilantro, water, garlic, honey, cumin, jalapeno pepper, salt and lemon juice until smooth. Over the chicken, drizzle sauce before serving.

Indian Butter Chicken

Servings: 6 | Ready in about: 30 min

INGREDIENTS

2 tbsp butter
1 large onion, minced
1 tsp salt
1 tbsp grated fresh ginger
1 tbsp minced fresh garlic
½ tsp ground turmeric
1 tbsp Kashmiri red chili powder
1 (14.5 ounces) can coconut milk, refrigerated overnight

2 pounds boneless, skinless chicken legs
3 Roma tomatoes, pureed in a blender
½ cup chopped fresh cilantro, divided
2 tbsp. Indian curry paste
2 tbsp dried fenugreek
2 tsp sugar
1 tsp garam masala
Salt to taste

DIRECTIONS

Set your Foodi to Sear/Sauté, set to Medium High, and choose Start/Stop to preheat the pot and melt butter.

Add in 1 tsp salt and onion. Cook for 2 to 3 minutes until fragrant. Stir in ginger, turmeric, garlic, and red chili powder to coat; cook for 2 more minutes.

Place water and coconut cream into separate bowls. Stir the water from the coconut milk can, pureed tomatoes, and chicken with the onion mixture. Seal the pressure lid, choose Pressure, set to High, and set the timer to 8 minutes. Press Start. When ready, release the pressure quickly.

Stir sugar, coconut cream, fenugreek, curry paste, half the cilantro, and garam masala through the chicken mixture; apply salt for seasoning. Simmer the mixture and cook for 10 minutes until the sauce thickens, on Sear/Sauté. Garnish with the rest of the cilantro before serving.

Chicken Chickpea Chili

Servings: 4 | Ready in about: 25 min

INGREDIENTS

1 tbsp olive oil
3 large serrano peppers, diced
1 onion, diced
1 jalapeño pepper, diced
1 pound boneless, skinless chicken breast, cubed
1 tsp ground cumin
1 tsp minced fresh garlic

1 tsp salt
2 (14.5 ounces) cans chickpeas, drained and rinsed
2 ½ cups water, divided
2 tbsp chili powder
½ cup chopped fresh cilantro
½ cup shredded Monterey Jack cheese
1 lime, cut into six wedges

DIRECTIONS

Warm oil on Sear/Sauté. Add in onion, serrano peppers, and jalapeno pepper and cook for 5 minutes until tender; add salt, cumin and garlic for seasoning.

Stir chicken with vegetable mixture; cook for 3 to 6 minutes until no longer pink; add 2 cups water and chickpeas.

Seal the pressure lid, choose Pressure, set to High, and set the timer to 5 minutes. Press Start. Release pressure naturally for 5 minutes. Press Start. Stir chili powder with remaining ½ cup water; mix in chili.

Press Sear/Sauté. Boil the chili as you stir and cook until slightly thickened. Divide chili into plates; garnish with cheese and cilantro. Over the chili, squeeze a lime wedge.

Paprika Buttered Chicken

Servings: 6 | Ready in about: 45 min

INGREDIENTS

1 cup chicken stock
½ cup white wine
½ onion, thinly sliced
2 cloves garlic, minced
3.5-pound whole chicken

1 tsp salt
½ tsp ground black pepper
½ tsp dried thyme
3 tbsp butter, melted
½ tsp paprika

DIRECTIONS

Into the Foodi, add onion, chicken stock, white wine, and garlic. Over the mixture, place the reversible rack.

Apply pepper, salt, and thyme to the chicken; lay onto reversible rack breast-side up.

Seal the pressure lid, choose Pressure, set to High, and set the timer to 26 minutes. Press Start. When ready, release the pressure quickly.

While pressure releases, preheat oven broiler. In a bowl, mix paprika and butter.

Remove the reversible rack with chicken from your pot. Get rid of onion and stock.

Onto the chicken, brush butter mixture and take the reversible rack back to the pot.

Cook under the broiler for 5 minutes until chicken skin is crispy and browned.

Set chicken to a cutting board to cool for about 5 minutes, then carve and transfer to a serving platter.

Buffalo Chicken and Navy Bean Chili

Servings: 6 | Ready in about: 45 min

INGREDIENTS

1 tbsp olive oil
1 shallot, diced
½ cup fennel, chopped
¼ cup minced garlic
1 tbsp smoked paprika
2 tsp chili powder
2 tsp ground cumin

½ tsp salt
½ tsp ground white pepper
1 (28 ounces) can crushed tomatoes
1 ½ pounds chicken sausage, sliced
1 (14 ounces) can diced tomatoes with green chilies
¾ cup Buffalo wing sauce
2 (14 ounces) cans navy beans, drained and rinsed

DIRECTIONS

Warm oil on Sear/Sauté. Add the sausages and brown for 5 minutes, turning frequently. Set aside on a plate.

In the same fat, sauté onion, roasted red peppers, fennel, and garlic for 4 minutes until soft; season with paprika, cumin, pepper, salt, and chili powder.

Stir in crushed tomatoes, diced tomatoes with green chilies, buffalo sauce, and navy beans. Return the sausages to the pot.

Seal the pressure lid, choose Pressure, set to High, and set the timer to 30 minutes. Press Start. When ready, do a quick pressure release. Spoon chili into bowls and serve warm.

Chicken in Tikka Masala Sauce

Servings: 4 | Ready in about: 40 min

INGREDIENTS

2 pounds boneless, skinless chicken thighs,
1 tsp salt
¼ tsp freshly ground black pepper
1½ tbsp olive oil
½ onion, chopped
2 garlic cloves, minced
3 tbsp tomato puree
1 tsp fresh ginger, minced
1 tbsp garam masala
2 tsp curry powder

1 tsp ground coriander
½ tsp ground cumin
⅛ tsp jalapeño pepper, seeded and chopped
29 ounces canned tomato sauce
3 tomatoes, chopped
½ cup natural yogurt
1 lemon, juiced
3 cups cooked basmati rice
¼ cup fresh chopped cilantro leaves
4 lemon wedges

DIRECTIONS

Apply black pepper and ½ tsp salt to the chicken.

Set your Foodi to Sear/Sauté, set to Medium High, and choose Start/Stop to preheat the pot. Warm oil.

Add garlic and onion and cook for 3 minutes until soft. Stir in tomato puree, garam masala, cumin, curry powder, ginger, coriander, and jalapeño pepper; cook for 30 seconds until fragrant.

Stir in remaining ½ tsp salt, tomato sauce, and tomatoes. Simmer the mixture as you scrape the bottom to get rid of any browned bits; stir in chicken to coat.

Seal the pressure lid, choose Pressure, set to High, and set the timer to 10 minutes. Press Start. When ready, release the pressure quickly. Press Sear/Sauté and simmer the sauce and cook for 3 to 5 minutes until thickened.

Stir lemon juice and yogurt through the sauce. Serve garnished with lemon wedges and cilantro.

Pesto Stuffed Chicken with Green Beans

Servings: 4 | Ready in about: 20 min

INGREDIENTS

4 chicken breasts
1 tbsp butter
1 tbsp olive oil
¼ cup dry white wine
¾ cup chicken stock
1 tsp salt
1 cup green beans, trimmed and cut into 1-inch pieces

For pesto:
1 cup fresh basil
1 garlic clove, smashed
2 tbsp. pine nuts
¼ cup Parmesan cheese
¼ cup extra virgin olive oil

DIRECTIONS

First make the pesto: in a bowl, mix fresh basil, pine nuts, garlic, salt, pepper and Parmesan and place in food processor. Add in oil and process until the desired consistency is attained. Adjust seasoning.

Apply a thin layer of pesto to one side of each chicken breast; tightly roll into a cylinder and fasten closed with small skewers. Press Sear/Sauté. Add oil and butter. Cook chicken rolls for 1 to 2 minutes per side until browned.

Add in wine cook until the wine has evaporated, about 3-4 minutes.

Add stock and salt into the pot. Top the chicken with green beans.

Seal the pressure lid, choose Pressure, set to High, and set the timer to 5 minutes. Press Start. When ready, release the pressure quickly.

Serve chicken rolls with cooking liquid and green beans.

Cajun Chicken with Rice and Peas

Servings: 4 | Ready in about: 30 min

INGREDIENTS

4 boneless, skinless chicken breasts, sliced
1 garlic clove, minced
½ tsp paprika
¼ tsp dried oregano
¼ tsp dried thyme
⅛ tsp cayenne pepper
⅛ tsp ground white pepper
Salt to taste

1 tbsp oil olive
1 onion, chopped
1 tbsp tomato puree
2 cups chicken broth, divided
1 cup long grain rice
1 celery stalk, diced
1 cup frozen green peas

DIRECTIONS

Season chicken with garlic powder, oregano, white pepper, thyme, paprika, cayenne pepper, and salt.

Warm the oil on Sear/Sauté. Add in onion and cook for 4 minutes until fragrant. Mix in tomato puree to coat.

Add ¼ cup chicken stock into the Foodi to deglaze the pan, scrape the pan's bottom to get rid of browned bits of food. Mix in celery, rice, and the seasoned chicken. Add in the remaining broth to the chicken mixture.

Seal the pressure lid, choose Pressure, set to High, and set the timer to 8 minutes. Press Start. Once ready, do a quick release.

Mix in green peas, cover with the lid and let sit for 5 minutes. Serve warm.

Spicy Chicken Wings with Lemon

Servings: 4 | Ready in about: 40 min

INGREDIENTS

2 tbsp olive oil
8 chicken wings
½ tsp chili powder
½ tsp garlic powder
½ tsp onion powder

½ dried oregano
½ tsp cayenne pepper
Sea salt and ground black pepper to taste
½ cup chicken broth
2 lemons, juiced

DIRECTIONS

Coat the chicken wings with olive oil; season with chili powder, onion powder, salt, oregano, garlic powder, cayenne, and pepper.

In the steel pot of the Foodi, add your wings and chicken broth.

Seal the pressure lid, choose Pressure, set to High, and set the timer to 4 minutes. Press Start. When ready, do a quick pressure release. Preheat an oven to high.

Onto a greased baking sheet, place the wings in a single layer and drizzle over the lemon juice. Bake for 5 minutes until skin is crispy.

Chicken with BBQ Sauce

Servings: 6 | Ready in about: 20 min

INGREDIENTS

2 pounds boneless skinless chicken breasts
1 tsp salt
1½ cups barbecue sauce

1 small onion, minced
1 cup carrots, thinly sliced
4 garlic cloves

DIRECTIONS

Apply a seasoning of salt to the chicken and place in the inner pot of the Foodi; add onion, carrots, garlic and barbeque sauce. Toss the chicken to coat.

Seal the pressure lid, choose Pressure, set to High, and set the timer to 15 minutes. Press Start. Once ready, do a quick release. Use two forks to shred chicken and stir into the sauce.

Spicy Salsa Chicken with Feta

Servings: 6 | Ready in about: 30 min

INGREDIENTS

2 pounds boneless skinless chicken drumsticks
¼ tsp salt
1 ½ cups hot tomato salsa

1 onion, chopped
1 cup feta cheese, crumbled

DIRECTIONS

Sprinkle salt over the chicken; set in the inner steel pot of Foodi. Stir in salsa to coat the chicken.

Seal the pressure lid, choose Pressure, set to High, and set the timer to 15 minutes. Press Start. When ready, do a quick pressure release. Press Sear/Sauté and cook for 5 to 10 minutes as you stir until excess liquid has evaporated.

Top with feta cheese and serve.

Chicken and Zucchini Pilaf

Servings: 4 | Ready in about: 40 min

INGREDIENTS

2 tsp olive oil
1 zucchini, chopped
1 cup leeks, chopped
2 garlic cloves, minced
1 tbsp chopped fresh rosemary

2 tsp chopped fresh thyme leaves
salt and ground black pepper to taste
2 cups chicken stock
1 pound boneless and skinless chicken legs
1 cup rice, rinsed

DIRECTIONS

Set your Foodi to Sear/Sauté, set to Medium High, and choose Start/Stop to preheat the pot. Warm oil. Add in zucchini and cook for 5 minutes until tender.

Stir in thyme, leeks, rosemary, pepper, salt and garlic. Cook the mixture for 3-4 minutes.

Add ½ cup chicken stock into the pot to deglaze, scrape the bottom to get rid of any browned bits of food.

When liquid stops simmering, add in the remaining stock, rice, and chicken with more pepper and salt.

Seal the pressure lid, choose Pressure, set to High, and set the timer to 5 minutes. Press Start. Once ready, do a quick release.

Chicken in Pineapple Gravy

Servings: 4 | Ready in about: 25 min

INGREDIENTS

1 tbsp olive oil
4 boneless, skinless chicken thighs,
¼ cup pineapple juice
2 tbsp ketchup
2 tbsp Worcestershire sauce

1 garlic clove, minced
1 tsp cornstarch
2 tsp water
A handful of fresh cilantro, chopped

DIRECTIONS

Warm oil on Sear/Sauté. In batches, sear chicken in oil for 3 minutes until golden brown; set aside on a plate.

Mix, pineapple juice, Worcestershire sauce, garlic, and ketchup; add to the pot to deglaze, scrape the bottom to get rid of any browned bits of food. Place the chicken into the sauce and stir well to coat.

Seal the pressure lid, choose Pressure, set to High, and set the timer to cook for 5 minutes. Press Start. When ready, release the pressure quickly.

In a small bowl, mix water and cornstarch until well dissolved. Press Start/Stop and set to Sear/Sauté. Stir the cornstarch slurry into the sauce; cook for 2 minutes until the sauce is well thickened. Set in serving bowls and cilantro to serve.

Salsa Verde Chicken with Salsa Verde

Servings: 4 | Ready in about: 50 min

INGREDIENTS

SALSA VERDE:

1 jalapeño pepper, deveined and sliced
½ cup capers
¼ cup parsley
1 lime, juiced
1 tsp salt

¼ cup extra virgin olive oil
Chicken:
4 boneless skinless chicken breasts
2 cups water
1 cup quinoa, rinsed

DIRECTIONS

In a blender, mix olive oil, salt, lime juice, jalapeño pepper, capers, and parsley and blend until smooth.

Arrange chicken breasts in the bottom of the Foodi pot. Over the chicken, add salsa verde mixture.

In a bowl that can fit in the cooker, mix quinoa and water. Set a reversible rack onto chicken and sauce. Set the bowl onto the reversible rack. Seal the pressure lid, choose Pressure, set to High, and set the timer to 20 minutes. Press Start.

When ready, release the pressure quickly. Remove the quinoa bowl and reversible rack. Using two forks, shred chicken into the sauce; stir to coat.

Divide the quinoa, between plates. Top with chicken and salsa verde before serving.

Chicken Meatballs in Tomato Sauce

Servings: 5 | Ready in about: 35 min

INGREDIENTS

1 pound ground chicken
3 tbsp red hot sauce
1 egg
⅓ cup crumbled blue cheese
¼ cup bread crumbs
¼ cup Pecorino cheese
1 tbsp ranch dressing

1 tsp dried basil
salt and ground black pepper to taste
15 ounces canned tomato sauce
1 cup chicken broth
2 tbsp olive oil
A handful of parsley, chopped

DIRECTIONS

In a bowl, mix ground chicken, egg, pecorino, basil, pepper, salt, ranch dressing, blue cheese, 3 tbsp hot sauce, and bread crumbs; shape the mixture into meatballs.

Warm oil on Sear/Sauté. Add in the meatballs and cook for 2 to 3 minutes until browned on all sides.

Add in tomato sauce and broth. Seal the pressure lid, choose Pressure, set to High, and set the timer to 7 minutes. Press Start.

When ready, release the pressure quickly. Remove meatballs carefully and place to a serving plate; top with parsley and serve.

Honey-Garlic Chicken and Okra

Servings: 4 | Ready in about: 25 min

INGREDIENTS

6 garlic cloves, grated
¼ cup tomato puree
½ cup soy sauce
⅓ cup honey
2 tbsp rice vinegar
1 tbsp olive oil
4 boneless, skinless chicken breasts, sliced
1 cup rice, rinsed

½ tsp salt
2 cups water
2 cups frozen okra
1 tbsp cornstarch
1 tbsp water
2 tsp toasted sesame seeds
4 spring onions, thinly sliced

DIRECTIONS

In the inner pot of the Foodi, mix garlic, tomato puree, vinegar, soy sauce, ginger, honey, and oil; toss in chicken to coat. In an ovenproof bowl, mix water, salt and rice.

Set the reversible rack on top of chicken. Lower the bowl onto the reversible rack.

Seal the pressure lid, choose Pressure, set to High, and set the timer to 10 minutes; press Start. Release pressure naturally for 5 minutes, release the remaining pressure quickly.

Use a fork to fluff the rice. Lay okra onto the rice. Allow the okra steam in the residual heat for 3 minutes. Take the trivet and bowl from the pot. Set the chicken to a plate.

Press Sear/Sauté. In a small bowl, mix 1 tbsp of water and cornstarch until smooth; stir into the sauce and cook for 3 to 4 minutes until thickened.

Divide the rice, chicken, and okra between 4 bowls. Drizzle sauce over each portion; garnish with spring onions and sesame seeds.

Shredded Chicken with Lentils and Rice

Servings: 4 | Ready in about: 45 min

INGREDIENTS

1 tsp olive oil
1 garlic clove, minced
1 small yellow onion, chopped
3 cups chicken broth, divided
4 boneless, skinless chicken thighs

1 cup white rice
½ cup dried lentils
Salt and ground black pepper to taste
Chopped fresh parsley for garnish

DIRECTIONS

Set your Foodi to Sear/Sauté, set to Medium High, and choose Start/Stop to preheat the pot. Warm oil. Add in onion and garlic and cook for 3 minutes until soft; add in broth, rice, lentils, and chicken. Season with pepper and salt.

Seal the pressure lid, choose Pressure, set to High, and set the timer to 15 minutes. Press Start.

Once ready, do a quick release. Remove and shred the chicken in a large bowl. Set the lentils and rice into serving plates, top with shredded chicken and parsley and serve.

Saucy Chicken Breasts

Servings: 4 | Ready in about: 45 min

INGREDIENTS

4 chicken breasts, boneless and skinless
salt and ground black pepper to taste
2 tbsp olive oil
2 tbsp soy sauce
2 tbsp tomato paste
2 tbsp honey

2 tbsp minced garlic
½ cup chicken broth
1 tbsp cornstarch
1 tbsp water
½ cup chives, sliced

DIRECTIONS

Season the chicken with pepper and salt. Warm oil on Sear/Sauté. Add in chicken and cook for 5 minutes until lightly browned.

In a small bowl, mix garlic, soy sauce, honey, and tomato paste; pour the mixture over the chicken. Stir in ½ cup broth. Seal the pressure lid, choose Pressure, set to High, and set the timer to 12 minutes. Press Start.

When ready, release the pressure quickly.

Set the chicken to a bowl. Mix water and cornstarch to create a slurry; briskly stir the mixture into the sauce that is remaining in the pan for 2 minutes until thickened. Serve the chicken with the sauce and chives.

Chicken with Tomatoes and Capers

Servings: 4 | Ready in about: 45 min

INGREDIENTS

4 chicken legs
sea salt and fresh ground black pepper to taste
2 tbsp olive oil
1 onion, diced
2 garlic cloves, minced

⅓ cup red wine
2 cups diced tomatoes
⅓ cup capers
¼ cup fresh basil
2 pickles, chopped

DIRECTIONS

Sprinkle pepper and salt over the chicken. Warm oil on Sear/Sauté. Add in onion and cook for 3 minutes until fragrant; add in garlic and cook for 30 seconds until softened.

Mix the chicken with vegetables and cook for 6 to 7 minutes until lightly browned.

Add red wine to the pan to deglaze, scrape the pan's bottom to get rid of any browned bits of food; stir in tomatoes. Seal the pressure lid, choose Pressure, set to High, and set the timer to 12 minutes; press Start. When ready, release the pressure quickly. To the chicken mixture, add basil, capers and pickles. Serve the chicken in plates covered with the tomato sauce mixture.

Winter Chicken Thighs with Cabbage

Servings: 4 | Ready in about: 35 min

INGREDIENTS

1 tbsp lard
4 slices pancetta, diced
4 chicken thighs, boneless skinless
salt and ground black pepper to taste

1 cup chicken broth
1 tbsp Dijon mustard
1 pound green cabbage, shredded
Fresh parsley, chopped

DIRECTIONS

Warm lard on Sear/Sauté. Fry pancetta for 5 minutes until crisp. Set aside. Season chicken with pepper and salt. Sear in Foodi for 2 minutes each side until browned. In a bowl, mix mustard and chicken broth.

In your Foodi, add pancetta and chicken broth mixture. Seal the pressure lid, choose Pressure, set to High, and set the timer to 6 minutes. Press Start. When ready, release the pressure quickly.

Open the lid, mix in green cabbage, seal again, and cook on High Pressure for 2 minutes. When ready, release the pressure quickly. Serve with sprinkled parsley.

Sriracha Chicken with Black Beans

Servings: 4 | Ready in about: 25 min

INGREDIENTS

½ cup soy sauce
½ cup chicken broth
3 tbsp honey
2 tbsp tomato paste
1 tbsp sriracha
1 (1 inch) piece fresh ginger, grated
3 garlic cloves, grated

4 boneless, skinless chicken drumsticks
1 tbsp cornstarch
1 tbsp water
2 tbsp toasted sesame seeds, divided
1 tbsp sesame oil
2 cups canned black beans
2 green onions, thinly sliced

DIRECTIONS

In your Foodi, mix the soy sauce, honey, ginger, tomato paste, chicken broth, sriracha, and garlic. Stir well until smooth; toss in the chicken to coat. Seal the pressure lid, choose Pressure, set to High, and set the timer to 3 minutes. Press Start. Release the pressure immediately.

Open the lid and Press Sear/Sauté. In a small bowl, mix water and cornstarch until no lumps remain; stir into the sauce and cook for 5 minutes until thickened.

Stir sesame oil and 1½ tbsp sesame seeds through the chicken mixture; garnish with extra sesame seeds and green onions. Serve with black beans.

Crunchy Chicken Schnitzels

Servings: 4 | Ready in about: 25 min

INGREDIENTS:

4 chicken breasts, boneless
1 cup flour
2 eggs, beaten
1 cup breadcrumbs
Salt and pepper to taste

2 tbsp fresh parsley, chopped
4 slices cold butter
4 slices lemon
Cooking spray

DIRECTIONS:

Combine the breadcrumbs with the parsley in a dish and set aside.

Season the chicken with salt and pepper. Coat in flour; shake off any excess. Dip the coated chicken into the beaten egg followed by breadcrumbs. Spray the schnitzels with cooking spray.

Put them into the Ninja Foodi basket, close the crisping lid and cook for 10 minutes at 380 F. After 5 minutes, turn the schnitzels over.

Arrange the schnitzels on a serving platter and place the butter and lemon slices over to serve.

Greek Turkey Meatballs

Servings: 6 | Ready in about: 30 min

INGREDIENTS

1 onion, minced and divided
½ cup plain bread crumbs
⅓ cup feta cheese, crumbled
2 tsp salt, divided
½ tsp dried oregano
¼ tsp ground black pepper
1 pound ground turkey

1 egg, lightly beaten
1 tbsp olive oil
1 carrot, minced
½ celery stalk, minced
3 cups tomato puree
2 cups water

DIRECTIONS

In a mixing bowl, thoroughly combine half the onion, oregano, ground turkey, salt, bread crumbs, pepper, and egg and stir until everything is well incorporated.

Heat oil on Sear/Sauté, and cook celery, remaining onion, and carrot for 5 minutes until soft. Pour in water, and tomato puree. Adjust the seasonings as necessary.

Roll the mixture into meatballs, and drop into the sauce. Seal the pressure lid, choose Pressure, set to High, and set the timer to 5 minutes. Press Start. Allow the cooker to cool and release pressure naturally for 20 minutes. Serve topped with feta cheese.

Potato and Ground Turkey Chili

Servings: 6 | Ready in about: 55 min

INGREDIENTS

1 tbsp olive oil
1 small onion, diced
2 garlic cloves, minced
1 pound ground turkey
2 bell peppers, chopped
6 potatoes, peeled and sliced
1cup carrots, chopped

1 cups fresh or frozen corn kernels, roasted
1 cups tomato puree
1 cups diced tomatoes
1 cup chicken broth
1 tbsp ground cumin
1 tbsp chili powder
salt and fresh ground black pepper

DIRECTIONS

Warm the olive on Sear/Sauté and stir-fry onions and garlic until soft, for about 3 minutes. Press Start. Stir in turkey and cook until thoroughly browned, about 5-6 minutes. Add the remaining ingredients, and stir to combine.

Seal the pressure lid, choose Pressure, set to High, and set the timer to 25 minutes; press Start. Once ready, do a quick release. Set on Sear/Sauté. Cook uncovered for 15 more minutes. Serve warm.

Sticky Drumsticks

Servings: 4 | Ready in about: 50 min

INGREDIENTS:

1 lb drumsticks
2 tbsp honey
2 tsp dijon mustard

Salt and pepper to taste
Cooking spray

DIRECTIONS:

Combine the honey, mustard, salt, and pepper in a large bowl. Add in the chicken and toss to coat.

Cover and put in the fridge for 30 minutes.

Preheat your Ninja Foodi to 380 degrees F. Grease the Ninja Foodi basket with cooking spray.

Arrange the drumsticks on the basket. Cook for 20 minutes on Air Crisp mode.

After 10 minutes, shake the drumsticks.

Turkey Meatballs with Rigatoni

Servings: 4 | Ready in about: 40 min

INGREDIENTS

2 tbsp canola oil
1 pound ground turkey
1 large egg
¼ cup bread crumbs
2 cloves garlic, minced

1 tsp dried oregano
salt and ground black pepper to taste
3 cups tomato sauce
ounces rigatoni
2 tbsp grated Grana Padano cheese

DIRECTIONS

In a bowl, combine ground turkey, bread crumbs, cumin, garlic, and egg. Season with oregano, salt, red pepper flakes, and pepper. Form the mixture into meatballs with well-oiled hands.

Warm the oil on Sear/Sauté. Cook the meatballs for 3 to 4 minutes until browned on all sides. Remove to a plate.

Add rigatoni to the Foodi and cover with tomato sauce. Pour water into the pot enough to cover the pasta. Stir well. Throw in the meatballs.

Seal the pressure lid, choose Pressure, set to High, and set the timer to 10 minutes; press Start. When ready, release the pressure quickly. Serve topped with Grana Padano cheese.

Spicy Turkey Casserole

Servings: 5 | Ready in about: 45 min

INGREDIENTS

1 tbsp olive oil
½ sweet onion, diced
3 cloves garlic, minced
1 jalapeno pepper, minced
1 pound turkey breast, cubed
2 (14 ounces) cans fire-roasted tomatoes
1½ cups water

1 cup salsa
2 bell peppers, cut into thick strips
2 tsp ancho chili powder
2 tsp chili powder
1 tsp ground cumin
Sea salt to taste
5 tbsp fresh oregano, chopped

DIRECTIONS

Warm the oil on Sear/Sauté. Add in garlic, onion and jalapeño and cook for 5 minutes until fragrant. Stir turkey into the pot; cook for 5-6 minutes until browned.

Add in salsa, tomatoes, bell peppers, and water; apply a seasoning of sea salt, ancho chili powder, cumin, and chili powder. Seal the pressure lid, choose Pressure, set to High, and set the timer to 10 minutes on High.

When ready, release the pressure quickly. Top with oregano and serve.

Chicken Fajitas with Avocado

Servings: 4 | Ready in about: 30 min

INGREDIENTS

4 chicken breasts, boneless and skinless
1 taco seasoning
1 tbsp olive oil
1 (24 ounces) can diced tomatoes
3 bell peppers, julienned
1 shallot, chopped

4 garlic cloves, minced
Juice of 1 lemon
salt and pepper to taste
4 flour tortillas
2 tbsp cilantro, chopped
1 avocado, sliced

DIRECTIONS

In a bowl, mix taco seasoning and chicken until evenly coated. Warm oil on Sear/Sauté.

Sear chicken for 2 minutes per side until browned. To the chicken, add tomatoes, shallot, lemon juice, garlic, and bell peppers; season with pepper and salt.

Seal the pressure lid, choose Pressure, set to High, and set the timer to 4 minutes. Press Start.

When ready, release the pressure quickly.

Move the bell peppers and chicken to tortillas. Add avocado slices and serve.

Chicken Burgers with Avocado

Servings: 8 | Ready in about: 15 min

INGREDIENTS:

1 lb ground chicken
1 red onion, chopped
1 egg, beaten
4 buns, halved
1 small red potato, shredded
A pinch of ground cumin
A pinch of ground chili

Fresh cilantro, chopped
Salt and pepper to taste
1 Avocado, sliced
½ cup mayonnaise
1 tomato, sliced
Cooking spray

DIRECTIONS:

Mix the chicken, onion, egg, potato, cumin, chili, cilantro, salt, and pepper in a large bowl with your hands until you have an even burger mixture.

Shape the mixture into 8 patties.

Grease your Ninja Foodi basket with cooking spray.

Arrange the burgers onto the basket. Close the crisping lid and cook for 10 minutes, at 360 F. After 5 minutes, shake the patties.

To assemble your burgers, spread mayonnaise on the bottom of each half of the buns, top with a chicken patty, then put over a tomato slice.

Cover with the other half of the buns and arrange on a serving platter to serve.

Hot Chicken Wings

Servings: 4 | Ready in about: 25 min

INGREDIENTS

8 chicken wings
1 tbsp ranch salad mix
1 tbsp garlic powder
1 tbsp onion powder

1 tbsp cayenne pepper
½ tsp paprika
Cooking spray

DIRECTIONS:

Combine the paprika, ranch salad mix, onion powder, garlic powder, and cayenne pepper in a bowl.

Pour the seasoning all over the chicken and oil with cooking spray.

Place in the Ninja Foodi basket, close the crisping lid and cook for 15 minutes at 380 F. After half of the cooking time, shake the wings. Oil the chicken again with cooking spray and continue cooking until the wings are crispy. Serve hot.

Basil & Cheddar Stuffed Chicken

Servings: 4 | Ready in about: 25 min

INGREDIENTS:

2 large chicken breasts, skinless
4 slices cheddar cheese
A handful of fresh basil leaves

4 cherry tomatoes, halved
Salt and pepper to taste
2 tbsp olive oil

DIRECTIONS:

With a sharp knife, cut a slit into the side of each chicken breast. Put 2 slices of cheese, 3-4 basil leaves, and 4 cherry tomato halves into each slit. Use toothpicks to keep the chicken breasts closed.

Season the meat with salt and pepper, and brush with some olive oil.

Grease the Ninja Foodi basket with the remaining olive oil and place the chicken breasts in the basket; close the crisping lid and cook for 12 minutes at 370 F.

After 6 minutes, turn the breasts over. Once ready, leave to sit the chicken breasts, then slice each one in half and serve with salad.

Spicy Buttered Turkey

Servings: 6 | Ready in about: 25 min

INGREDIENTS:

6 turkey breasts, boneless and skinless
2 cups panko breadcrumbs
1 tsp salt

½ tsp cayenne pepper
½ tsp black pepper
1 stick butter, melted

DIRECTIONS:

In a bowl, combine the panko breadcrumbs, half of the black pepper, the cayenne pepper, and half of the salt.

In another bowl, combine the melted butter with salt and pepper. Brush the butter mixture over the turkey breast.

Coat the turkey with the panko mixture. Arrange on a lined Ninja Foodi basket. Close the crisping lid and cook for 15 minutes at 390 F on Air Crisp mode, flipping the meat after 8 minutes.

Chicken with Prunes

Servings: 6 | Ready in about: 55 min

INGREDIENTS:

1 whole chicken, 3 lb
½ cup pitted prunes
3 minced cloves of garlic
2 tbsp capers
2 bay leaves
2 tbsp red wine vinegar

2 tbsp olive oil
1 tbsp dried oregano
¼ cup packed brown sugar
1 tbsp chopped fresh parsley
Salt and black pepper to taste

DIRECTIONS:

In a big and deep bowl, mix the prunes, olives, capers, garlic, olive oil, bay leaves, oregano, vinegar, salt, and pepper.

Spread the mixture on the bottom of a baking tray, and place the chicken.

Preheat the Ninja Foodi to 360° F. Sprinkle a little bit of brown sugar on top of the chicken, close the crisping lid and cook for 45-55 minutes on Air Crisp mode.

When ready, garnish with fresh parsley.

Tom Yum Wings

Servings: 2 | Ready in about: 4 hours 20 min

INGREDIENTS:

8 chicken wings
1 tbsp water
2 tbsp potato starch

2 tbsp cornstarch
2 tbsp tom yum paste
½ tsp baking powder

DIRECTIONS:

Combine the tom yum paste and water, in a small bowl.

Place the wings in a large bowl, add the tom yum mixture and coat well.

Cover the bowl and refrigerate for 4 hours.

Preheat the Ninja Foodi to 370 degrees F.

Combine the baking powder, cornstarch, and potato starch. Dip each wing in the starch mixture.

Place on a lined baking dish in the Ninja Foodi and cook for 7 minutes on Air Crisp mode. Flip over and cook for 5 to 7 minutes more.

Honey-Glazed Chicken Kabobs

Servings: 4 | Ready in about: 20 min

INGREDIENTS:

4 chicken breasts, skinless and cubed
4 tbsp honey
Juice from 1 Lime

½ tsp ground paprika
Salt and pepper to taste

DIRECTIONS:

In a large bowl, combine the honey, soy sauce, lime juice, paprika, salt, and pepper.

Add in the chicken cubes and toss to coat.

Load 8 small skewers with honey-glazed chicken. Lay the kabobs into the Ninja Foodi basket, close the crisping lid and cook for 15 minutes at 360 F.

After 8 minutes, turn the kabobs over. Drizzle the remaining honey sauce and serve with sautéed veggies.

Cordon Bleu Chicken

Servings: 4 | Ready in about: 40 min

INGREDIENTS:

4 skinless and boneless chicken breasts
4 slices ham
4 slices Swiss cheese
3 tbsp all-purpose flour
4 tbsp butter

1 tsp paprika
1 tsp chicken bouillon granules
½ cup dry white wine
1 cup heavy whipping cream

DIRECTIONS:

Pound the chicken breasts and put a slice of ham and then a slice of swiss cheese on each of the breasts.

Fold the edges over the filling and secure the sides with toothpicks.

In a medium bowl, combine the paprika and the flour and coat the chicken pieces.

Close the crisping lid and fry the chicken for 20 minutes on Air Crisp mode at 380 F.

Meanwhile, in a large skillet over medium heat, melt the butter and add the bouillon and the wine. Reduce the heat to low.

Add in the heavy cream and let simmer for 20-25 minutes. When the chicken is done, remove to a serving platter and drizzle with the sauce; serve hot.

Rosemary Lemon Chicken

Servings: 2 | Ready in about: 60 min

INGREDIENTS:

2 chicken breasts
1 tsp minced ginger
2 rosemary sprigs
½ lemon, cut into wedges

1 tbsp soy sauce
½ tbsp olive oil
1 tbsp oyster sauce
3 tbsp brown sugar

DIRECTIONS:

Place the ginger, soy sauce, and olive oil, in a bowl. Add the chicken and coat well.

Cover the bowl and refrigerate for 30 minutes.

Transfer the marinated chicken to the Ninja Foodi basket.

Close the crisping lid and cook for about 6 minutes on Air Crisp mode at 370 F.

Mix the oyster sauce, rosemary and brown sugar in a small bowl. Pour the sauce over the chicken. Arrange the lemon wedges in the dish. Return to the Ninja Foodi and cook for 13 more minutes on Air Crisp mode.

Greek-Style Chicken

Servings: 6 | Ready in about: 45 min

INGREDIENTS:

1 whole chicken (3 lb), cut in pieces
3 garlic cloves, minced
½ cup olive oil
½ cup white wine
1 tbsp fresh rosemary

1 tbsp chopped fresh oregano
1 tbsp fresh thyme
Juice from 1 lemon
Salt and black pepper, to taste

DIRECTIONS:

In a large bowl, combine the garlic, rosemary, thyme, olive oil, lemon juice, oregano, salt, and pepper.

Mix all ingredients very well and spread the mixture into the Ninja Foodi basket.

Stir in the chicken. Sprinkle with wine and cook for 45 minutes on Air Crisp mode at 380 F.

Asian-Style Chicken

Servings: 4 | Ready in about: 35 min

INGREDIENTS:

1 lb chicken, cut in stripes
2 tomatoes, cubed
3 green peppers, cut in stripes
1 tbsp cumin powder
1 large onion

2 tbsp oil
1 tbsp mustard
1 pinch ginger
1 pinch fresh and chopped coriander
Salt and black pepper

DIRECTIONS:

Heat the oil in a deep pan. Add in the mustard, onion, ginger, cumin and green chili peppers. Sauté the mixture for 2-3 minutes. Then, add the tomatoes, coriander, and salt and keep stirring.

Coat the chicken with oil, salt, and pepper and cook for 25 minutes on Air Crisp mode at 380 F.

Remove from the Ninja Foodi and pour the sauce over and around.

Crumbed Sage Chicken Scallopini

Servings: 4 | Ready in about: 12 min

INGREDIENTS:

4 chicken breasts, skinless and boneless
3 oz breadcrumbs
2 tbsp grated Parmesan cheese
2 oz flour

2 eggs, beaten
1 tbsp fresh, chopped sage
Cooking spray

DIRECTIONS:

Place some plastic wrap underneath and on top of the chicken breasts. Using a rolling pin beat the meat until it becomes fragile. In a small bowl, combine the Parmesan, sage, and breadcrumbs. Dip the chicken in the egg first, and then in the sage mixture.

Spray with cooking oil and arrange the meat in the Ninja Foodi. Cook for 7 minutes on Air Crisp mode at 370 F.

Chicken Tenders with Broccoli & Rice

Servings: 3 | Ready in about: 60 min

INGREDIENTS:

1 pound chicken tenderloins
1 package instant long grain rice
1 cup chopped broccoli

2 cups water
1 can condensed cream chicken soup
1 tbsp minced garlic

DIRECTIONS:

Place the chicken quarters in the Ninja Foodi.

Season with salt, pepper and a tbsp of oil and cook for 30 minutes on Roast mode at 390 F. Meanwhile, in a bowl, mix rice, water, minced garlic, soup, and broccoli. Combine the mixture very well. Remove the chicken from the Ninja Foodi and place it on a platter to drain.

Spread the rice mixture on the bottom of the dish and place the chicken on top of the rice. Close the crisping lid and cook for 30 minutes on Roast mode at 390 F.

Buttermilk Chicken Thighs

Servings: 6 | Ready in about: 4 hours 40 min

INGREDIENTS:

1 ½ lb chicken thighs
1 tsp cayenne pepper
3 tsp salt divided
2 cups flour

2 tsp black pepper
1 tbsp paprika
1 tbsp baking powder
2 cups buttermilk

DIRECTIONS:

Rinse and pat dry the chicken thighs. Place the chicken thighs in a bowl. Add cayenne pepper, 2 tsp salt, black pepper, and buttermilk, and stir to coat well. Refrigerate for 4 hours. Preheat the Ninja Foodi to 350 degrees F.

In another bowl, mix the flour, paprika, 1 tsp salt, and baking powder.

Dredge half of the chicken thighs, one at a time, in the flour, and then place on a lined dish. Close the crisping lid and cook for 18 minutes on Air Crisp mode, flipping once halfway through. Repeat with the other batch.

Korean-Style Barbecued Satay

Servings: 4 | Ready in about: 4h 15 min

INGREDIENTS:

1 lb boneless,skinless chicken tenders
4 cloves garlic, chopped
4 scallions, chopped
2 tsp sesame seeds, toasted
1 tsp fresh ginger, grated

½ cup pineapple juice
½ cup soy sauce
⅓ cup sesame oil
1 pinch black pepper

DIRECTIONS:

Skew each tender and trim any excess fat. Mix the other ingredients in one large bowl. Add the skewered chicken and place in the fridge for 4 to 24 hours.

Preheat the Ninja Foodi to 370 degrees F. Using a paper towel, pat the chicken dry. Fry for 10 minutes on Air Crisp mode.

Sweet Garlicky Chicken Wings

Servings: 4 | Ready in about: 20 min

INGREDIENTS:

16 chicken wings
¼ cup butter
¼ cup honey

½ tsp salt
4 garlic cloves, minced
¾ cup potato starch

DIRECTIONS:

Rinse and pat dry the wings, and place them in a bowl.

Add the starch to the bowl, and mix to coat the chicken.

Place the chicken in a baking dish that has been previously coated lightly with cooking oil. Close the crisping lid and cook for 5 minutes on Air Crisp mode at 370 F. Meanwhile, whisk the rest of the ingredients together in a bowl.

Pour the sauce over the wings and cook for another 10 minutes.

Thyme Turkey Nuggets

Servings: 2 | Ready in about: 20 min

INGREDIENTS:

8 oz turkey breast, boneless and skinless
1 egg, beaten
1 cup breadcrumbs

1 tbsp dried thyme
½ tsp dried parsley
Salt and pepper, to taste

DIRECTIONS:

Mince the turkey in a food processor. Transfer to a bowl.

Stir in the thyme and parsley, and season with salt and pepper.

Take a nugget-sized piece of the turkey mixture and shape it into a ball, or another form. Dip it in the breadcrumbs, then egg, then in the breadcrumbs again. Place the nuggets onto a prepared baking dish.

Close the crisping lid and cook for 10 minutes on Air Crisp mode at 350 F.

Spicy Chicken Wings

Servings: 2 | Ready in about: 25 min

INGREDIENTS:

10 chicken wings
2 tbsp hot chili sauce
½ tbsp lime juice

½ tbsp honey
½ tsp kosher salt
½ tsp black pepper

DIRECTIONS:

Mix the lime juice, honey, and chili sauce.

Toss the mixture over the chicken wings.

Put the wings in the fryer's basket, close the crisping lid and cook for 25 minutes on Air Crisp mode at 350 F. Shake the basket every 5 minutes.

Herby Chicken with Asparagus Sauce

Servings: 4 | Ready in about: 1 hr

INGREDIENTS

1 (3 ½ pounds) Young Whole Chicken
4 garlic cloves, minced
1 tsp olive oil
4 fresh thyme, minced
3 fresh rosemary, minced
2 lemons, zested and quartered
salt and freshly ground black pepper to taste
2 tbsp olive oil

8 ounces asparagus, trimmed and chopped
1 onion, chopped
1 cup chicken stock
1 tbsp soy sauce
1 fresh thyme sprig
Cooking spray
1 tbsp flour
Chopped parsley to garnish

DIRECTIONS

Rub all sides of the chicken with garlic, rosemary, black pepper, lemon zest, minced thyme, and salt. Into the chicken cavity, insert lemon wedges.

Warm oil on Sear/Sauté. Add in onion and asparagus, and cook for 5 minutes until softened. Mix in chicken stock, 1 thyme sprig, black pepper, soy sauce, and salt.

Into the inner pot, set trivet over asparagus mixture. On top of the trivet, place your chicken with breast-side up.

Seal the pressure lid, choose Pressure, set to High, and set the timer to 20 minutes. Press Start. Once ready, do a quick release. Remove the chicken to a serving platter.

In the inner pot, sprinkle flour over asparagus mixture and blend the sauce with an immersion blender until desired consistency. Top the chicken with asparagus sauce and garnish with parsley.

Greek-Style Chicken with Potatoes

Servings: 4 | Ready in about: 40 min

INGREDIENTS

4 potatoes, peeled and quartered
4 cups water
2 lemons, zested and juiced
1 tbsp olive oil
2 tsp fresh oregano
Salt to taste
¼ tsp freshly ground black pepper
2 Serrano peppers, stemmed, cored, and chopped
4 boneless skinless chicken drumsticks

3 tbsp finely chopped parsley
1 cup packed watercress
1 cucumber, thinly sliced
½ cup cherry tomatoes, quartered
¼ cup Kalamata olives, pitted
¼ cup hummus
¼ cup feta cheese, crumbled
Lemon wedges, for serving

DIRECTIONS

In the cooker, add water and potatoes. Set trivet over them. In a baking bowl, mix lemon juice, olive oil, black pepper, oregano, zest, salt, and red pepper flakes. Add chicken drumsticks in the marinade and stir to coat.

Set the bowl with chicken on the trivet in the inner pot. Seal the lid, select Pressure and set the time to 15 minutes on High pressure. Press Start.

When ready, do a quick pressure release. Take out the bowl with chicken and the trivet from the pot. Drain potatoes and add parsley and salt.

Split the potatoes among four serving plates and top with watercress, cucumber slices, hummus, cherry tomatoes, chicken, olives, and feta cheese. Each bowl should be garnished with a lemon wedge.

Chicken Stroganoff with Fetucini

Servings: 4 | Ready in about: 35 min

INGREDIENTS

2 large boneless skinless chicken breasts
1½ tsp salt
2 tbsp butter
½ cup sliced onion
1 tbsp flour
½ cup dry white wine
1 ½ cups water

2 cups chicken stock
8 ounces fettucini
½ tsp Worcestershire sauce
1 cup sautéed mushrooms
¼ cup heavy cream
2 tbsp chopped fresh dill to garnish

DIRECTIONS

Season the chicken on both sides with salt and set aside. Choose Sear/Sauté and adjust to Medium. Press Start to preheat the pot. Melt the butter and sauté the onion until brown, about 3 minutes.

Mix in the flour to make a roux, about 2 minutes and gradually pour in the dry white wine while stirring and scraping the bottom of the pot to release any browned bits. Allow the white wine to simmer and to reduce by two-thirds.

Pour in the water, chicken stock, 1 tablespoon of salt, and fettucini. Mix and arrange the chicken on top of the fettucini.

Lock the pressure lid to Seal. Choose Pressure; adjust the pressure to High and the cook time to 5 minutes; press Start. When done pressure-cooking, perform a quick pressure release.

Transfer the chicken breasts to a cutting board to cool slightly, and then cut into bite-size chunks. Return the chicken to the pot and stir in the Worcestershire sauce and mushrooms. Add the heavy cream and cook until the mixture stops simmering.

Ladle the stroganoff into bowls and garnish with dill.

Tuscany-Style Turkey Soup

Servings: 4 | Ready in about: 40 min

INGREDIENTS

1 pound hot turkey sausage
2 tbsp olive oil
2 tbsp melted butter
3 celery stalks, chopped
3 garlic cloves, chopped
1 red onion, chopped
1 tsp salt
½ cup dry white wine
4 cups chicken broth

½ tsp fennel seeds
1 (15-oz) can cannellini beans, rinsed
9 ounces refrigerated tortellini
1 Parmesan cheese rind
2 cups chopped spinach
4 Italian bread slices
½ cup grated Parmesan cheese
Cooking spray

DIRECTIONS

On the Foodi, choose Sear/Sauté and adjust to Medium. Press Start to preheat the inner pot. Heat olive oil and cook the sausage for 4 minutes, while stirring occasionally until golden brown.

Stir in the celery, garlic, and onion, season with the salt and cook for 2 to 3 minutes, stirring occasionally. Pour in the wine and bring the mixture to a boil until the wine reduces by half. Scrape the bottom of the pot to let off any browned bits. Add the chicken stock, fennel seeds, tortellini, Parmesan rind, cannellini beans, and spinach.

Lock the pressure lid into place and to seal. Select Pressure; adjust the pressure to High and the cook time to 5 minutes; press Start. Brush the butter on the bread slices, and sprinkle with half of the cheese. Once the timer is over, perform a natural pressure release for 5 minutes.

Grease the reversible rack with cooking spray and fix in the upper position of the pot. Lay the bread slices on the rack.

Close the crisping lid and Choose Broil. Adjust the cook time to 5 minutes; press Start. When the bread has browned and crisp, transfer from the rack to a cutting board and let cool for a couple of minutes. Cut the slices into cubes.

Ladle the soup into bowls and sprinkle with the remaining cheese. Share the croutons among the bowls and serve.

Turkey and Brown Rice Salad with Peanuts

Servings: 4 | Ready in about: 60 min

INGREDIENTS

4 cups water
1 cup brown rice
2¼ tsp salt
1 pound turkey tenderloins
3 tsp peanut oil, divided
3 tbsp apple cider vinegar

⅛ tsp freshly ground black pepper
¼ tsp celery seeds
A pinch of sugar
½ cup peanuts, toasted
3 celery stalks, thinly sliced
1 apple, cored and cubed

DIRECTIONS

Pour the water into the inner pot. Stir in the brown rice and 1 teaspoon of salt. Lock the pressure lid into the Seal position. Choose Pressure; adjust the pressure to High and the cook time to 10 minutes. Press Start.

Season the turkey on both sides with salt; set aside. After cooking the brown rice, perform a natural pressure release for 10 minutes. Carefully open the lid and spoon the rice into a large bowl to cool completely.

Put the turkey in the Crisping Basket and brush with 2 teaspoons of peanut oil. Fix in the basket. Close the crisping lid and Choose Bake/Roast; adjust the temperature to 375°F and the cook time to 12 minutes; press Start.

Pour the remaining peanut oil and the vinegar into a jar with a tight-fitting lid. Add the black pepper, celery seeds, salt, and sugar. Close the jar and shake until the ingredients properly combined. When the turkey is ready, transfer to a plate to cool for several minutes. Cut it into bite-size chunks and add to the rice along with the peanuts, celery, and apple.

Pour half the dressing over the salad and toss gently to coat, adding more dressing as desired. Proceed to serve the salad.

RICE, GRAINS & PASTA

Indian-Style Beef with Rice

Servings: 5 | Ready in about: 40 min

INGREDIENTS

¼ cup yogurt
2 cloves garlic, smashed
1 tbsp olive oil
1 lime, juiced
Salt and black pepper to taste
2 pounds beef stew meat, cut into bite-sized cubes
1 tbsp garam masala
1 tbsp fresh ginger, grated
1 ½ tsp smoked paprika
1 tsp ground cumin

¼ tsp cayenne pepper
3 tbsp butter
1 onion, chopped
1 (14-ounce) can puréed tomatoes
½ cup beef broth
2 cups basmati rice, rinsed
2 cups water
½ cup heavy cream
½ bunch fresh cilantro, chopped

DIRECTIONS

In a bowl, mix garlic, lime juice, olive oil, pepper, salt and yogurt. Stir in the beef to coat.

In a different bowl, thoroughly mix paprika, garam masala, cumin, ginger, and cayenne pepper.

Melt butter on Sear/Sauté; stir-fry the onion for 7 to 9 minutes, until translucent. Sprinkle spice mixture over onion; cook for about 30 seconds until soft.

To the onion, add in the beef-yogurt mixture; cook for 3 to 4 minutes until meat is slightly cooked. Mix in broth and puréed tomatoes. Set trivet over beef in the pressure cooker's inner pot.

In an oven-proof bowl, mix water and rice. Set the bowl onto the trivet. Seal the pressure lid, press Pressure, set to High, and set the timer to 10 minutes; press Start. When ready, release pressure quickly.

Remove the bowl with rice and trivet. Add pepper, salt and cream into beef and stir. Use a fork to fluff rice and divide into serving plates; apply a topping of beef. Use cilantro to garnish.

Creamed Kale Parmesan Farro

Servings: 2 | Ready in about: 35 min

INGREDIENTS

1 tbsp butter
1 small onion, diced
1 cup pearl barley, rinsed and drained
2 garlic cloves, smashed
2 cups vegetable broth

½ cup grated Parmesan cheese, plus 1 tbsp for topping
1 cup kale, chopped
Juice of ½ lemon, juiced
Salt and freshly ground black pepper to taste

DIRECTIONS

Warm butter on Sear/Sauté. Add in onion and cook for 3 minutes until soft. Stir in garlic and barley, and cook for 1-2 minutes until barley is toasted; mix in broth. Seal the pressure lid, choose Pressure, set to High, and set the timer to 9 minutes. Press Start. Release pressure naturally for 10 minutes, then quick-release the remaining pressure.

Add Parmesan cheese into barley mixture and stir until fully melted. Just before serving, add lemon juice and kale into barley mixture. Add pepper and salt for seasoning.

Veggie Quinoa Bowls with Pesto

Servings: 2 | Ready in about: 30 min

INGREDIENTS

1 cup quinoa, rinsed and drained
2 cups vegetable broth
Salt and ground black pepper to taste
1 potato, peeled, cubed
1 head broccoli, cut into small florets
1 bunch baby heirloom carrots, peeled

¼ cabbage, sliced
2 eggs
1 avocado, thinly sliced
¼ cup pesto sauce
Lemon wedges, for serving

DIRECTIONS

In the Foodi, mix broth, pepper, quinoa and salt. Set trivet to the inner pot on top of quinoa and add a steamer basket to the top of the trivet. Mix carrots, potato, eggs and broccoli in the steamer basket. Add pepper and salt for seasoning.

Seal the pressure lid, choose Pressure, set to High, and set the timer to 1 minute. Press Start. Quick-release the pressure.

Take away the trivet and steamer basket from pot. Set the eggs in a bowl of ice water. Then peel and halve the eggs. Use a fork to fluff quinoa. Adjust the seasonings.

In two bowls, equally divide avocado, quinoa, broccoli, eggs, carrots, potato, and a dollop of pesto. Serve alongside a lemon wedge.

Shrimp Risotto with Vegetables

Servings: 4 | Ready in about: 1 hr 15 min

INGREDIENTS

1 tbsp avocado oil
1 pound asparagus, trimmed and roughly chopped
1 cup spinach, chopped
1½ cups mushrooms, sliced
1 cup rice, rinsed and drained
1¼ cups chicken broth

¾ cup coconut milk
1 tbsp coconut oil
16 shrimp, cleaned and deveined
Salt and ground black pepper to taste
¾ cup Parmesan cheese, shredded

DIRECTIONS

Warm the oil on Sear/Sauté. Add spinach, mushrooms and asparagus and cook for 10 minutes until cooked through; press Start. Add rice, coconut milk and broth to the pot as you stir.

Seal the pressure lid, choose Pressure, set to High, and set the timer to 40 minutes. Press Start. Do a quick release, open the lid and put the rice on a serving plate.

Take back the empty pot to the Foodi, add coconut oil and press Sear/Sauté. Add shrimp and cook each side taking 4 minutes until cooked through and turns pink.

Set the shrimp over rice, add pepper and salt for seasoning. Serve topped with shredded parmesan cheese.

Baked Garbanzo Beans and Pancetta

Servings: 6 | Ready in about: 50 min

INGREDIENTS

3 strips pancetta, cut into strips
1 onion, diced
15 oz canned garbanzo beans
2 cups water
1 cup apple cider
2 garlic cloves, minced

½ cup ketchup
¼ cup sugar
1 tsp ground mustard powder
1 tsp salt
1 tsp ground black pepper
Fresh parsley to garnish

DIRECTIONS

Set your Foodi to Sear/Sauté, set to Medium High, and choose Start/Stop to preheat the pot. Cook pancetta for 5 minutes until crispy. Add onion and garlic, and cook for 3 minutes until soft.

Mix in garbanzo beans, ketchup, sugar, salt, apple cider, mustard powder, water, and pepper.

Seal the pressure lid, press Pressure, set to High, and set the timer to 30 minutes; press Start.

Once done, release pressure naturally for 10 minutes, then turn steam vent valve to Venting to release the remaining pressure quickly. Serve in bowls garnished with parsley.

Black Beans Tacos

Servings: 6 | Ready in about: 1 hr 30 min

INGREDIENTS

2 cups black beans, soaked overnight
1 cup shallots, chopped
4 cups water
1 tbsp dried oregano
1 tsp chili powder

6 soft Taco tortillas
1 avocado, sliced
Salt to taste
Fresh Cilantro for garnish

DIRECTIONS

Drain the beans and add to the Foodi. Mix in the onion, oregano and chili powder. Pour water.

Seal the pressure lid, choose Pressure, set to High, and set the timer to 60 minutes. Press Start. Do a quick release, carefully open the lid and Allow cooling for a few minutes. Serve with taco tortillas, avocado slices and cilantro.

Herby Millet with Cherry Tomatoes

Servings: 8 | Ready in about: 1 hr 15 min

INGREDIENTS

2 cups millet, rinsed and drained
4 cups vegetable stock
½ sweet onion, chopped
1 cup cherry tomatoes, cut into halves

1 tbsp fresh sage, chopped
1 tsp fresh thyme, chopped
1 tsp fresh parsley, chopped
Salt and ground black pepper to taste

DIRECTIONS

Add millet, onion, and vegetable stock the inner pot of Foodi. Seal the pressure lid, choose Pressure, set to High, and set the timer to 10 minutes; press Start. When ready, release pressure quickly. Fluff the millet with a fork, add in herbs and tomatoes and apply a seasoning of pepper and salt.

Spicy Lentils with Chorizo

Servings: 10 | Ready in about: 50 min

INGREDIENTS

2 cups lentils, drained and rinsed

7 ounces chorizo, sliced

1 onion, diced

2 garlic cloves, crushed

2 cups tomato sauce

2 cups vegetable broth

½ cup mustard

½ cup cider vinegar

3 tbsp Worcestershire sauce

2 tbsp maple syrup

2 tbsp liquid smoke

1 tbsp lime juice

2 cups brown sugar

1 tbsp salt

1 tbsp black pepper

1 tsp chili powder

1 tsp paprika

¼ tsp cayenne pepper

DIRECTIONS

Set on Sear/Sauté, set to Medium High, and choose Start/Stop to preheat the pot; add in chorizo and cook for 3 minutes as you stir until crisp; add garlic and onion and cook for 2 more minutes until translucent.

Mix tomato sauce, broth, cider vinegar, liquid smoke, Worcestershire sauce, lime juice, mustard, and maple syrup in a mixing bowl. Pour the mixture in the Foodi to deglaze the pan, scrape the bottom of the pan to do away with any browned bits of food. Add pepper, chili powder, brown sugar, paprika, salt, and cayenne into the sauce mixture as you stir to mix.

Stir in lentils to coat. Seal the pressure lid, choose Pressure, set to High, and set the timer to 30 minutes. Press Start.

Release pressure naturally for 10 minutes.

Red Lentil and Spinach Dhal

Servings: 6 | Ready in about: 35 min

INGREDIENTS

2 tbsp olive oil

1 red jalapeño, seeded and minced

1 cup spinach, chopped

4 cloves garlic, minced

1 tsp fresh ginger, peeled and grated

1 tbsp cumin seeds

1 tbsp coriander seeds

1 tsp ground turmeric

¼ tsp cayenne pepper

3 cups water

1½ cups red lentils

1 tomato, diced

¼ cup lemon juice

Salt to taste

Fresh Cilantro, chopped for garnish

Natural yogurt for garnish

DIRECTIONS

Heat oil on Sear/Sauté, add cayenne pepper, jalapeño pepper, ginger, turmeric, cumin, and garlic, and coriander and cook for 2-3 minutes until seeds become fragrant and begin to pop.

Pour in water, tomato, and lentils into pot and stir. Seal the pressure lid, choose Pressure, set to High, and set the timer to 10 minutes; press Start. Release pressure naturally for 10 minutes, then turn steam vent valve to Venting to release the remaining pressure quickly.

Stir in spinach until wilted. Add lemon juice and season to taste. Divide lentils between bowls and garnish with yogurt and cilantro.

Parsley-Lime Bulgur Bowl

Servings: 4 | Ready in about: 30 min

INGREDIENTS

1 tbsp olive oil
1small onion, chopped
2 cloves garlic, minced
1 cup bulgur wheat
1 pinch salt

2 ½ cups vegetable broth
1 tbsp lime juice, or more to taste
1 handful fresh parsley, roughly chopped
10 black olives to garnish
Salt and black pepper to taste

DIRECTIONS

Heat oil on Sear/Sauté, stir in garlic and onion and cook for 10 to 13 minutes until golden brown. Add in cilantro, bulgur, salt, 1 tbsp lime juice, and vegetable broth.

Seal the pressure lid, choose Pressure, set to High, and set the timer to 1 minute.

Once ready, do a quick release. Use a fork to fluff bulgur. Add fresh parsley as you stir. Season with additional lime salt, juice, and pepper if desired. Serve in bowls topped with black olives.

Spinach and Kidney Bean Stew

Servings: 4 | Ready in about: 45 min

INGREDIENTS

2 tbsp olive oil
1 onion, chopped
2 cloves garlic, minced
2 carrots, peeled and sliced
1 cup celery, chopped
4 cups vegetable broth
1 cup white kidney beans, soaked, drained, rinsed

1 tsp dried thyme
1 tsp dried rosemary
1 bay leaf
A pinch of salt
1 cup spinach, torn into pieces
Salt and black pepper to taste

DIRECTIONS

Set your Foodi to Sear/Sauté, set to Medium High, and choose Start/Stop to preheat the pot. Warm olive oil; stir in garlic and onion and cook for 3 minutes until tender and fragrant. Mix in celery and carrots and cook for 2 to 3 minutes more until they start to soften. To the Foodi, add vegetable broth, bay leaf, thyme, rosemary, kidney beans, and salt.

Seal the pressure lid, choose Pressure, set to High, and set the timer to 30 minutes. Press Start. Quick release the pressure and add spinach to the beans as you stir and allow sit for 2 to 4 minutes until the spinach wilts; add pepper and salt for seasoning.

Tri-Color Quinoa and Pinto Bean Bowl

Servings: 5 | Ready in about: 30 min

INGREDIENTS

1 tsp extra-virgin olive oil
1 green bell pepper, diced
1 onion, diced
1 tsp ground cumin
½ tsp salt

14 ounces canned pinto beans, drained and rinsed
1 cup organic Tri-Color Quinoa, rinsed
1 cup red salsa
1 cup vegetable broth

DIRECTIONS

Warm oil on Sear/Sauté. Add red onion and green bell pepper as you stir. Add salt and cumin for seasoning and cook for 7-8 minutes until fragrant.

To the vegetable mixture, add quinoa, broth, salsa, and pinto beans.

Seal the pressure lid, choose Pressure, set to High, and set the timer to 12 minutes. Press Start. When ready, do a quick pressure release.

Use a fork to fluff quinoa and divide between serving bowls to serve.

Simple Brown Rice

Servings: 6 | Ready in about: 30 min

INGREDIENTS

1 ½ cups brown rice
3 cups chicken broth
2 tsp lemon juice

2 tsp sesame olive oil
1 tbsp toasted sunflower seeds

DIRECTIONS

Add broth and brown rice to the Foodi.

Seal the pressure lid, choose Pressure, set to High, and set the timer to 15 minutes. Press Start. When ready, release the pressure quickly.

Do not open the lid for an additional 5 minutes. Use a fork to fluff rice. Add lemon juice, sunflower seeds and oil.

Creamy Grana Padano Risotto

Servings: 6 | Ready in about: 25 min

INGREDIENTS

1 tbsp olive oil
1 white onion, chopped
1 tbsp butter
2 cups Carnaroli rice, rinsed
¼ cup dry white wine

4 cups chicken stock
1 tsp salt
½ tsp ground white pepper
2 tbsp Grana Padano cheese, grated
¼ tbsp Grana Padano cheese, flakes

DIRECTIONS

Warm oil on Sear/Sauté. Stir-fry onion for 3 minutes until soft and translucent. Add in butter and rice and cook for 5 minutes stirring occasionally.

Pour wine into the pot to deglaze, scrape away any browned bits of food from the pan. Stir in stock, pepper, and salt to the pot.

Seal the pressure lid, choose Pressure, set to High, and set the timer to 15 minutes. Press Start. When ready, release the pressure quickly.

Sprinkle with grated Parmesan cheese and stir well. Top with flaked cheese for garnish before serving.

Lemony Wild Rice Pilaf

Servings: 6 | Ready in about: 25 min

INGREDIENTS

4 cups vegetable broth
2 cups white wild rice, rinsed and drained
1 tbsp butter

Zest and juice from 1 lemon
½ tsp salt
½ tsp ground black pepper

DIRECTIONS

In your Foodi, mix rice, lemon zest, butter, and water.

Seal the pressure lid, choose Pressure, set to High, and set the timer to 3 minutes. Press Start. When ready, release pressure naturally for 10 minutes.

Sprinkle salt, lemon juice, and pepper over the pilaf and use a fork to gently fluff.

Rice Pilaf with Mushrooms

Servings: 6 | Ready in about: 35 min

INGREDIENTS

1 tbsp olive oil
2 cloves garlic, minced
1 yellow onion, finely chopped
2 cups button mushrooms, thinly sliced

4 cups vegetable stock
2 cups white rice
1 tsp salt
2 sprigs parsley, chopped

DIRECTIONS

Select Sear/Sauté, set to Medium High, choose Start/Stop to preheat the pot and heat oil.

Add mushrooms, onion, and garlic, and stir-fry for 5 minutes until tender. Mix in rice, stock, and salt. Seal the pressure lid, choose Pressure, set to High, and set the timer to 20 minutes. Press Start. When ready, release pressure naturally for 10 minutes.

Use a fork to fluff the rice and add parsley for garnishing before serving.

Quinoa with Carrots and Onion

Servings: 6 | Ready in about: 15 min

INGREDIENTS

1 cup quinoa, rinsed until the water runs clear
2 cups water
2 carrots, cut into sticks
1 large onion, sliced

2 tbsp olive oil
Salt to taste
Fresh cilantro, chopped for garnish

DIRECTIONS

Heat oil on Sear/Sauté. Add in onion and carrots and stir-fry for about 10 minutes until tender and crispy; remove to a plate. Add water, salt and quinoa to the steel pot of the Foodi.

Seal the pressure lid, choose Pressure, set to High, and set the timer to 1 minute. Press Start.

Once ready, do a quick release. Fluff the cooked quinoa with a fork. Transfer to a serving plate and top with the carrots and onion. Serve scattered with cilantro.

Three-Bean Veggie Chili

Servings: 8 | Ready in about: 1 hr

INGREDIENTS

1 tbsp canola oil
1 onion, chopped
3 stalks of celery, chopped
1 green bell pepper, chopped
1 head broccoli, chopped into florets
2 tbsp minced garlic
2 tbsp chili powder
2 tsp ground cumin
4 cups vegetable broth

1 (28 ounces) can tomatoes, crushed
½ cup dried pinto beans, soaked, drained and rinsed
½ cup dried black beans, soaked, drained and rinsed
½ cup dried cannellini beans, soaked, drained and rinsed
1 bay leaf
Salt to taste
Fresh parsley, chopped for garnish

DIRECTIONS

Warm oil on Sear/Sauté. Add onion and bell pepper, broccoli, and celery, and cook for about 8 minutes until softened. Mix in cumin, chili powder, and garlic and cook for another 1 minute.

Add vegetable broth, tomatoes, black beans, salt, cannellini beans, pinto beans, and bay leaf to the pot.

Seal the pressure lid, choose Pressure, set to High, and set the timer to 25 minutes. Press Start. When ready, do a quick pressure release.

Dispose of the bay leaf. Taste and adjust the seasonings. Sprinkle with fresh parsley and serve.

Black-Eyed Peas with Kale

Servings: 6 | Ready in about: 30 min

INGREDIENTS

1 tsp olive oil
1 onion, thinly sliced
2 garlic cloves, minced
1 cup fire-roasted red peppers, diced
½ tsp ground allspice
½ tsp red pepper, crushed

Salt to taste
1 ½ cups dried black-eyed peas, soaked and rinsed
1 ½ cups vegetable broth
1 bay leaf
1 (15 ounces) can fire roasted tomatoes
2 cups chopped kale

DIRECTIONS

Warm oil on Sear/Sauté. Add onion and cook for 5 minutes until fragrant; add garlic and fire roasted red peppers and cook for 1 more minute until softened.

To the vegetable mixture, add a seasoning of salt, crushed red pepper, and allspice.

Add vegetable broth, bay leaf, and black-eyed peas to the pot.

Seal the pressure lid, choose Pressure, set to High, and set the timer to 5 minutes. Press Start. When ready, do a quick pressure release.

Remove the bay leaf and discard. Mix the peas with kale and tomatoes.

Seal the pressure lid again, choose Pressure, set to High, and set the timer to 1 minute. Press Start. When ready, release the pressure quickly. Adjust the seasoning and serve.

Easy Vegan Sloppy Joes

Servings: 6 | Ready in about: 45 min

INGREDIENTS

2 cups water
1 cup pearl barley, rinsed
1 cup green onion, chopped
1 clove garlic, minced
2 cups tomato sauce
2 tbsp brown sugar

2 tbsp Worcestershire sauce
1 tsp Dijon mustard
1 tsp smoked paprika
1 tsp chili powder
6 brioche buns
Dill Pickles for garnish

DIRECTIONS

In the pot, mix Worcestershire sauce, water, onion, garlic, brown sugar, barley, tomato sauce, and spices.

Seal the pressure lid, choose Pressure, set to High, and set the timer to 25 minutes. Press Start. When ready, release the pressure quickly.

Press Sear/Sauté and cook until the mixture becomes thick.

Transfer the sloppy joe mixture to the brioche buns and add a topping of dill pickles.

Indian Yellow Lentils

Servings: 6 | Ready in about: 30 min

INGREDIENTS

1 tbsp ghee
2 tsp cumin seeds
1 onion, chopped
4 garlic cloves, minced
1-inch piece of ginger, peeled, minced
Sea salt salt
1 tomato, chopped

2 cups split yellow lentils, soaked and drained
2 tbsp garam masala
½ tsp ground turmeric
½ tsp cayenne pepper
6 cups water
1 tbsp fresh cilantro, finely chopped

DIRECTIONS

Warm ghee on Sear/Sauté, set to Medium High, and choose Start/Stop to preheat the pot. Press Start. Add cumin seeds and cook for 10 seconds until they begin to pop; stir in onion and cook for 2 to 3 minutes until softened. Mix in ginger and garlic and cook for 1 minute as you stir. Add salt for seasoning.

Mix in tomato and cook for 3 to 5 minutes until the mixture breaks down. Stir in turmeric, lentils, garam masala, and cayenne and cover with water. Seal the pressure lid, choose Pressure, set to High, and set the timer to 8 minutes. Press Start.

When ready, release pressure quickly. Serve in bowls sprinkled with fresh cilantro.

Cherry Tomato-Basil Linguine

Servings: 4 | Ready in about: 22 min

INGREDIENTS

2 tbsp olive oil
1 small onion, diced
2 garlic cloves, minced
1 cup cherry tomatoes, halved

1 ½ cups vegetable stock
¼ cup julienned basil leaves
1 tsp salt
½ tsp ground black pepper

¼ tsp red chili flakes
1 pound Linguine noodles, halved

Fresh basil leaves for garnish
½ cup Parmigiano-Reggiano cheese, grated

DIRECTIONS

Warm oil on Sear/Sauté. Add onion and cook for 2 minutes until soft. Mix garlic and tomatoes and sauté for 4 minutes. To the pot, add vegetable stock, salt, julienned basil, red chili flakes and pepper.

Add linguine to the tomato mixture until covered. Seal the pressure lid, choose Pressure, set to High, and set the timer to 5 minutes. Press Start.

When ready, naturally release the pressure for 5 minutes. Stir the mixture to ensure it is broken down. Divide into plates. Top with basil and Parmigiano-Reggiano cheese and serve.

South American Black Bean Chili

Servings: 8 | Ready in about: 1 hr 10 min

INGREDIENTS

1 tsp olive oil
1 onion, chopped
3 cloves garlic, minced
6 cups vegetable broth
2 cups dried black beans, soaked, drained and rinsed
1 jalapeño pepper, deseeded and diced

1 tsp dried oregano
1 tsp dried chili flakes
Salt to taste
Cotija Cheese, crumbled for garnish
Fresh cilantro for garnish

DIRECTIONS

Warm oil on Sear/Sauté. Add in garlic and onion and cook for 3 to 4 minutes until fragrant. Add beans, vegetable broth, oregano, chili flakes, salt and jalapeño pepper.

Seal the pressure lid, choose Pressure, set to High, and set the timer to 35 minutes. Press Start. When ready, quick-release pressure. Divide between serving plates. Apply a topping of cilantro and cotija cheese to serve.

Spicy Pinto Bean and Corn Stew

Servings: 6 | Ready in about: 1 hr 5 min

INGREDIENTS

2 tbsp olive oil
1 onion, chopped
1 red bell pepper, chopped
1 tbsp dried oregano
1 tbsp ground cumin
1 tsp red pepper flakes
3 cups vegetable stock

2 cups dried pinto beans, rinsed
14 ounces canned tomatoes, chopped
1 tsp sea salt
1 tbsp white wine vinegar
½ cup fresh chives, chopped
¼ cup fresh corn kernels

DIRECTIONS

Set your Foodi to Sear/Sauté, set to Medium High, and choose Start/Stop to preheat the pot. Press Start. Stir in oil, bell pepper, pepper flakes, oregano, onion, and cumin. Cook for 3 minutes until soft.

Mix in pinto beans, vegetable stock, and tomatoes. Seal the pressure lid, choose Pressure, set to High, and set the timer to 30 minutes. Press Start. Release pressure naturally for 20 minutes. Add in salt and vinegar. Divide in serving plates and top with corn and fresh chives.

Simple Jasmine Rice

Servings: 4 | Ready in about: 25 min

INGREDIENTS

2 cups jasmine rice
3 ½ cups of water

Salt and black pepper to taste

DIRECTIONS

Stir rice and water together in the Foodi. Season with salt to taste. Seal the pressure lid, press Pressure, set to High, and set the timer to 15 minutes; press Start. When ready, release pressure naturally for 10 minutes. Use a fork to fluff rice. Season with black pepper before serving.

Chili-Garlic Rice Noodles with Tofu

Servings: 6 | Ready in about: 20 min

INGREDIENTS

2 cups water
½ cup soy sauce
2 tbsp brown sugar
2 tbsp rice vinegar
1 tbsp sweet chili sauce

1 tbsp sesame oil
1 tsp fresh minced garlic
20 ounces extra firm tofu, pressed and cubed
8 ounces rice noodles
1/4 cup chopped fresh chives, for garnish

DIRECTIONS

Heat the oil on Sear/Sauté and fry the tofu for 5 minutes until golden brown. Set aside.

To the pot, add water, garlic, olive oil, vinegar, brown sugar, soy sauce, and chili sauce and mix well until smooth; stir in rice noodles.

Seal the pressure lid, choose Pressure, set to High, and set the timer to 3 minutes. Press Start. When ready, release the pressure quickly. Split the noodles between bowls. Top with fried tofu and sprinkle with fresh chives before serving.

Rigatoni with Sausage and Spinach

Servings: 4 | Ready in about: 45 min

INGREDIENTS

1 tbsp butter
½ cup diced red bell pepper
1 onion, chopped
3 cups vegetable broth
¼ cup tomato purée
4 sausage links, sliced

2 tsp chili powder
salt and ground black pepper to taste
12 ounces rigatoni pasta
1 cup baby spinach
½ cup Parmesan cheese

DIRECTIONS

Warm the butter on Sear/Sauté. Add red bell pepper, onion, and sausage, and cook for 5 minutes.

Mix in vegetable broth, chili powder, tomato paste, salt, and pepper to combine. Stir in rigatoni pasta.

Seal the pressure lid, choose Pressure, set to High, and set the timer to 12 minutes. Press Start. When ready, naturally release pressure for 20 minutes. Stir in spinach and let simmer until wilted. Top with Parmesan cheese and serve.

Chicken and Chickpea Stew

Servings: 6 | Ready in about: 40 min

INGREDIENTS

1 pound boneless, skinless chicken legs

2 tsp ground cumin

1 tsp salt

½ tsp cayenne pepper

2 tbsp olive oil

1 onion, minced

2 jalapeño peppers, deseeded and minced

3 garlic cloves, crushed

2 tsp freshly grated ginger

¼ cup chicken stock

1 (24 ounces) can crushed tomatoes

2 (14 ounces) cans chickpeas, drained and rinsed

Salt to taste

⅔ cup coconut milk

¼ cup fresh parsley, chopped

2 cups hot cooked basmati rice

DIRECTIONS

Season the chicken with 1 tsp salt, cayenne pepper, and cumin.

Set your Foodi to Sear/Sauté, set to Medium High, and choose Start/Stop to preheat the pot. Warm oil.

Add in jalapeño peppers and onion and cook for 5 minutes until soft; mix in ginger and garlic and cook for 3 minutes until tender.

Add ¼ cup chicken stock into the Foodi to ensure the pan is deglazed, from the pan's bottom scrape any browned bits of food.

Mix the onion mixture with chickpeas, tomatoes, and salt. Stir in the chicken to coat in sauce.

Seal the pressure lid, choose Pressure, set to High, and set the timer to 20 minutes. Press Start. When ready, release the pressure quickly.

Transfer the chicken from the cooker and slice into chunks.

Into the remaining sauce, mix in coconut milk; simmer for 5 minutes on Keep Warm.

Split rice into 6 bowls. Top with chicken, then sauce and add cilantro for garnish.

Shrimp Lo Mein

Servings: 2 | Ready in about: 20 min

INGREDIENTS

1 tbsp sesame oil

1 lb shrimp, peeled and deveined

½ cup diced onion

2 cloves garlic, minced

1 cup carrots, cut into strips

1 cup green beans, washed

2 cups vegetable stock

3 tbsp soy sauce

2 tbsp rice wine vinegar

10 ounces lo mein egg noodles

½ tsp toasted sesame seeds

Sea salt and ground black pepper to taste

DIRECTIONS

Warm oil on Sear/Sauté. Stir-fry the shrimp for 5 minutes. Remove to a plate and set aside.

Add in garlic and onion and cook for 3 minutes until fragrant. Mix in soy sauce, carrots, vegetable stock, green beans, and rice wine vinegar. Add noodles into the mixture and ensure they are covered. Season with pepper and salt.

Seal the pressure lid, choose Pressure, set to High, and set the timer to 5 minutes. Press Start. When ready, release the pressure quickly. Plate the lo mein, add the reserved shrimp, sprinkle with sesame seeds, and serve.

Beef-Stuffed Pasta Shells

Servings: 4 | Ready in about: 35 min

INGREDIENTS

2 tbsp olive oil
1 pound ground beef
16 ounces pasta shells
2 cups water
15 ounces tomato sauce
15-ounce can black beans, drained and rinsed
15-ounces canned corn, drained

10 ounces red enchilada sauce
4 ounces diced green chiles
1 cup shredded mozzarella cheese
salt and ground black pepper to taste
additional cheese for topping if desired
Finely chopped parsley for garnish

DIRECTIONS

Heat oil on Sear/Sauté. Add ground beef and cook for 7 minutes until it starts to brown.

Mix in pasta, tomato sauce, enchilada sauce, black beans, water, corn, and green chiles and stir to coat well. Add more water if desired.

Seal the pressure lid, choose Pressure, set to High, and set the timer to 10 minutes. Press Start. When ready, do a quick pressure release. Into the pasta mixture, mix in mozzarella cheese until melted; add black pepper and salt. Garnish with parsley to serve.

Turkey Fajita Tortiglioni

Servings: 6 | Ready in about: 35 min

INGREDIENTS

2 tsp chili powder
1 tsp salt
1 tsp cumin
1 tsp onion powder
1 tsp garlic powder
½ tsp thyme
1 ½ pounds turkey breast, cut into strips
1 tbsp olive oil
1 medium red onion, cut into wedges
4 garlic cloves, minced

3 cups chicken broth
1 cup salsa
16 ounces tortiglioni
1 red bell pepper, sliced diagonally
1 yellow bell pepper, sliced diagonally
1 green bell pepper, sliced diagonally
1 cup shredded Gouda cheese
½ cup sour cream
½ cup chopped parsley

DIRECTIONS

In a bowl, mix chili powder, cumin, garlic powder, onion powder, salt, and oregano. Reserve 1 tsp seasoning. Coat turkey with the remaining seasoning.

Warm the oil on Sear/Sauté. Add in turkey strips and cook for 4 to 5 minutes until browned. Place the turkey in a bowl.

Cook the onion and garlic lightly for 1 minute until soft.

In the Foodi, mix salsa and chicken broth, scrape the bottom of any brown bits.

Into the broth mixture, stir in tortiglioni pasta and cover with bell peppers and turkey.

Seal the pressure lid, choose Pressure, set to High, and set the timer to 5 minutes. Press Start. When ready, do a quick pressure release. Open the lid and sprinkle with shredded gouda cheese and reserved seasoning and stir well. Add more salt if desired. Divide into plates and top with sour cream. Add parsley for garnishing and serve.

Chipotle Mac and Cheese

Servings: 6 | Ready in about: 15 min

INGREDIENTS

12 ounces macaroni
4 cups cold water
1 tsp salt
2 eggs
1 tbsp chipotle chili powder
½ tsp ground black pepper

4 tbsp butter
1½ cup milk
4 cups sharp Cheddar cheese, grated
2 cups Pecorino Romano cheese, grated
Salt and black pepper to taste

DIRECTIONS

In your Foodi, add salt, water and macaroni. Seal the pressure lid, choose Pressure, set to High, and set the timer to 4 minutes. Press Start.

As the pasta cooks, take a bowl and beat eggs, chipotle chili powder, and black pepper, to mix well.

When ready, release the pressure quickly. Add butter to the pasta and stir until melts. Stir in milk and egg mixture.

Pour in Pecorino Romano and Cheddar cheeses until well melted. You can do so in batches.

Add pepper and salt to season.

Chicken Ragù Bolognese

Servings: 8 | Ready in about: 50 min

INGREDIENTS

2 tbsp olive oil
6 ounces bacon, cubed
1 onion, minced
1 carrot, minced
1 celery stalk, minced
2 garlic cloves, crushed
¼ cup tomato paste

¼ tsp crushed red pepper flakes
1 ½ pounds ground chicken
½ cup white wine
1 cup milk
1 cup chicken broth
Salt to taste
1 pound spaghetti

DIRECTIONS

Warm oil on Sear/Sauté. Add in bacon and fry for 5 minutes until crispy.

Add celery, carrot, garlic and onion and cook for 5 minutes until fragrant. Mix in red pepper flakes and tomato paste and cook for 2 minutes. Break chicken into small pieces and place in the pot. Cook for 10 minutes as you stir until browned. Pour in wine and simmer for 2 minutes. Add in chicken broth and milk.

Seal the pressure lid, choose Pressure, set to High, and set the timer to 15 minutes. Press Start. When ready, release the pressure quickly.

Add in the spaghetti and stir. Seal the pressure lid again, choose Pressure, set to High, and set the timer to another 5 minutes. Press Start.

When ready, release the pressure quickly. Check the pasta for doneness. If necessary press Sear/Sauté and cook for an additional 2 minutes. Adjust the seasoning and serve right away.

Pasta Caprese Ricotta-Basil Fusilli

Servings: 3 | Ready in about: 15 min

INGREDIENTS

1 tbsp olive oil
1 onion, thinly sliced
6 garlic cloves, minced
1 tsp red pepper flakes
2 ½ cups dried fusilli
1 (15 ounces) can tomato sauce

1 cup tomatoes, halved
1 cup water
¼ cup basil leaves
1 tsp salt
1 cup Ricotta cheese, crumbled
2 tbsp chopped fresh basil

DIRECTIONS

Warm the oil on Sear/Sauté. Add in red pepper flakes, garlic and onion and cook for 3 minutes until soft.

Mix in fusilli, tomatoes, half of the basil leaves, water, tomato sauce, and salt.

Seal the pressure lid, choose Pressure, set to High, and set the timer to 4 minutes. Press Start. When ready, release the pressure quickly.

Transfer the pasta to a serving platter and top with the crumbled ricotta and remaining chopped basil.

Cheese and Spinach Stuffed Shells

Servings: 6 | Ready in about: 1 hr

INGREDIENTS

2 cups onion, chopped
1 cup carrot, chopped
3 garlic cloves, minced
3 ½ tbsp olive oil,
1 (28 ounces) canned tomatoes, crushed
12 ounces jumbo shell pasta
1 tbsp olive oil
2 cups ricotta cheese, crumbled

1 ½ cup feta cheese, crumbled
2 cups spinach, chopped
¾ cup grated Pecorino Romano cheese
2 tbsp chopped fresh chives
1 tbsp chopped fresh dill
Salt and ground black pepper to taste
1 cup shredded cheddar cheese

DIRECTIONS

Warm olive oil on Sear/Sauté. Add in onion, carrot, and garlic, and cook for 5 minutes until tender; stir in tomatoes and cook for another 10 minutes. Remove to a bowl and set aside.

Wipe the pot with a damp cloth, add pasta and cover with enough water. Seal the pressure lid, choose Pressure, set to High, and set the timer to 5 minutes. Press Start.

Do a quick pressure and drain the pasta. Lightly grease olive oil to a baking sheet.

In a bowl, combine feta and ricotta cheese. Add in spinach, Pecorino Romano cheese, dill, and chives, and stir well. Adjust the seasonings. Using a spoon, fill the shells with the mixture.

Spread 4 cups tomato sauce on the baking sheet. Place the stuffed shells over with seam-sides down and sprinkle cheddar cheese atop. Use aluminum foil to the cover the baking dish.

Pour 1 cup of water in the pot of the Foodi and insert the trivet. Lower the baking dish onto the trivet.

Seal the pressure lid, choose Pressure, set to High, and set the timer to 15 minutes. Press Start. Once ready, do a quick release. Take away the foil.

Place the stuffed shells to serving plates and top with tomato sauce before serving.

Pomodoro Sauce with Rigatoni and Kale

Servings: 6 | Ready in about: 15 min

INGREDIENTS

1 pound rigatoni pasta
15 ounces canned tomato sauce
3 garlic cloves, minced
1 tsp chili flakes
2 tsp salt

2 tbsp extra-virgin olive oil
1 handful fresh basil, minced
1 cup kale, chopped
¼ cup Parmesan cheese

DIRECTIONS

In your Foodi, mix tomato sauce, salt, pasta, chili flakes, and garlic powder. Cover with water.

Seal lid and cook for 5 minutes on Low Pressure. When ready, release the pressure quickly. Stir in kale until wilted.

Plate the pasta and top with the parmesan and basil. Drizzle olive oil over the pasta.

Pork Spaghetti with Spinach and Tomatoes

Servings: 4 | Ready in about: 35 min

INGREDIENTS

2 tbsp olive oil
½ cup onion, chopped
1 garlic clove, minced
1 pound pork sausage meat
2 cups water
1 (14 ounces) can diced tomatoes, drained
½ cup sun-dried tomatoes

1 tbsp dried oregano
1 tsp Italian seasoning
1 fresh jalapeño chile, stemmed, seeded, and minced
1 tsp salt
8 ounces dried spaghetti, halved
1 cup spinach

DIRECTIONS

Warm oil on Sear/Sauté. Add in onion and garlic and cook for 2 minutes until softened.

Stir in sausage meat and cook for 5 minutes. Stir in jalapeño, water, sun-dried tomatoes, Italian seasoning, oregano, diced tomatoes, and salt; mix spaghetti and press to submerge into the sauce.

Seal the pressure lid, choose Pressure, set to High, and set the timer to 9 minutes. Press Start. When ready, release the pressure quickly.

Stir in spinach, close lid again, and simmer on Keep Warm for 5 minutes until spinach is wilted.

Ground Beef Stuffed Empanadas

Servings: 2 | Ready in about: 60 min

INGREDIENTS

1 tbsp olive oil
1 garlic clove, minced
½ white onion, chopped
¼ pound ground beef
6 green olives, pitted and chopped
¼ tsp cumin powder

¼ tsp paprika
⅛ tsp cinnamon powder
2 small tomatoes, chopped
8 square gyoza wrappers
1 egg, beaten

DIRECTIONS

Choose Sear/Sauté on the pot and set to Medium High. Choose Start/Stop to preheat the pot.

Put the oil, garlic, onion, and beef in the preheated pot and cook for 5 minutes, stirring occasionally, until the fragrant and the beef is no longer pink.

Stir in the olives, cumin, paprika, and cinnamon and cook for an additional 3 minutes. Add the tomatoes and cook for 1 more minute.

Spoon the beef mixture into a plate and allow cooling for a few minutes.

Meanwhile, put the Crisping Basket in the pot. Close the crisping lid; choose Air Crisp, set the temperature to 400°F, and the time to 5 minutes. Press Start.

Lay the gyoza wrappers on a flat surface. Place 1 to 2 tablespoons of the beef mixture in the middle of each wrapper. Brush the edges of the wrapper with egg and fold in half to form a triangle. Pinch the edges together to seal.

Place 4 empanadas in a single layer in the preheated Basket.

Close the crisping lid. Choose Air Crisp, set the temperature to 400°F, and set the time to 7 minutes. Choose Start/Stop to begin frying.

Once the timer is done, remove the empanadas from the basket and transfer to a plate. Repeat with the remaining empanadas.

Smoky Horseradish Spare Ribs

Servings: 4 | Ready in about: 55 min

INGREDIENTS

1 spare rack ribs
1 tsp salt

1 cup smoky horseradish sauce

DIRECTIONS

Season all sides of the rack with salt and cut into 3 pieces. Cut the rack into 3 pieces.

Pour 1 cup of water into the Foodi's inner pot. Fix the reversible rack in the pot in the lower position and put the ribs on top, bone-side down.

Seal the pressure lid, choose Pressure; adjust the pressure to High and the cook time to 18 minutes. Press Start. After cooking, perform a quick pressure release and carefully open the lid.

Take out the rack with ribs and pour out the water from the pot. Return the inner pot to the base. Set the reversible rack and ribs in the pot in the lower position. Close the crisping lid and Choose Air Crisp; adjust the temperature to 400°F and the cook time to 20 minutes. Press Start.

After 10 minutes, open the lid and turn the ribs. Lightly baste the bony side of the ribs with the smoky horseradish sauce and close the lid to cook further. After 4 minutes, open the lid and turn the ribs again. Baste the meat side with the remaining sauce and close the lid to cook until the ribs are done.

Teriyaki Pork Noodles

Servings: 4 | Ready in about: 60 min

INGREDIENTS

8 ounces egg noodles
1 pound green beans, trimmed
1 tbsp olive oil
¼ tsp salt
¼ tsp black pepper

1 pork tenderloin, trimmed and cut into 1-inch pieces
1 cup teriyaki sauce
Cooking spray
Sesame seeds, for garnish

DIRECTIONS

Pour the egg noodles and cover with egough water in the pot. Seal the pressure lid, choose Pressure, set to High, and set the time to 2 minutes. Choose Start/Stop.

In a large bowl, toss the green beans with the olive oil, salt, and black pepper. In another bowl, toss the pork with the teriyaki sauce.

When the egg noodles are ready, perform a quick pressure release, and carefully open the lid.

Fix the reversible rack in the upper position of the pot, which will be over the egg noodles. Oil the rack with cooking spray and place the pork in the rack. Also, lay the green beans around the pork.

Close the crisping lid. Choose Broil and set the time to 12 minutes. Press Start/Stop to begin cooking the pork and vegetables.

When done cooking, check for your desired crispiness and take the rack out of the pot. Serve the pork and green beans over the drained egg noodles and garnish with sesame seeds.

Greek Beef Gyros

Servings: 4 | Ready in about: 55 min

INGREDIENTS

1 pound beef sirloin, cut into thin strips
1 onion, thinly sliced
⅓ cup beef broth
2 tbsp fresh lemon juice
2 tbsp olive oil
2 tsp dry oregano

1 clove garlic, minced
salt and ground black pepper to taste
4 slices pita bread
1 cup Greek yogurt
2 tbsp fresh dill, chopped

DIRECTIONS

In the Foodi, mix beef, beef broth, oregano, garlic, lemon juice, pepper, onion, olive oil, and salt.

Seal the pressure lid, choose Pressure, set to High, and set the timer to 30 minutes. Press Start. Release pressure naturally for 15 minutes, then turn steam vent valve to Venting to release the remaining pressure quickly.

Divide the beef mixture between the pita bread slices, top with yogurt and dill, and roll up to serve.

Sweet Gingery Beef and Broccoli

Servings: 4 | Ready in about: 70 min

INGREDIENTS

1 tbsp olive oil
2 pounds skirt steak, cut into strips
4 garlic cloves, minced
½ cup coconut aminos
½ cup water, plus 3 tbsp

⅔ cup dark brown sugar
½ tsp ginger puree
2 tbsp cornstarch
1 head broccoli, trimmed into florets
3 scallions, thinly sliced

DIRECTIONS

Choose Sear/Sauté on the pot and set to Medium High; hit Start/Stop to preheat the pot.

Pour the oil and beef in the preheated pot and brown the beef strips on both sides, about 5 minutes in total. Remove the beef from the pot and set aside.

Add the garlic to the oil and Sear/Sauté for 1 minute or until fragrant.

Stir in the coconut aminos, ½ cup of water, brown sugar, and ginger to the pot. Mix evenly and add the beef. Seal the pressure lid, choose Pressure, set to High, and set the time to 10 minutes. Choose Start/Stop to begin cooking.

Meanwhile, in a small bowl whisk combine the cornstarch and the remaining water.

When done cooking, perform a quick pressure release. Choose Sear/Sauté and set to Medium Low. Choose Start/Stop. Pour in the cornstarch mixture and stir continuously until the sauce becomes syrupy. Add the broccoli, stir to coat in the sauce, and cook for another 5 minutes.

Once ready, garnish with scallions, and serve.

Bolognese-Style Pizza

Servings: 4 | Ready in about: 70 min

INGREDIENTS

4 pizza crusts
Cooking spray
½ cup canned crushed tomatoes
1 yellow bell pepper, sliced, divided

½ lb ground pork, meat cooked and crumbled
1 cup shredded mozzarella cheese
1 tsp red chili flakes, divided.
1 tbsp chopped fresh basil, for garnish

DIRECTIONS

Place the reversible rack in the pot. Close the crisping lid; choose Air Crisp, set the temperature to 400°F, and the time to 5 minutes.

Grease one side of a pizza crust with cooking spray and lay on the preheated rack, oiled side up. Close the crisping lid. Choose Air Crisp, set the temperature to 400°F, and set the time to 4 minutes. Choose Start/Stop to begin baking.

Remove the crust from the rack and flip so the crispy side is down. Top the crust with 2 tablespoons of crushed tomatoes, a quarter of bell pepper, 2 ounces of ground pork, ¼ cup of mozzarella cheese, and ¼ tablespoon of red chili flakes.

Close the crisping lid. Choose Broil and set the time to 3 minutes. Choose Start/Stop to continue baking.

When done baking and crispy as desired, remove the pizza from the rack. Repeat with the remaining pizza crusts and ingredients. Top each pizza with some basil and serve.

Juicy Barbecue Pork Chops

Servings: 4 | Ready in about: 100 min

INGREDIENTS

3 tbsp brown sugar
1 tbsp salt
1½ tbsp smoked paprika
2 tsp garlic powder
1 tbsp freshly ground black pepper

4 bone-in pork chops
1 tbsp olive oil
1½ cups chicken broth
4 tbsp barbecue sauce

DIRECTIONS

Choose Sear/Sauté and set to High. Choose Start/Stop to preheat the pot. In a small bowl, mix the brown sugar, salt, paprika, garlic powder, and black pepper. Season both sides of the pork with the rub.

Heat the oil in the preheated pot and sear the pork chops, one at a time, on both sides, about 5 minutes per chop. Set aside.

Pour the chicken broth into the pot and with a wooden spoon, scrape the bottom of the pot of any browned bits. Place the Crisping Basket in the upper position of the pot. Put the pork chops in the basket and brush with 2 tablespoons of barbecue sauce.

Seal the pressure lid, choose Pressure and set to High. Set the time to 5 minutes, then Choose Start/Stop to begin cooking. When the timer is done, perform a natural pressure release for 10 minutes, then a quick pressure release, and carefully open the lid.

Apply the remaining barbecue sauce on both sides of the pork and close the crisping lid. Choose Broil and set the time to 3 minutes. Press Start/Stop to begin. When ready, check for your desired crispiness and remove the pork from the basket.

Baked Rigatoni with Beef Tomato Sauce

Servings: 4 | Ready in about: 75 min

INGREDIENTS

1 tbsp butter
2 pounds ground beef
2 (24-ounce) cans tomato sauce
1 cup water
1 cup dry red wine
16-ounce dry rigatoni

½ tsp garlic powder
½ tsp salt
1 cup cottage cheese
1 cup shredded mozzarella cheese
½ cup chopped fresh parsley

DIRECTIONS

Choose Sear/Sauté and set to High. Choose Start/Stop to preheat the pot. Melt the butter, add the beef and cook for 5 minutes, or until browned and cooked well.

Stir in the tomato sauce, water, wine, and rigatoni; season with the garlic powder and salt.

Put the pressure lid together and lock in the Seal position. Choose Pressure, set to Low, and set the time to 2 minutes. Choose Start/Stop to begin cooking.

When the timer is done, perform a natural pressure release for 10 minutes, then a quick pressure release and carefully open the lid. Stir in the cottage cheese and evenly sprinkle the top of the pasta with the mozzarella cheese. Close the crisping lid. Choose Broil, and set the time to 3 minutes. Choose Start/Stop to begin. Cook for 3 minutes, or until the cheese has melted, slightly browned, and bubbly.

Garnish with the parsley and serve immediately.

Honey Short Ribs with Rosemary Potatoes

Servings: 4 | Ready in about: 105 min

INGREDIENTS

4 bone-in beef short ribs, silver skin
1 tsp salt
1 tsp black pepper
2 tbsp olive oil
1 onion, chopped

2 tbsp honey
½ cup beef broth
2 tbsp minced fresh rosemary
3 garlic cloves, minced
2 potatoes, peeled and cut into 1-inch pieces

DIRECTIONS

Choose Sear/Sauté on the pot and set to High. Choose Start/Stop to preheat the pot. Season the short ribs on all sides with ½ teaspoon of salt and ½ teaspoon of pepper.

Heat 1 tablespoon of olive oil and brown the ribs on all sides, about 10 minutes total. Stir in the onion, honey, broth, 1 tablespoon of rosemary, and garlic.

Seal the pressure lid, choose Pressure, set to High, and set the time to 40 minutes. Choose Start/Stop to begin. In a large bowl, toss the potatoes with the remaining oil, rosemary, salt, and black pepper.

When the ribs are ready, perform a quick pressure release and carefully open the lid.

Fix the reversible rack in the higher position of the pot, which is over the ribs. Put the potatoes on the rack. Close the crisping lid. Choose Bake/Roast, set the temperature to 350°F, and set the time to 15 minutes. Choose Start/Stop to begin roasting.

Once the potatoes are tender and roasted, use tongs to pick the potatoes and the short ribs into a plate; set aside. Choose Sear/Sauté and set to High. Simmer the sauce for 5 minutes and spoon the sauce into a bowl.

Allow sitting for 2 minutes and scoop off the fat that forms on top. Serve the ribs with the potatoes and sauce.

Thai Roasted Beef

Servings: 2 | Ready in about: 4 hours 20 min

INGREDIENTS:

1 lb ground beef
½ tsp salt
2 tbsp soy sauce
½ tsp pepper
Thumb-sized piece of ginger, chopped
3 chilies, deseeded and chopped
4 garlic cloves, chopped

1 tsp brown sugar
Juice of 1 lime
2 tbsp mirin
2 tbsp coriander, chopped
2 tbsp basil, chopped
2 tbsp oil
2 tbsp fish sauce

DIRECTIONS:

Place all ingredients, except beef, salt, and pepper, in a blender; pulse until smooth.

Season the beef with salt and pepper. Place the meat and Thai mixture in a zipper bag. Shake well to combine and let marinate in the fridge for about 4 hours.

Place the beef in the Ninja Foodi basket and cook for about 12 minutes, or a little more for well done, on Air Crisp mode at 350 F. Let sit for 5 minutes before serving.

Steak and Chips

Servings: 4 | Ready in about: 50 min

INGREDIENTS

4 potatoes, cut into wedges
1 tsp sweet paprika
1 tbsp olive oil
1 tsp salt, divided

1 tsp ground black pepper
4 rib eye steaks
Cooking spray

DIRECTIONS

Put the Crisping Basket in the pot. Close the crisping lid. Choose Air Crisp, set the temperature to 390°F, and set the time to 5 minutes. Press Start.

Meanwhile, rub all over with olive oil. Put the potatoes in the preheated Crisping Basket and season with ½ teaspoon of salt and ½ teaspoon of black pepper and sweet paprika.

Close the crisping lid. Choose Air Crisp, set the temperature to 400°F, and set the time to 35 minutes. Choose Start/Stop to begin baking.

Season the steak on both sides with the remaining salt and black pepper. When done cooking, remove potatoes to a plate.

Grease the Crisping Basket with cooking spray and put the steaks in the basket.

Close the crisping lid. Choose Air Crisp, set the temperature to 400°F, and set the time to 8 minutes. Choose Start/Stop to begin grilling.

When ready, check the steaks for your preferred doneness and cook for a few more minutes if needed. Take out the steaks from the basket and rest for 5 minutes.

Serve the steaks with the potato wedges and the steak sauce.

Sticky BBQ Baby Back Ribs

Servings: 4 | Ready in about: 35 min

INGREDIENTS

1½ tbsp smoked paprika
3 tbsp brown sugar
2 tsp garlic powder
1 tbsp salt

1 tbsp black pepper
1 (3-pound) rack baby back ribs, cut into quarters
1 cup beer
1 cup barbecue sauce

DIRECTIONS

In a bowl, mix the paprika, brown sugar, garlic, salt, and black pepper. Season all sides of the ribs with the rub.

Pour the beer into the pot, put the ribs in the Crisping Basket, and place the basket in the pot. Seal the pressure lid, choose Pressure, set to High, and set the time to 10 minutes. Choose Start/Stop.

When done cooking, perform a quick pressure release, and carefully the open the lid.

Close the crisping lid. Choose Air Crisp, set the temperature to 400°F, and the time to 15 minutes. Choose Start/Stop to begin crisping.

After 10 minutes, open the lid, and brush the ribs with the barbecue sauce. Close the lid to cook further for 5 minutes.

Winter Pot Roast with Biscuits

Servings: 6 | Ready in about: 75 min

INGREDIENTS

2 tbsp olive oil
1 (3-pound) chuck roast
1½ tsp salt
⅔ cup dry red wine
⅔ cup beef broth
1 tsp dried oregano leaves
1 bay leaf

¼ tsp black pepper
1 small red onion, peeled and quartered
1 pound small butternut squash, diced
2 carrots, peeled and cut into 1-inch pieces
¾ cup frozen pearl onions
6 refrigerated biscuits

DIRECTIONS

On the Foodi, choose Sear/Sauté and adjust to Medium-High. Press Start to preheat the pot.

Heat the olive oil until shimmering. Season the beef on both sides with salt and add to the pot. Cook, undisturbed, for 3 minutes or until deeply browned. Flip the roast over and brown the other side for 3 minutes. Transfer the beef to a wire rack.

Pour the oil out of the pot and add the wine to the pot. Stir with a wooden spoon, scraping the bottom of the pot to let off any browned bits. Bring to a boil and cook for 1 to 2 minutes or until the wine has reduced by half.

Mix in the beef broth, oregano, bay leaf, black pepper, and red onion. Stir to combine and add the beef with its juices. Seal the pressure lid and choose Pressure; adjust the pressure to High and the cook time to 35 minutes. Press Start to begin cooking.

After cooking, perform a quick pressure release. Carefully open the pressure lid.

Add the butternut squash, carrots, and pearl onions to the pot.

Lock the pressure lid into place, set to Seal position and Choose Pressure; adjust the pressure to High and the cook time to 2 minutes. Press Start to cook the vegetables.

After cooking, perform a quick pressure release, and open the lid. Transfer the beef to a cutting board and cover with aluminum foil.

Put the reversible rack in the upper position of the pot and cover with a circular piece of aluminum foil. Put the biscuits on the rack and put the rack in the pot.

Close the crisping lid and Choose Bake/Roast; adjust the temperature to 300°F and the cook time to 15 minutes. Press Start. After 8 minutes, open the lid and carefully flip the biscuits over. After baking, remove the rack and biscuits. Allow the biscuits to cool for a few minutes before serving.

While the biscuits cook, remove the foil from the beef and cut it against the grain into slices. Remove and discard the bay leaf and transfer the beef to a serving platter.

Spoon the vegetables and the sauce over the beef. Serve with the biscuits.

Beef Carnitas

Servings: 4 | Ready in about: 55 min

INGREDIENTS

2½ pounds bone-in country ribs
1 tsp salt
¼ cup orange juice
2 tbsp beef stock

1 tbsp lime juice
1 small onion, cut into 8 wedges
3 garlic cloves, smashed and peeled
Cooking spray

DIRECTIONS

Season the ribs with salt on all sides.

In the Foodi's inner pot, combine the orange juice, stock, and lime juice. Drop in the onion and garlic; stir. Put the ribs in the pot,

Seal the pressure lid, choose Pressure; adjust the pressure to High and the cook time to 25 minutes. Press Start/Stop to begin cooking.

After cooking, do a natural pressure release for 12 minutes. Transfer the ribs to a plate to cool slightly. Remove and discard the bones.

Run the juice in the pot through a fat separator and set aside for a few minutes. Pour the sauce back into the pot and reserve the fat.

Close the crisping lid and Choose Air Crisp; adjust the temperature to 400°F and the time to 3 minutes to preheat; press Start. Oil the reversible rack with cooking spray and lay the ribs in a single layer on the rack. Baste with the reserved fat.

When the Foodi is heated, put the rack in the pot in the upper position. Close the crisping lid and Choose Air Crisp; adjust the temperature to 375°F and the cook time to 6 minutes; press Start.

After crisping, put the beef back in the sauce and use long forks to shred the meat. Stir the beef into the sauce. Serve the carnitas with flat bread or on rice.

Classic Carbonnade Flamande

Servings: 4 | Ready in about: 70 min

INGREDIENTS

2 pounds brisket, cut into 2 or 3 pieces	¼ tsp dried rosemary leaves
½ tsp salt	¼ cup beef broth
1 tbsp olive oil	½ tsp Dijon-style mustard
1 large onion, sliced	½ tsp brown sugar to taste
8 fluid ounces stout	2 tbsp chopped fresh chervil

DIRECTIONS

Season the brisket with salt on all sides. On the Foodi, choose Sear/Sauté and adjust to Medium to preheat the inner pot. Press Start. Allow the pot to preheat for 5 minutes.

Heat the olive oil in the pot until shimmering and sear the brisket. Cook, without turning, for 4 minutes or until browned. Use tongs to turn the beef and move to the side.

Add the onion on the other side. Cook, stirring, for 1 to 2 minutes or until slightly softened. Pour in the stout, scraping off any browned bits from the bottom of the pot. Simmer and cook until the stout has reduced by about half. Stir in the rosemary and broth.

Seal the pressure lid, choose pressure; adjust the pressure to High and the cook time to 35 minutes; press Start. After cooking, perform a natural pressure release for 10 minutes, then a quick release and carefully open the pressure lid.

Remove the beef onto a cutting board. Scoop off any excess fat on the sauce and stir in the mustard and brown sugar.

Choose Sear/Sauté and adjust to Medium. Press Start. Simmer the sauce and cook until reduced to a thin gravy. Taste and adjust the seasoning.

Slice the beef and return to the sauce to reheat. Serve over mashed potatoes or noodles and garnish with chervil.

Sausage with Noodles and Braised Cabbage

Servings: 4 | Ready in about: 35 min

INGREDIENTS

3 ounces serrano ham, diced
1 small onion, sliced
⅓ cup dry white wine
1 cup chicken stock
1 tsp salt

¼ tsp black pepper
5 ounces wide egg noodles
4 cups shredded green cabbage
1½ pounds smoked sausage, cut into 4 pieces
Cooking spray

DIRECTIONS

On the Foodi, choose Sear/Sauté and adjust to Medium. Press Start to preheat the pot for 5 minutes.

Put the ham in the pot and cook for 6 minutes until crisp. Using a slotted spoon, transfer the ham to a paper towel-lined plate to drain, leaving the fat in the pot.

Sauté the onion to the pot for about 2 minutes or until the onion starts to soften. Pour in the wine and simmer until the wine reduces slightly while scraping the bottom of the pot with a wooden spoon to let off any browned bits.

Pour in the chicken stock, salt, black pepper, and noodles. Stir, while pushing the noodles as much as possible into the sauce. Put the cabbage on top of the noodles and the sausages on the cabbage.

Lock the pressure lid into place and seal. Choose Pressure; adjust the pressure to High and the cook time to 3 minutes.

When the cooking time is over, do a quick pressure release, and carefully open the lid.

Stir the noodles and cabbage and adjust the taste with seasoning.

Grease the reversible rack with cooking spray and fix in the upper position of the pot. Transfer the sausages to the rack.

Close the crisping lid and Choose Bake/Roast; adjust the temperature to 390°F and the cook time to 8 minutes; press Start.

After 4 minutes, open the lid and check the sausages. When browned, turn the sausages, close the lid, and cook to brown the other side.

Ladle the cabbage and noodles into a bowl and top with the bacon. Serve with the sausages.

Ragu with Pork and Rigatoni

Servings: 6 | Ready in about: 70 min

INGREDIENTS

1 pound boneless pork shoulder
1 tsp salt
2 tbsp olive oil
4 oz sweet and hot Italian sausage, casings removed
1 medium onion, chopped
2 garlic cloves, minced or pressed
1 medium carrot, peeled and chopped
1 celery stalk, diced
½ cup dry red wine

⅛ tsp red pepper flakes
1 (28-ounce) can crushed tomatoes
2 tbsp tomato paste
2 tsp dried Italian herb mix
1 cup water, divided
12 ounces rigatoni
½ cup grated Parmesan cheese, plus more for serving

DIRECTIONS

Season the pork shoulder with ½ teaspoon of salt.

On the Foodi, choose Sear/Sauté and adjust to Medium. Press Start to preheat the pot for 5 minutes.

Heat in the olive oil in the pot until shimmering and add the pork. Sear on one side for 4 minutes or until browned. Then, add the sausage, the onion, garlic, carrot, and celery. Sauté for 2 minutes or until the vegetables just start softening.

Stir in the wine, use a wooden spoon to scrape the bottom of any browned bits. Cook for 2 to 3 minutes until the wine has reduced by half. Add the red prepper flakes, tomatoes, tomato paste, remaining salt, and the dried herbs. Stir to combine.

Lock the pressure lid into place and Seal. Choose Pressure; adjust the pressure to High, and the cook time to 20 minutes. Press Start to continue cooking.

After cooking, perform a natural pressure release for 10 minutes, then a quick pressure release. Carefully open the lid. Mix the sauce and shred the pork with two forks and break the sausage apart. Add the water and the rigatoni.

Lock the pressure lid into place again and set to Seal. Choose Pressure; adjust the pressure to High and the cook time to 4 minutes. Press Start to boil the rigatoni.

After cooking, perform a quick pressure release, and carefully open the lid.

Sprinkle the cheese over the sauce and pasta. Close the crisping lid and Choose Broil. Adjust the time to 7 minutes. Press Start to broil the cheese.

After cooking, open the lid; the cheese should be brown and crispy. Cool slightly and serve.

Beef and Broccoli Sauce

Servings: 4 | Ready in about: 35 min

INGREDIENTS:

2 lb chuck roast, boneless and cut into thin strips	1 cup beef broth
4 cloves garlic, minced	1 tbsp cornstarch
7 cups broccoli florets	¾ cup soy sauce
1 tbsp olive oil	Salt to taste

DIRECTIONS:

Open the lid of Ninja Foodi, and select Sear/Sauté mode.

Add the olive oil, and once heated, add the beef and minced garlic. Cook the meat until brown. Stir in soy sauce and beef broth.

Close the lid, secure the pressure valve, and select Pressure mode on High pressure for 10 minutes. Press Start/Stop to start cooking.

Once the timer has ended, do a quick pressure release and remove the meat and set aside.

Use a soup spoon to fetch out a quarter of the liquid into a bowl, add the cornstarch, and mix it until it is well dissolved.

Pour the starch mixture into the pot and place the reversible rack. Place the broccoli florets on it and seal the pressure lid. Select Steam mode on LOW for 5 minutes.

When ready, do a quick pressure release and open the lid. Remove the rack, stir the sauce, add the meat and close the crisping lid.

Cook for 5 minutes on Broil mode. The sauce should be thick enough when you finish cooking. Dish the beef broccoli sauce into a serving bowl and serve with a side of cooked pasta.

Chorizo Stuffed Yellow Bell Peppers

Servings: 4 | Ready in about: 40 min

INGREDIENTS

4 large yellow bell peppers
2 tsp olive oil
¾ pound chorizo
1 small onion, diced

⅔ cup diced fresh tomatoes
1½ cups cooked rice
1 cup shredded Mexican blend cheese, divided

DIRECTIONS

Cut about ¼ to ⅓ inch off the top of each pepper. Cut through the ribs inside the peppers and pull out the core and remove as much of the ribs as possible.

On the Foodi, choose Sear/Sauté and adjust to Medium. Press Start to preheat the inner pot for 5 minutes. Heat the oil in the pot until shimmering and cook in the chorizo while breaking the meat with a spatula. Cook until just starting to brown, about 2 minutes.

Add the onion and sauté until the vegetables soften and the chorizo has now browned, about 3 minutes.

Turn the Foodi off and scoop the chorizo and vegetables into a medium bowl. Add the tomatoes, rice, and ½ cup of cheese to the bowl. Mix to combine well.

Spoon the filling mixture into the bell peppers to the brim.

Clean the inner pot with a paper towel and return the pot to the base. Pour 1 cup of water into the pot and fix the rack in the pot in the lower position. Put the peppers on the rack and cover the tops loosely with a piece of foil.

Lock the pressure lid into place and set to Seal. Choose Pressure; adjust the pressure to High and the time to 12 minutes. Press Start.

After cooking, perform a quick pressure release and carefully open the lid.

Remove the foil from the top of the peppers and sprinkle the remaining ½ cup of cheese on the peppers.

Close the crisping lid; choose Broil, adjust the time to 5 minutes, and press Start to broil the cheese.

After 4 minutes, open the lid and check the peppers. The cheese should have melted and browned a bit. If not, close the lid and continue cooking. Let the peppers cool for several minutes before serving.

Calzones with Sausage and Mozzarella

Servings: 4 | Ready in about: 35 min

INGREDIENTS

2 tbsp olive oil
1 small green bell pepper, seeded and chopped
2 or 3 Italian sausages

1 pound frozen bread dough
¼ cup tomato sauce
1 cup shredded mozzarella cheese

DIRECTIONS

On your Foodi, choose Sear/Sauté, and adjust to Medium-High to preheat the inner pot. Press Start to preheat the pot.

Heat 1 tbsp of olive oil in the pot and sauté the bell pepper for 1 minute or until just starting to soften. Remove the pepper into a plate and set aside. Brown the sausages for 2 to 3 minutes on one side. Turn the sausages and brown the other side.

Add ¾ cup of water to the inner pot. Then, lock the pressure lid into place and set to seal. Choose Pressure; adjust the pressure to High and the cook time to 4 minutes. Press Start.

After cooking, perform a quick pressure release and carefully open the pressure lid.

Remove the sausages from the pot onto a cutting board and cool for several minutes. Discard the water in the pot, wipe the pot dry with a clean napkin, and return the pot to the base. When the sausages have cooled, slice into ¼-inch rounds.

Cut four pieces of parchment paper about 8 inches and divide the dough into four equal pieces. One at a time and on a piece of parchment, use your hands to press each dough into a circle about 6 to 7 inches in diameter.

Close the crisping lid. Choose Bake/Roast and adjust the temperature to 400°F. Press Start to preheat the pot for 5 minutes.

While the preheats, make the calzones. One after the other, spread 1 tablespoon of tomato sauce over half a dough circle, leaving a ½-inch clear border. Arrange the sausage rounds in a single layer and sprinkle a quarter of the green peppers over the top. Top with a quarter cup of cheese. Use the parchment to pull the other side of the dough over the filling and pinch the edges together to seal. Repeat the process with another dough.

Cut the parchment around each calzone, so it is about ½ inch larger than the calzone. Brush the calzones with some of the remaining olive oil. With a large spatula, transfer the two calzones to the reversible rack set in the lower position in the pot. Open the lid and place the rack in the pot.

Close the crisping lid and choose Bake/Roast; adjust the temperature to 400°F and the cook time to 12 minutes. Press Start.

After 6 minutes, check the calzones, which will be a dark golden brown. Remove the rack and turn the calzones over. Remove the parchment paper and brush the tops with a little olive oil. Return the rack to the pot. Close the lid and continue cooking for the last 6 minutes.

While the first two calzones bake, assemble the remaining two.

When the first set of calzones are done, transfer to a wire rack to cool and bake the second batch.

Sweet Potato Gratin with Peas and Bacon

Servings: 4 | Ready in about: 30 min

INGREDIENTS

1½ pounds sweet potatoes, peeled and quartered
½ tsp salt or to taste
⅛ tsp freshly ground black pepper
½ cup heavy cream, or more to taste
1 cup shredded Provolone cheese

10 ounces prosciutto, cooked and diced
¾ cup frozen peas, thawed
½ cup grated Pecorino Romano
3 tbsp chopped fresh chives

DIRECTIONS

Place the sweet potatoes on the reversible rack. Pour 1 cup of water into the inner pot and put the rack in the lower position in the pot.

Seal the pressure lid, choose Pressure; adjust the pressure to High and the cook time to 4 minutes. Press Start to begin cooking.

After cooking, perform a quick pressure release, and carefully open the lid.

Remove the rack. Empty the water out of the pot and return the pot to the base. Put the potatoes back in the pot and season with the salt and pepper. Use a large fork to break the potatoes into pieces about ½ inch on a side. Mix in the heavy cream, Provolone cheese, and prosciutto. Gently stir in the peas. Sprinkle the mixture with the Pecorino Romano.

Close the crisping lid and Choose Bake/Roast; adjust the temperature to 400°F and the cook time to 10 minutes. Press Start to begin browning. When the top of the gratin has browned, sprinkle with chives and serve.

Peanut Sauce Beef Satay

Servings: 4 | Ready in about: 60 min

INGREDIENTS

1 pound flank steak
½ tsp salt
1 tbsp lime juice

1½ tsp red curry paste
1 tbsp coconut aminos
1 tbsp coconut oil

For the Cucumber Relish

½ cucumber
½ cup rice vinegar
¼ cup water

2 tbsp sugar
1 tsp salt
1 serrano chile, cut into thin rounds

For the Sauce

1 tbsp coconut oil
1 tbsp onion, minced
1 tsp garlic, minced
1 cup coconut milk
2 tsp red curry paste

1 tsp brown sugar
⅓ cup water
½ cup peanut butter
1 tbsp lime juice

DIRECTIONS

Season both sides of the steak with salt. Put in a resealable plastic bag, set aside, and make the marinade.

In a small bowl, whisk the lime juice, curry paste, coconut aminos, and coconut oil. Pour the marinade over the steak, seal the bag, and massage the bag to coat the meat. Set aside for 20 minutes. While the steak marinates, cut the cucumber into ¼-inch slices, then into quarters.

In a bowl, whisk the vinegar, water, sugar, and salt until the sugar and salt dissolve. Add the cucumber pieces. Refrigerate until needed.

To make the sauce, on the Foodi, choose Sear/Sauté and adjust to Medium-High. Press Start to preheat the pot for 5 minutes. Then, heat the coconut oil until shimmering and sauté the onion and garlic in the pot. Cook for 1 to 2 minutes or until fragrant. Stir in the coconut milk, curry paste, and brown sugar.

Seal the pressure lid, choose Pressure; adjust the pressure to High and the cook time to 0 minutes. Press Start.

After cooking, perform a quick pressure release, and carefully open the lid. Pour in the water and mix.

Remove the meat from the marinade, holding the meat above the bag for a while to drain the excess marinade, put on the reversible rack, and put the rack with the steak in the upper position of the pot above the sauce.

Close the crisping lid; choose Broil, adjust the cook time to 14 minutes, and press Start to begin cooking. After about 7 minutes, open the lid and turn the steak. Close the lid and begin broiling.

Transfer the steak to a cutting board and allow resting for a few minutes.

While the steak cools, mix the peanut butter and lime juice into the sauce. Taste and adjust the seasoning. Cut the steak into thin slices and serve with the peanut sauce and cucumber relish.

Beef and Pepperoncini Peppers

Servings: 4 | Ready in about: 55 min

INGREDIENTS:

2 lb beef roast, cut into cubes
14 oz jar pepperoncini peppers, with liquid
1 pack brown gravy mix

½ cup water
1 pack Italian salad dressing mix

DIRECTIONS:

Place the beef, pepperoncini peppers, brown gravy mix, Italian salad dressing mix, and water, in Ninja Foodi's inner pot.

Close the lid, secure the pressure valve, and select Pressure mode on High pressure for 35 minutes. Press Start/Stop to start cooking.

Once the timer has stopped, do a quick pressure release, and open the pot.

Close the crisping lid and cook on Bake/Roast mode for 15 to 20 minutes at 380 F, until nice and tender.

When ready, dish the ingredients into a bowl and use two forks to shred the beef. Serve beef sauce in plates with a side of a veggie mash, or bread.

Chunky Pork Meatloaf with Mashed Potatoes

Servings: 4 | Ready in about: 55 min

INGREDIENTS

1 tbsp olive oil
1 cup chopped white onion
2 garlic cloves, minced
12 ounces pork meatloaf
2 tsp salt
½ tsp black pepper
3 tbsp chopped fresh cilantro
¼ tsp dried rosemary
12 individual saltine crackers, crushed

1¾ cups full cream milk, divided
2 large eggs
1 tsp yellow mustard
1 tsp Worcestershire sauce
½ cup heavy cream
2 pounds potatoes, cut into large chunks
3 tbsp unsalted butter
¼ cup barbecue sauce

DIRECTIONS

Select Sear/Sauté and adjust to Medium. Press Start to preheat the pot for 5 minutes. Heat the olive oil until shimmering and sauté the onion and garlic in the oil. Cook for about 2 minutes until the onion softens. Transfer the onion and garlic to a plate and set aside.

In a bowl, crumble the meatloaf mix into small pieces. Sprinkle with 1 teaspoon of salt, the pepper, cilantro, and thyme. Add the sautéed onion and garlic. Sprinkle the crushed saltine crackers over the meat and seasonings.

In a small bowl, beat ¼ cup of milk, the eggs, mustard, and Worcestershire sauce. Pour the mixture on the layered cracker crumbs and gently mix the ingredients in the bowl with your hands. Shape the meat mixture into an 8-inch round.

Cover the reversible rack with aluminum foil and carefully lift the meatloaf into the rack.

Pour the remaining 1½ cups of milk and the heavy cream into the inner pot. Add the potatoes, butter, and remaining salt. Place the rack with meatloaf over the potatoes in the upper position in the pot.

Seal the pressure lid, choose Pressure; adjust the pressure to High and the cook time to 25 minutes; press Start. After cooking, perform a quick pressure release, and carefully open the pressure lid. Brush the meatloaf with the barbecue sauce.

Close the crisping lid; choose Broil and adjust the cook time to 7 minutes. Press Start to begin grilling. When the top has browned, remove the rack, and transfer the meatloaf to a serving platter. Mash the potatoes in the pot.

Slice the meatloaf and serve with the mashed potatoes.

Short Ribs with Egg Noodles

Servings: 4 | Ready in about: 65 min

INGREDIENTS

4 pounds bone-in short ribs
2½ tsp salt
Low-sodium beef broth
6 ounces egg noodles
2 tbsp prepared horseradish

6 tbsp Dijon mustard
1 garlic clove, minced
½ tsp freshly ground black pepper
3 tbsp melted unsalted butter
1½ cups panko bread crumbs

DIRECTIONS

Season the short ribs on all sides with 1½ teaspoons of salt. Pour 1 cup of broth into the inner pot. Put the reversible rack in the lower position in the pot, and place the short ribs on top.

Seal the pressure lid, choose Pressure; adjust the pressure to High and the time to 25 minutes; press Start. After cooking, perform a natural pressure release for 5 minutes, then a quick pressure release, and carefully open the lid. Remove the rack and short ribs.

Pour the cooking liquid into a measuring cup to get 2 cups. If lesser than 2 cups, add more broth and season with salt and pepper.

Add the egg noodles and the remaining salt. Stir and submerge the noodles as much as possible. Seal the pressure lid, choose Pressure; adjust the pressure to High and the cook time to 4 minutes; press Start.

In a bowl, combine the horseradish, Dijon mustard, garlic, and black pepper. Brush the sauce on all sides of the short ribs and reserve any extra sauce.

In a bowl, mix the butter and breadcrumbs. Coat the ribs with the crumbs. Put the ribs back on the rack. After cooking, do a quick pressure release, and carefully open the lid. Stir the noodles, which may not be quite done but will continue cooking.

Return the rack and beef to the pot in the upper position.

Close the crisping lid and Choose Bake/Roast; adjust the temperature to 400°F and the cook time to 15 minutes. Press Start. After 8 minutes, open the lid and turn the ribs over. Close the lid and continue cooking.

Serve the beef and noodles, with the extra sauce on the side, if desired.

Beef and Cabbage Stew

Servings: 4 | Ready in about: 30 min

INGREDIENTS:

1 cup rice
1 large head cabbage, cut in chunks
1 lb ground beef
Salt and black pepper to taste
½ cup chopped onion
4 cloves garlic, minced
2 tbsp butter
1 bay leaf

1 cup diced tomatoes
1 ½ cup beef broth
¼ cup Plain vinegar
2 tbsp Worcestershire sauce
1 tbsp paprika powder
1 tbsp dried oregano
Chopped parsley to garnish

DIRECTIONS:

Set the Ninja Foodi on Sear/Sauté mode. Melt the butter and add the beef. Brown it for about 6 minutes and add in the onions, garlic, and bay leaf. Stir and cook for 2 more minutes.

Stir in the oregano, paprika, salt, pepper, rice, cabbage, vinegar, broth, and Worcestershire sauce. Cook for 3 minutes, stirring occassionally. Add the tomatoes but don't stir. Close the lid, secure the pressure valve, and select Pressure Cook mode on High for 5 minutes. Press Start/Stop.

Once the timer is done, let the pot sit closed for 5 minutes and then do a quick pressure. Open the lid. Stir the sauce, remove the bay leaf, and adjust the seasoning with salt. Dish the cabbage sauce in serving bowls and serve with bread rolls.

Cheeseburgers in Hoagies

Servings: 4 | Ready in about: 65 min

INGREDIENTS:

1 tbsp olive oil
1 (14 oz) can French onion soup
1 lb chuck beef roast
1 onion, sliced
2 tbsp Worcestershire sauce
2 Cups beef broth

Salt and black pepper to taste
1 tsp garlic powder
3 slices Provolone cheese
3 hoagies, halved
3 tsp mayonnaise

DIRECTIONS:

Season the beef with garlic powder, salt, and pepper.

On Ninja Foodi, select Sear/Sauté mode. Heat the olive oil and brown the beef on both sides for about 5 minutes. Remove the meat onto a plate.

Into the pot, add the onions and cook until soft. Then, pour the beef broth and stir, while scraping the bottom off every stuck bit. Add the onion soup, Worcestershire sauce, and beef. Close the lid, secure the pressure valve, and select Pressure mode on High pressure for 20 minutes. Press Start/Stop.

Once the timer has stopped, do a natural pressure release for 10-15 minutes, and then a quick pressure release to let out any remaining steam.

Use two forks to shred the meat. Close the crisping lid and cook on Bake/Roast for 10 minutes at 350 F.

When ready, open the lid and strain the juice of the pot through a sieve into a bowl. Assemble the burgers by slathering mayo on halved hoagies, spoon the shredded meat over and top each hoagie with cheese.

Herbed Lamb Chops

Servings: 4 | Ready in about: 30 min

INGREDIENTS:

4 lamb chops
1 garlic clove, peeled
1 tbsp plus
2 tsp olive oil

½ tbsp oregano
½ tbsp thyme
½ tsp salt
¼ tsp black pepper

DIRECTIONS:

Coat the garlic clove with 1 tsp of olive oil and cook in the Ninja Foodi for 10 minutes on Air Crisp mode.

Meanwhile, mix the herbs and seasonings with the remaining olive oil.

Using a towel, squeeze the hot roasted garlic clove into the herb mixture and stir to combine. Coat the lamb chops with the mixture well, and place in the Ninja Foodi.

Close the crisping lid and cook for about 8 to 12 minutes on Air Crisp mode at 390 F, until crispy on the outside.

Beef and Bell Pepper with Onion Sauce

Servings: 6 | Ready in about: 62 min

INGREDIENTS:

2 lb round steak pieces, about 6 to 8 pieces
½ green bell pepper, finely chopped
½ red bell pepper, finely chopped
½ yellow bell pepper, finely chopped
1 yellow onion, finely chopped

2 cloves garlic, minced
Salt and pepper, to taste
¼ cup flour
2 tbsp olive oil
½ cup water

DIRECTIONS:

Wrap the steaks in plastic wrap, place on a cutting board, and use a rolling pin to pound flat of about 2-inch thickness.

Remove the plastic wrap and season them with salt and pepper. Set aside.

Put the chopped peppers, onion, and garlic in a bowl, and mix them evenly.

Spoon the bell pepper mixture onto the flattened steaks and roll them to have the peppers inside.

Use some toothpicks to secure the beef rolls and dredge the steaks in all-purpose flour while shaking off any excess flour. Place them in a plate.

Select Sear/Sauté mode on Ninja Foodi and heat the oil. Add the beef rolls and brown them on both sides, for about 6 minutes.

Pour the water over the meat, close the lid, secure the pressure valve, and select Pressure mode on High pressure for 20 minutes. Press Start/Stop.

Once the timer has stopped, do a natural pressure release for 10 minutes. Close the crisping lid and cook for 10 minutes on Broil mode.

When ready, Remove the meat to a plate and spoon the sauce from the pot over. Serve the stuffed meat rolls with a side of steamed veggies.

Beef Soup with Tortillas

Servings: 8 | Ready in about: 30 min

INGREDIENTS:

2 tbsp olive oil
6 green bell pepper, diced
2 medium yellow onion, chopped
3 lb ground beef, grass fed
Salt and black pepper to taste
3 tbsp chili powder
2 tbsp cumin powder
2 tsp paprika

1 tsp garlic powder
1 tsp cinnamon
1 tsp onion powder
6 cups chopped tomatoes
½ cup chopped green chilies
3 cups bone broth
3 cups milk

Topping:
Chopped Jalapenos, cilantro and green onions, sliced
Avocados, lime juice

DIRECTIONS:

Select Sear/Sauté mode and set High on your Ninja Foodi. Pour in the oil, once it has heated, add the yellow onion and green peppers.

Sauté until they are soft for about 5 minutes. Include the ground beef, stir the ingredients, and let the beef cook for about 8 minutes until it browns.

Next, add the chili powder, cumin powder, black pepper, paprika, cinnamon, garlic powder, onion powder, and green chilies. Give them a good stir.

Top with tomatoes, milk, and bone broth. Close the lid, secure the pressure valve, and select Pressure mode on High for 20 minutes. Press Start.

Once the timer has ended, do a quick pressure release. Adjust the taste with salt and pepper. Dish the taco soup into serving bowls and add the toppings.

Serve warm with a side of tortillas.

Asian Beef Curry

Servings: 4 | Ready in about: 40 min

INGREDIENTS:

1 ½ lb beef brisket, cut in cubes
1 tbsp olive oil
2 cloves garlic, minced
¼-inch ginger, peeled and sliced
2 bay leaves
2 star anises
1 large carrot, chopped
1 medium onion, chopped

2 tbsp red curry paste
1 cup milk
1 Potato, peeled and chopped
1 tbsp sugar
2 tsp oyster sauce
2 tsp flour
3 tbsp water

DIRECTIONS:

Select Sear/Sauté mode. Heat oil, add garlic, ginger, and red curry paste.

Stir-fry them for 1 minute. Stir in onion and beef. Cook for 4 minutes.

Add the carrots, bay leaves, potato, star anises, sugar, and water. Stir.

Close the lid, secure the pressure valve, and select Pressure mode on High for 25 minutes. Press Start/Stop to start cooking.

Once the timer goes off, do a quick pressure release.

In a bowl, add the flour and 4 tablespoons of milk. Mix well with a spoon and pour it in the pot along with the oyster sauce and remaining milk. Stir it gently not to break the potato.

Close the crisping lid and cook on Broil mode for about 3 minutes, until the sauce thickens and meat is tender. After, turn off the pot.

Spoon the sauce into soup bowls and serve with a side of rice.

Beef and Green Bell Pepper Pot

Servings: 4 | Ready in about: 55 min

INGREDIENTS:

2 lb beef chuck roast
1 tbsp onion powder
1 tbsp garlic powder
1 tbsp Italian Seasoning
Salt and black pepper to taste, cut in 4 pieces

1 cup beef broth
1 medium white onion, sliced
1 green bell pepper, seeded and sliced
1 red bell pepper, seeded and sliced
2 tbsp olive oil

DIRECTIONS:

Rub the beef with pepper, salt, garlic powder, Italian seasoning, and onion powder. Select Sear/Sauté mode on Ninja Foodi.

Heat 1 tbsp oil, add the beef pieces and sear them on both sides until brown, for about 5 minutes. Use a pair of tongs to remove them onto a plate after. (You can do this in 2 batches).

Pour the beef broth and fish sauce into the pot to deglaze the bottom while you use a spoon to scrape any stuck beef bit at the bottom. Add the meat back to the pot, close the lid, secure the pressure valve, and select Pressure mode on High pressure for 30 minutes. Press Start/Stop.

Once the timer has stopped, do a quick pressure release, and open the pot.

Use two forks to shred the beef, inside the pot. Close the crisping lid and select Broil mode for 10 minutes. When ready, set aside the meat and discard the liquid. Wipe clean the pot.

Select Sear/Sauté mode, heat the remaining oil, add the beef with onions and peppers. Sauté them for 3 minutes and season with salt and pepper.

Turn off the pot and dish the stir-fried beef into serving plates. Serve as a side to rice with sauce dish.

Classic Beef Bourguignon

Servings: 4 | Ready in about: 45 min

INGREDIENTS:

2 lb stewing beef, cut in large chunks
Salt and pepper, to taste
2 ½ tbsp olive oil
¼ tsp red wine vinegar
¼ cup pearl onion
3 tsp tomato paste
½ lb mushrooms, sliced
2 carrots, peeled and chopped

1 onion, sliced
2 cloves garlic, crushed
1 cup red wine
2 cups beef broth
1 bunch thyme
½ cup cognac
2 tbsp flour

DIRECTIONS:

Select Sear/Sauté mode. Season the beef with salt, pepper, and a light sprinkle of flour. Heat the oil in the pot, and brown the meat on all sides.

Pour the cognac into the pot and stir the mixture with a spoon to deglaze the bottom. Stir in thyme, red wine, broth, paste, garlic, mushrooms, onion, and pearl onions.

Close the lid, secure the pressure valve, and select Pressure mode on High for 25 minutes. Press Start/Stop.

Once the timer is off, do a natural pressure release for 10 minutes, then a quick pressure release to let out the remaining steam. Close the crisping lid and cook for 10 minutes on Broil mode. When ready, open the lid.

Use the spoon to remove the thyme, adjust the taste with salt and pepper, and add the vinegar. Stir the sauce and serve hot, with a side of rice.

Beef and Cheese Stuffed Mushrooms

Servings: 3 | Ready in about: 10 min

INGREDIENTS:

6 large white mushrooms, stems removed
2 cups cooked leftover beef, cut in very small cubes
2 tsp garlic salt
½ cup vegetable broth

2 oz cream cheese, softened
1 cup shredded Cheddar cheese
1 tsp olive oil

DIRECTIONS:

In a bowl, add the beef, garlic salt, cream cheese, and cheddar cheese. Use a spoon to mix them.

Spoon the beef mixture into the mushrooms and place the mushrooms in the inner pot of Ninja Foodi. Drizzle them with olive oil, and add the broth.

Close the lid, secure the pressure valve, and select Pressure mode on High pressure for 3 minutes. Press Start/Stop to start cooking.

Once the timer is off, do a quick pressure release and open the pressure lid, discard the liquid, and remove the mushrooms.

Place the reversible rack and lay the mushrooms on it. Close the crisping lid and cook for 2 to 3 minutes on Air Crisp mode at 350 F. Remove the stuffed mushrooms onto a plate, and serve hot with a side of steamed green veggies.

Pot Roast with Broccoli

Servings: 4 | Ready in about: 35 min

INGREDIENTS:

2 lb beef chuck roast
3 tbsp olive oil, divided into 2
Salt to taste
1 cup beef broth

1 packet onion soup mix
1 cup chopped broccoli
2 red bell peppers, seeded and quartered
1 yellow onion, quartered

DIRECTIONS:

Season the chuck roast with salt and set aside. Select Sear/Sauté mode on the Ninja Foodi cooker.

Add the olive oil, and once heated, add the chuck roast. Sear for 5 minutes on each side. Then, pour in the beef broth.

In a zipper bag, add broccoli, onions, peppers, the remaining olive oil, and onion soup.

Close the bag and shake the mixture to coat the vegetables well. Use tongs to remove the vegetables into the pot and stir with a spoon.

Close the lid, secure the pressure valve, and select Pressure mode on High pressure for 18 minutes. Press Start/Stop.

Once the timer has stopped, do a quick pressure release, and open the pressure lid. Make cuts on the meat inside the pot and close the crisping lid.

Cook on Air Crisp mode for about 10 minutes, at 380 F, until nice and crispy. Plate and serve with the vegetables and a drizzle of the sauce in the pot.

Beef Stew with Beer

Servings: 4 | Ready in about: 60 min

INGREDIENTS:

2 lb beef stewed meat, cut into bite-size pieces
Salt and black pepper to taste
¼ cup flour
3 tbsp butter
2 tbsp Worcestershire sauce

2 cloves garlic, minced
1 packet dry onion soup mix
2 cups beef broth
1 medium bottle beer
1 tbsp tomato paste

DIRECTIONS:

In a zipper bag, add beef, salt, all-purpose flour, and pepper. Close the bag up and shake it to coat the meat well with the mixture.

Select Sear/Sauté mode on the Ninja Foodi. Melt the butter, and brown the beef on both sides, for 5 minutes.

Pour the broth to deglaze the bottom of the pot. Stir in tomato paste, beer, Worcestershire sauce, and the onion soup mix.

Close the lid, secure the pressure valve, and select Pressure mode on High pressure for 25 minutes. Press Start/Stop to start cooking.

Once the timer is done, do a natural pressure release for 10 minutes, and then a quick pressure release to let out any remaining steam.

Open the pressure lid and close the crisping lid. Cook on Broil mode for 10 minutes.

Spoon the beef stew into serving bowls and serve with over a bed of vegetable mash with steamed greens.

Meatballs with Spaqhuetti Sauce

Servings: 6 | Ready in about: 20 min

INGREDIENTS:

2 lb ground beef
1 cup breadcrumbs
1 onion, finely chopped
2 cloves garlic, minced
Salt and pepper, to taste
1 tsp dried oregano

3 tbsp milk
1 cup water
1 cup grated Parmesan cheese
2 eggs, cracked into a bowl
4 cups spaghetti sauce
1 tbsp olive oil

DIRECTIONS:

In a bowl, add beef, onion, breadcrumbs, parmesan, eggs, garlic, milk, salt, oregano, and pepper. Mix well with hands and shape bite-size balls.

Open the pot, and add the spaghetti sauce, water and the meatballs.

Close the lid, secure the pressure valve, and select Steam mode on High pressure for 6 minutes. Press Start/Stop.

Once the timer is done, do a natural pressure release for 5 minutes, then do a quick pressure release to let out any extra steam, and open the lid.

Dish the meatball sauce over cooked pasta and serve.

Cheddar Cheeseburgers

Servings: 4 | Ready in about: 20 min

INGREDIENTS:

1 lb ground beef
1 (1 oz) packet dry onion soup mix
1 cup water
4 burger buns
4 tomato slices

4 Cheddar cheese slices
4 small leaves lettuce
Mayonnaise
Mustard
Ketchup

DIRECTIONS:

In a bowl, add beef and onion mix, and mix well with hands. Shape in 4 patties and wrap each in foil paper.

Pour the water into the inner steel insert of Ninja Foodi, and fit in the steamer rack. Place the wrapped patties on the trivet, close the lid, and secure the pressure valve, and cook on 10 minutes on Pressure mode on High pressure.

Once the timer has stopped, do a natural pressure release for 5 minutes, then a quick pressure release to let out the remaining steam.

Use a set of tongs to remove the wrapped beef onto a flat surface and carefully unwrap the patties.

To assemble the burgers:

In each half of the buns, put a lettuce leaf, then a beef patty, a slice of cheese, and a slice of tomato. Top it with the other halves of buns.

Serve with some ketchup, mayonnaise, and mustard.

Beef Roast with Peanut Satay Sauce

Servings: 4 | Ready in about: 40 min

INGREDIENTS:

1 lb beef roast, cut into cubes
Salt and black pepper to taste
½ cup coconut milk, light

½ cup Peanut Satay sauce
2 cups diced carrots

DIRECTIONS:

Place the beef inside Ninja Foodi. In a bowl, mix in coconut milk, salt, pepper, and satay sauce. Pour over the beef. Add the carrots too.

Close the lid, secure the pressure valve, and select Pressure mode on High pressure for 15 minutes. Press Start/Stop to start cooking.

Once the timer has ended, do a natural pressure release, then a quick pressure release to let out any remaining steam, and open the pot.

Give it a stir and close the crisping lid. Cook for 10 minutes on Bake/Roast mode at 400 F.

Use a spoon to dish the meat into a serving plate, and serve with a side of steamed greens.

Spiced Beef Chili

Servings: 4 | Ready in about: 40 min

INGREDIENTS:

2 lb ground beef
2 tbsp olive oil
1 large red bell pepper, seeded and chopped
1 large yellow bell pepper, seeded and chopped
1 white onion, chopped
2 cups chopped tomatoes
2 cups beef broth
2 carrots, cut in little bits

2 tsp onion powder
2 tsp garlic powder
5 tsp chili powder
2 tbsp Worcestershire sauce
2 tsp paprika
½ tsp cumin powder
2 tbsp chopped parsley
Salt and black pepper to taste

DIRECTIONS:

Select Sear/Sauté mode, and add the olive oil and ground beef. Cook the meat until brown, stirring occasionally, for about 8 minutes.

Top with the remaining ingredients and mix well. Seal the lid, and cook on Pressure mode on High for 15 minutes. Press Start/Stop to start cooking.

Once the timer has ended, do a quick pressure release, and open the lid.

Stir the stew and close the crisping lid. Cook on Broil mode for 10 minutes.

Dish into serving bowls. Serve this beef chili with crackers or potato mash.

Beef and Vegetable Stew

Servings: 4 | Ready in about: 70 min

INGREDIENTS:

2 lb brisket, cut into 2-inch pieces
4 cups beef broth
Salt and black pepper to taste
1 tbsp Dijon mustard
1 tbsp olive oil
1 lb small potato, quartered
¼ lb carrots, cut in 2-inch pieces

1 large red onion, quartered
3 cloves garlic, minced
1 bay leaf
2 fresh thyme sprigs
2 tbsp cornstarch
3 tbsp chopped cilantro to garnish

DIRECTIONS:

Pour broth, cornstarch, mustard, ½ teaspoon salt, and ½ teaspoon pepper in a bowl. Whisk them and set aside. Season the beef with salt and pepper.

On the Ninja Foodi, select Sear/Sauté mode.

Add the olive oil, and once heated, add the beef strips. Flip halfway through to brown evenly. That should take 7 to 10 minutes.

Then, add potato, carrots, onion, garlic, thyme, mustard mixture, and bay leaf. Stir once more. Close the lid, secure the pressure valve, and select Pressure mode on High pressure for 35 minutes. Press Start/Stop.

Once the timer has ended, do a quick pressure release.

Stir the stew and remove the bay leaf. Season the stew with pepper and salt.

Close the crisping lid and cook for 10 minutes on Broil mode. Serve the soup with a bread of your choice.

Beef and Garbanzo Bean Chili

Servings: 10 | Ready in about: 45 min

INGREDIENTS

1 pound garbanzo beans, soaked overnight, rinsed
1 tbsp olive oil
2 onions, finely chopped
2 ½ pounds ground beef
1 small jalapeño with seeds, minced
6 garlic cloves, minced
¼ cup chili powder
2 tbsp ground cumin

2 tsp salt
1 tsp smoked paprika
1 tsp dried oregano
1 tsp garlic powder
¼ tsp cayenne pepper
2 ½ cups beef broth
1 (6 ounces) can tomato puree

DIRECTIONS

Add the garbanzo beans to the Foodi and pour in cold water to cover 1 inch. Seal the pressure lid, choose Pressure, set to High, and set the timer to 20 minutes.Press Start. When ready, release the pressure quickly.

Drain beans and rinse with cold water. Set aside. Wipe clean the Foodi and set to Sear/Sauté, set to Medium High, and choose Start/Stop to preheat the pot. Press Start. Warm olive oil, add in onion, and cook for 3 minutes until soft.

Add jalapeño, ground beef, and minced garlic, and stir-fry for 5 minutes until everything is cooked through.

Stir in chili powder, kosher salt, garlic powder, paprika, cumin, oregano, and cayenne pepper, and cook until soft, about 30 seconds. Pour beef broth, garbanzo beans, and tomato paste into the pot.

Seal the pressure lid, choose Pressure, set to High, and set the timer to 20 minutes; press Start. When ready, release pressure naturally for about 10 minutes. Open the lid, press Sear/Sauté, and cook as you stir until desired consistency is attained. Spoon chili into bowls and serve.

Chipotle Beef Brisket

Servings: 4 | Ready in about: 1 hr 10 min

INGREDIENTS

2 tsp smoked paprika
½ tsp dried oregano
½ tsp salt
½ tsp ground black pepper
1 tbsp Worcestershire sauce
½ tsp ground cumin
½ tsp garlic powder

1 tsp chipotle powder
¼ tsp cayenne pepper
2 pounds, beef brisket
2 tbsp olive oil
1 cup beef broth
¼ cup red wine
A handful of parsley, chopped

DIRECTIONS

In a bowl, combine oregano, cumin, cayenne pepper, garlic powder, salt, paprika, pepper, Worcestershire sauce and chipotle powder; rub the seasoning mixture on the beef to coat.

Warm olive oil on Sear/Sauté. Add in beef and cook for 3 to 4 minutes each side until browned completely. Pour in beef broth and red wine.

Seal the pressure lid, choose Pressure, set to High, and set the timer to 50 minutes. Press Start. Release the pressure naturally, for about 10 minutes.

Place the beef on a cutting board and Allow cooling for 10 minutes before slicing. Arrange the beef slices on a serving platter, pour the cooking sauce over and scatter with parsley to serve.

Beef Bourguignon

Servings: 5 | Ready in about: 40 min

INGREDIENTS

1 pound boneless chuck steak, trimmed and cut chunks
¼ cup flour
1 tsp salt
1 tsp ground black pepper
1 cup pancetta, chopped
½ cup red burgundy wine

1¼ cup beef broth
1 carrot, diced
2 cups Portobello mushrooms, quartered
4 shallots, sliced
3 garlic cloves, crushed
A handful of parsley, chopped

DIRECTIONS

Toss beef with black pepper, salt, and flour in a large bowl to coat.

Set your Foodi on Sear/Sauté, set to Medium High, and choose Start/Stop to preheat the pot. Press Start. Cook pancetta for 5 minutes until brown and crispy.

Pour in approximately half the beef and cook for 5 minutes each side until browned all over. Transfer the pancetta and beef to a plate.

Sear remaining beef and transfer to the plate.

Add in beef broth and wine to deglaze the pan, scrape the pan's bottom to get rid of any browned bits of food. Return beef and pancetta to cooker; stir in garlic, carrot, shallots, and mushrooms.

Seal the pressure lid, choose Pressure, set to High, and set the timer to 32 minutes. Press Start. When ready, release the pressure quickly.

Garnish with fresh chopped parsley and serve.

Beef and Cherry Tagine

Servings: 4 | Ready in about: 1 hr 20 min

INGREDIENTS

2 tbsp olive oil
1 onion, chopped
1 ½ pounds stewing beef, trimmed
1 tsp ground cinnamon
½ tsp paprika
½ tsp turmeric
½ tsp salt

¼ tsp ground ginger
¼ tsp ground allspice
1-star anise
1 cup water
1 tbsp honey
1 cup dried cherries, halved
¼ cup toasted almonds, slivered

DIRECTIONS

Set your Foodi to Sear/Sauté, set to Medium High, and choose Start/Stop to preheat the pot. Warm olive oil. Add in onions and cook for 3 minutes until fragrant. Mix in beef and cook for 2 minutes each side until browned.

Stir in anise, cinnamon, turmeric, allspice, salt, paprika, and ginger; cook for 2 minutes until aromatic.

Add in honey and water. Seal the pressure lid, choose Pressure, set to High, and set the timer to 50 minutes. Press Start.

Meanwhile, in a bowl, soak dried cherries in hot water until softened.

Once ready, release pressure naturally for 15 minutes. Drain cherries and stir into the tagine. Top with toasted almonds before serving.

Beef and Bacon Chili

Servings: 6 | Ready in about: 1 hr

INGREDIENTS

2 pounds stewing beef, trimmed
4 tsp salt, divided
4 ounces smoked bacon, cut into strips
1 tsp freshly ground black pepper, divided
2 tsp olive oil, divided
1 onion, diced
2 bell peppers, diced
3 garlic cloves, minced

1 tbsp ground cumin
1 tsp chili powder
½ tsp cayenne pepper
1 chipotle in adobo sauce, finely chopped
2 cups beef broth
29 ounces canned whole tomatoes
15 ounces canned kidney beans, drained and rinsed

DIRECTIONS

Set on Sear/Sauté, set to Medium High, and choose Start/Stop to preheat the pot and fry the bacon until crispy, about 5 minutes. Set aside.

Rub the beef with ½ tsp black pepper and 1 tsp salt.

In the bacon fat, brown beef for 5-6 minutes; transfer to a plate.

Warm the oil. Add in garlic, peppers and onion and cook for 3 to 4 minutes until soft. Stir in cumin, cayenne pepper, the extra pepper and salt, chopped chipotle, and chili powder and cook for 30 seconds until soft.

Return beef and bacon to the pot with vegetables and spices; add in tomatoes and broth.

Seal the pressure lid, choose Pressure, set to High, and set the timer to 45 minutes. Press Start. When ready, release the pressure quickly.

Stir in beans. Let simmer on Keep Warm for 10 minutes until flavors combine.

Beef and Pumpkin Stew

Servings: 6 | Ready in about: 35 min

INGREDIENTS

2 tbsp canola oil
2 pounds stew beef, cut into 1-inch chunks
1 cup red wine
1 onion, chopped
1 tsp garlic powder
1 tsp salt

3 whole cloves
1 bay leaf
3 carrots, sliced
½ butternut pumpkin, sliced
2 tbsp cornstarch
3 tbsp water

DIRECTIONS

Warm oil on Sear/Sauté. Add beef and brown for 5 minutes on each side.

Deglaze the pot with wine, scrape the bottom to get rid of any browned beef bits. Add in onion, salt, bay leaf, cloves, and garlic powder. Seal the pressure lid, choose Pressure, set to High, and set the timer to 15 minutes. Press Start.

When ready, release the pressure quickly. Add in pumpkin and carrots without stirring. Seal the pressure lid again, choose Pressure, set to High, and set the timer to 5 minutes. Press Start.

When ready, release the pressure quickly.

In a bowl, mix water and cornstarch until cornstarch dissolves completely; mix into the stew. Allow the stew to simmer while uncovered on Keep Warm for 5 minutes until you attain the desired thickness.

Caribbean Ropa Vieja

Servings: 6 | Ready in about: 1 hr 10 min

INGREDIENTS

Salt and ground black pepper to taste
2 pounds beef skirt steak
3½ cups beef stock
2 bay leaves
¼ cup olive oil
1 red onion, halved and thinly sliced
1 green bell pepper, thinly sliced
1 red bell pepper, thinly sliced

¼ cup minced garlic
1 tsp dried oregano
1 tsp ground cumin
1 cup tomato sauce
1 cup dry red wine
1 tbsp vinegar
¼ cup cheddar cheese, shredded

DIRECTIONS

Season the skirt steak with pepper and salt. Add water into Foodi; mix in bay leaves and flank steak.

Seal the pressure lid, choose Pressure, set to High, and set the timer to 35 minutes. Press Start. When ready, release the pressure quickly.

Remove skirt steak to a cutting board and allow to sit for about 5 minutes. Press Start. When cooled, shred the beef using two forks. Drain the pressure cooker, and reserve the bay leaves and 1 cup liquid.

Warm the oil on Sear/Sauté. Add onion, red bell pepper, cumin, garlic, green bell pepper, and oregano and continue cooking for 5 minutes until vegetables are softened.

Stir in reserved liquid, tomato sauce, bay leaves and red wine. Return shredded beef to the pot with vinegar; season with pepper and salt.

Seal the pressure lid, choose Pressure, set to High, and set the timer to 15 minutes. Press Start. Release pressure naturally for 10 minutes, then turn steam vent valve to Venting to release the remaining pressure quickly. Serve with shredded cheese.

Beef Pho with Swiss Chard

Servings: 6 | Ready in about: 1 hr 10 min

INGREDIENTS

2 tbsp coconut oil
1 yellow onion, quartered
¼ cup minced fresh ginger
2 tsp coriander seeds
2 tsp ground cinnamon
2 tsp ground cloves
9 cups water
2 pounds Beef Neck Bones
2 ½ tsp kosher salt

8 ounces rice noodles
3 tbsp sugar
2 tbsp fish sauce
10 ounces sirloin steak
A handful of fresh cilantro, chopped
2 scallions, chopped
2 jalapeño peppers, sliced
2 cups Swiss chard, chopped
Freshly ground black pepper to taste

DIRECTIONS

Melt the oil on Sear/Sauté. Add ginger and onions and cook for 4 minutes until the onions are softened. Stir in cloves, cinnamon and coriander seeds and cook for 1 minute until soft. Add in water, salt, beef meat and bones. Seal the pressure lid, choose Pressure, set to High, and set the timer to 30 minutes. Press Start. Release pressure naturally for 10 minutes.

Transfer the meat to a large bowl; cover with it enough water and soak for 10 minutes. Drain the water and slice the beef. In hot water, soak rice noodles for 8 minutes until softened and pliable; drain and rinse with cold water. Drain liquid from cooker into a separate pot through a fine-mesh strainer; get rid of any solids.

Add fish sauce and sugar to the broth; transfer into the Foodi and simmer on Sear/Sauté.

Place the noodles in four separate soup bowls. Top with steak slices, scallions, swiss chard, sliced jalapeño pepper, cilantro, red onion, and pepper. Spoon the broth over each bowl to serve.

Brisket Chili con Carne

Servings: 6 | Ready in about: 1 hr 25 min

INGREDIENTS

1 tbsp ground black pepper
2 tsp salt
1 tsp sweet paprika
1 tsp cayenne pepper
1 tsp chili powder
½ tsp garlic salt

½ tsp onion powder
1 (4 pounds) beef brisket
1 cup beef broth
2 bay leaves
2 tbsp Worcestershire sauce
14 ounces canned black beans, drained and rinsed

DIRECTIONS

In a bowl, combine pepper, paprika, chili powder, cayenne pepper, salt, onion powder and garlic salt; rub onto brisket pieces to coat.

Add the brisket to your Foodi. Cover with Worcestershire sauce and water.

Seal the pressure lid, choose Pressure, set to High, and set the timer to 50 minutes. Press Start. Release pressure naturally for 10 minutes.

Transfer the brisket to a cutting board. Drain any liquid present in the pot using a fine-mesh strainer; get rid of any solids and fat.

Slice brisket, arrange the slices onto a platter add the black beans on side and spoon the cooking liquid over the slices and beans to serve.

Meatballs with Marinara Sauce

Servings: 6 | Ready in about: 35 min

INGREDIENTS

1½ pounds ground beef
⅓ cup warm water
¾ cup grated Parmigiano-Reggiano cheese
½ cup bread crumbs
1 egg
2 tbsp fresh parsley

¼ tsp garlic powder
¼ tsp dried oregano
salt and ground black pepper to taste
1/2 cup capers
1 tsp olive oil
3 cups marinara sauce

DIRECTIONS

In a large bowl, mix ground beef, garlic powder, pepper, oregano, bread crumbs, egg, and salt; shape into meatballs. Warm the oil on Sear/Sauté. Add meatballs to the oil and brown for 2-3 minutes and all sides.

Pour water and marinara sauce over the meatballs. Seal the pressure lid, choose Pressure, set to High, and set the timer to 10 minutes. Press Start.

When ready, release the pressure quickly. Serve in large bowls topped with capers and Parmigiano-Reggiano cheese.

Beer-Braised Short Ribs with Mushrooms

Servings: 4 | Ready in about: 1 hr

INGREDIENTS

2 pounds beef short ribs
1 tsp smoked paprika
½ tsp dried oregano
½ tsp cayenne pepper
salt and ground black pepper to taste
1 tbsp olive oil
1 small onion, sliced

4 garlic cloves, smashed
1 cup beer
⅓ cup beef broth
1 cup crimini mushrooms, sliced
1 tbsp soy sauce
1 bell pepper, diced

DIRECTIONS

In a small bowl, combine pepper, paprika, cayenne pepper, salt, and oregano. Rub the seasoning mixture on all sides of the short ribs.

Warm oil on Sear/Sauté. Add mushrooms and cook until browned, about 6-8 minutes; set aside. Add short ribs to the Foodi, and cook for 3 minutes for each side until browned; set aside on a plate.

Throw in garlic and onion to the oil and stir-fry for 2 minutes until fragrant.

Add in beer to deglaze, scrape the pot's bottom to get rid of any browned bits of food; bring to a simmer and cook for 2 minutes until reduced slightly.

Stir in soy sauce, bell pepper and beef broth. Dip short ribs into the liquid in a single layer.

Seal the pressure lid, choose Pressure, set to High, and set the timer to 40 minutes. Press Start.

Release pressure naturally for about 10 minutes. Divide the ribs with the sauce into bowls and top with fried mushrooms.

Beef and Turnip Chili

Servings: 6 | Ready in about: 30 min

INGREDIENTS

1 tbsp olive oil
1 yellow onion, chopped
salt to taste
4 garlic cloves, minced
2 tbsp tomato puree
1 tbsp chili powder
2 tsp ground cumin
1 tsp dried oregano

½ tsp ground turmeric
1 pinch cayenne pepper
1 pound ground beef meat
1 (28 ounces) can whole tomatoes
2 cups beef stock
1 pound turnips, peeled and cubed
2 tomatoes, chopped
1 bell pepper, chopped

DIRECTIONS

Warm oil on Sear/Sauté. Add in onion with a pinch of salt and cook for 3 to 5 minutes until softened.

Stir in garlic, chili powder, turmeric, cumin, tomato puree, oregano, and cayenne pepper; cook for 2 to 3 minutes as you stir until very soft and sticks to the pot's bottom; add beef and cook for 5 minutes until completely browned. Mix in tomatoes, turnips, bell pepper, and beef stock.

Seal the pressure lid, choose Pressure, set to High, and set the timer to 15 minutes; press Start.

When ready, release the pressure quickly.

Italian-Style Pot Roast

Servings: 5 | Ready in about: 1 hr 30 min

INGREDIENTS

2 ½ pounds beef brisket, trimmed
salt and freshly ground black pepper
2 tbsp olive oil
1 onion, chopped
3 garlic cloves, minced
1 cup beef broth
¾ cup dry red wine

2 fresh thyme sprigs
2 fresh rosemary sprigs
4 ounces pancetta, chopped
6 carrots, chopped
1 bay leaf
A handful of parsley, chopped

DIRECTIONS

Warm olive oil on Sear/Sauté. Fry the pancetta for 4-5 minutes until crispy. Set aside. Season the beef with pepper and salt and add it to the pot and brown for 5 to 7 minutes for each; remove and set aside on a plate.

In the same oil, fry garlic and onion for 3 minutes until softened. Pour in red wine and beef broth to deglaze the bottom, scrape the bottom of the pot to get rid of any browned bits of food.

Return the beef and pancetta to the Foodi and add rosemary sprigs and thyme. Seal the pressure lid, choose Pressure, set to High, and set the timer to 50 minutes. Press Start.

When ready, release the pressure quickly. Add carrots and bay leaf to the pot. Seal the pressure lid again, choose Pressure, set to High, and set the timer to an additional 4 minutes. Press Start.

When ready, release the pressure quickly. Get rid of the thyme, bay leaf and rosemary sprigs. Place beef on a serving plate and sprinkle with parsley to serve.

Mississippi Pot Roast with Potatoes

Servings: 6 | Ready in about: 1 hr 40 min

INGREDIENTS

1 tbsp canola oil
2 pounds chuck roast
2 tsp salt
½ tsp black pepper
¼ cup butter
1 onion, finely chopped
1 tsp onion powder
1 tsp garlic powder

½ tsp dried thyme
½ tsp dried parsley
6 cups beef broth
½ cup pepperoncini juice
10 pepperoncini
5 potatoes, peeled and sliced
2 bay leaves

DIRECTIONS

Warm oil on Sear/Sauté. Season chuck roast with pepper and salt, then sear in the hot oil for 2 to 4 minutes for each side until browned. Set aside.

Melt butter and cook onion for 3 minutes until fragrant. Sprinkle with dried parsley, onion powder, dried thyme, and garlic powder and stir for 30 seconds.

Into the pot, stir bay leaves, beef broth, pepperoncini juice, and pepperoncini. Nestle chuck roast down into the liquid. Seal the pressure lid, choose Pressure, set to High, and set the timer to 60 minutes. Press Start.

Release pressure naturally for about 10 minutes. Set the chuck roast to a cutting board and use two forks to shred. Serve immediately.

Traditional Beef Stroganoff

Servings: 6 | Ready in about: 1 hr 15 min

INGREDIENTS

¼ cup flour
salt and ground black pepper to taste
2 pounds beef stew meat
2 tbsp olive oil
1 onion, chopped
2 garlic cloves, minced

1 cup beef broth
3 cups fresh mushrooms, chopped
8 ounces sour cream
1 tbsp chopped fresh parsley
1 cup long-grain rice, cooked

DIRECTIONS

In a large bowl, combine salt, pepper and flour. Add beef and massage to coat beef in flour mixture.

Warm oil on Sear/Sauté. Brown the beef for 4 to 5 minutes. Add garlic and onion and cook for 3 minutes until fragrant. Add beef broth to the pot.

Seal the pressure lid, choose Pressure, set to High, and set the timer to 35 minutes. Press Start.

When ready, release the pressure quickly.

Open the lid and stir mushrooms and sour cream into the beef mixture.

Seal the pressure lid again, choose Pressure, set to High, and set the timer to 2 minutes. Press Start.

When ready, release the pressure quickly. Season the stroganoff with pepper and salt; scoop over cooked rice before serving.

Beef Stew with Veggies

Servings: 6 | Ready in about: 1 hr 15 min

INGREDIENTS

¼ cup flour
2 tsp salt, divided
1 tsp paprika
1 tsp ground black pepper
2 pounds beef chuck, cubed
2 tbsp olive oil
2 tbsp butter
1 onion, diced
3 garlic cloves, minced
1 cup dry red wine

2 cups beef stock
1 tbsp dried Italian seasoning
2 tsp Worcestershire sauce
4 cups potatoes, diced
2 celery stalks, chopped
3 cups carrots, chopped
3 tomatoes, chopped
2 bell pepper, thinly sliced
salt and ground black pepper to taste
A handful of fresh parsley, chopped

DIRECTIONS

In a bowl, mix black pepper, beef, flour, paprika, and 1 tsp salt. Toss the ingredients and ensure the beef is coated. Warm butter and oil on Sear/Sautét. Add in beef and cook for 8- 10 minutes until browned. Set aside on a plate.

To the same fat, add garlic, onion, and celery, bell peppers, and cook for 4-5 minutes until tender.

Deglaze with wine, scrape the bottom to get rid of any browned beef bits. Pour in remaining salt, beef stock, Worcestershire sauce, and Italian seasoning.

Return beef to the pot; add carrots, tomatoes, and potatoes.

Seal the pressure lid, choose Pressure, set to High, and set the timer to 35 minutes. Press Start. Release pressure naturally for 10 minutes. Taste and adjust the seasonings as necessary. Serve on plates and scatter over the parsley.

Meatloaf and Cheesy Mashed Potatoes

Servings: 6 | Ready in about: 45 min

INGREDIENTS

Meatloaf:
1 ½ pounds ground beef
1 onion, diced
1 egg
1 potato, grated
1/4 cup tomato puree
1 tsp garlic powder
1 tsp salt
1 tsp ground black pepper

Mashed Potatoes:
4 potatoes, chopped
2 cups water
½ cup milk
2 tbsp butter
1 tsp salt
½ tsp ground black pepper
1 cup ricotta cheese

DIRECTIONS

In a bowl, combine ground beef, eggs, 1 tsp pepper, garlic powder, potato, onion, tomato puree, and 1 tsp salt to obtain a consistent texture. Shape the mixture into a meatloaf and place onto an aluminum foil. Arrange potatoes into Foodi pot and pour water over them.

Place a trivet onto potatoes and set the foil sheet with meatloaf onto the trivet.

Seal the pressure lid, choose Pressure, set to High, and set the timer to 22 minutes. Press Start.

When ready, release the pressure quickly.

Take the meatloaf from the pot and set on a cutting board to cool before slicing.

Drain the liquid out of the pot. Mash potatoes in the pot with ½ tsp pepper, milk, ricotta cheese, 1 tsp salt, and butter until smooth and all the liquid is absorbed.

Divide potatoes into serving plates and lean a meatloaf slice to one side of the potato pile before serving.

Spiced Beef Shapes

Servings: 12 | Ready in about: 40 min

INGREDIENTS:

1 ½ lb ground beef
½ cup minced onion
2 tbsp chopped mint leaves
3 garlic cloves, minced
2 tsp paprika
2 tsp coriander seeds

½ tsp cayenne pepper
1 tsp salt
1 tbsp chopped parsley
2 tsp cumin
½ tsp ground ginger

DIRECTIONS:

Soak 24 skewers in water, until ready to use.

Combine all ingredients in a large bowl.

Make sure to mix well with your hands until the herbs and spices are evenly distributed, and the mixture is well incorporated.

Shape the beef mixture into 12 shapes around 2 skewers.

Close the crisping lid and cook for 12 - 15 minutes on Air Crisp mode at 330 F, or until preferred doneness. Serve with tzatziki sauce and enjoy.

BBQ Sticky Baby Back Ribs with

Servings: 6 | Ready in about: 40 min

INGREDIENTS

2 tbsp olive oil
1 reversible rack baby back ribs, cut into bones
½ tsp salt
1 tbsp mustard powder
1 tbsp smoked paprika

1 tbsp dried oregano
½ tsp ground black pepper
1/3 cup ketchup
1 cup barbecue sauce
½ cup apple cider

DIRECTIONS

In a bowl, thoroughly combine salt, mustard powder, smoked paprika, oregano, and black pepper. Rub the mixture over the ribs. Warm oil on Sear/Sauté.

Add in the ribs and sear for 1 to 2 minutes for each side until browned.

Pour apple cider and barbecue sauce into the pot. Turn the ribs to coat.

Seal the pressure lid, choose Pressure, set to High, and set the timer to 30 minutes. Press Start. When ready, release the pressure quickly.

Place the Cook & Crisp Basket in the pot. Close the crisping lid, choose Air Crisp, set the temperature to 390°F, and the time to 5 minutes.

Place the ribs with the sauce in the Cook & Crisp Basket. Close the Crisping Lid. Preheat the unit by selecting Air Crisp, setting the temperature to 390°F, and setting the time to 7 minutes. Press Start. When ready, the ribs should be sticky with a brown dark color.

Transfer the ribs to a serving plate. Baste with the sauce to serve.

Apple and Onion Topped Pork Chops

Servings: 3 | Ready in about: 25 min

INGREDIENTS:

Topping:
1 small onion, sliced
2 tbsp olive oil
1 tbsp apple cider vinegar
2 tsp thyme

¼ tsp brown sugar
1 cup sliced apples
2 tsp rosemary

Meat:
¼ tsp smoked paprika
1 tbsp olive oil
3 pork chops

1 tbsp apple cider vinegar
Salt and pepper, to taste

DIRECTIONS:

Place all topping ingredients in a baking dish, and then in the Ninja Foodi.

Cook for 4 minutes on Air Crisp mode. Meanwhile, place the pork chops in a bowl. Add olive oil, vinegar, paprika, and season with salt and pepper. Stir to coat them well. Remove the topping from the dish.

Add the pork chops in the dish, close the crisping lid and cook for 10 minutes on Air Crisp mode at 350 F.

Place the topping on top, return to the Ninja Foodi and cook for 5 more minutes.

Swedish Meatballs with Mashed Cauliflower

Servings: 6 | Ready in about: 1 hr

INGREDIENTS

¾ pound ground beef
¾ pound ground pork
1 large egg, beaten
½ onion, minced
¼ cup bread crumbs
1 tbsp water
salt and freshly ground black pepper to taste
4 tbsp butter, divided

2 cups beef stock
3 tbsp flour
½ tsp red wine vinegar
1 ¾ cup heavy cream, divided
1 head cauliflower, cut into florets
¼ cup sour cream
¼ cup fresh chopped parsley

DIRECTIONS

In a mixing bowl, mix ground beef, onion, salt, bread crumbs, ground pork, egg, water, and pepper; shape meatballs. Warm 2 tbsp of butter on Sear/Sauté.

Add meatballs and cook until browned, about 5-6 minutes. Set aside to a plate.

Pour beef stock in the pot to deglaze, scrape the pan to get rid of browned bits of food.

Stir vinegar and flour with the liquid in the pot until smooth; bring to a boil. Stir ¾ cup heavy cream into the liquid. Arrange meatballs into the gravy. Place trivet onto meatballs. Arrange cauliflower florets onto the trivet.

Seal the pressure lid, choose Pressure, set to High, and set the timer to 8 minutes. Press Start.

When ready, release the pressure quickly.

Set the cauliflower in a mixing bowl. Add in the remaining 1 cup heavy cream, pepper, sour cream, salt, and 2 tbsp butter and use a potato masher to mash the mixture until smooth.

Spoon the mashed cauliflower onto serving bowls; place a topping of gravy and meatballs. Add parsley for garnishing.

Peppercorn Meatloaf

Servings: 8 | Ready in about: 35 min

INGREDIENTS:

4 lb ground beef
1 tbsp basil
1 tbsp oregano
1 tbsp parsley
1 onion, diced
1 tbsp Worcestershire sauce

3 tbsp ketchup
½ tsp salt
1 tsp ground peppercorns
10 whole peppercorns, for garnishing
1 cup breadcrumbs

DIRECTIONS:

Place the beef in a large bowl.

Add all of the ingredients except the whole peppercorns and the breadcrumbs.

Mix with your hand until well combined. Stir in the breadcrumbs.

Put the meatloaf on a lined baking dish.

Insert in the Ninja Foodi, close the crisping lid and cook for 25 minutes on Air Crisp mode at 350 F.

Garnish the meatloaf with the whole peppercorns and let cool slightly before serving.

Braised Short Ribs with Creamy Sauce

Servings: 6 | Ready in about: 1 hr 55 min

INGREDIENTS

3 pounds beef short ribs
2 tsp salt, divided
1½ tsp freshly ground black pepper, divided
2 tbsp olive oil
1 onion, chopped
1 large carrot, chopped
1 celery stalk, chopped
3 garlic cloves, chopped

2 cups beef broth
1 (14.5 ounces) can diced tomatoes
½ cup dry red wine
¼ cup red wine vinegar
2 bay leaves
¼ tsp red pepper flakes
2 tbsp chopped parsley
1/2 cup cheese cream

DIRECTIONS

Season your short ribs with 1 tsp black pepper and 1 tsp salt. Warm olive oil on Sear/Sauté.

Add in short ribs and sear for 3 minutes each side until browned. Set aside on a bowl.

Drain everything only to be left with 1 tbsp of the remaining fat from the pot.

Set on Sear/Sauté, and stir-fry garlic, carrot, onion, and celery in the hot fat for 4 to 6 minutes until fragrant.

Stir in broth, wine, red pepper flakes, vinegar, tomatoes, bay leaves, and remaining pepper and salt; turn the Foodi to Sear/Sauté on Low and bring the mixture to a boil.

With the bone-side up, lay short ribs into the braising liquid.

Seal the pressure lid, choose Pressure, set to High, and set the timer to 40 minutes. Press Start.

When ready, release the pressure quickly.

Set the short ribs on a plate. Get rid of bay leaves. Skim and get rid of the fat from the surface of braising liquid.

Using an immersion blender, blend the liquid for 1 minute; add cream cheese, pepper and salt and blitz until smooth Arrange the ribs onto a serving plate, pour the sauce over and top with parsley.

Italian Beef Sandwiches with Pesto

Servings: 4 | Ready in about: 1 hr

INGREDIENTS

1 1/2 pounds beef steak, cut into strips
salt and ground black pepper
1 tbsp olive oil
1/4 cup dry red wine
1 cup beef broth
1 tbsp oregano

1 tsp onion powder
1 tsp garlic powder
4 hoagie rolls, halved
8 slices mozzarella cheese
1/2 cup sliced pepperoncini peppers
4 tbsp pesto

DIRECTIONS

Sprinkle pepper and salt to season the beef cubes and bring to room temperature. Warm oil on Sear/Sauté.

Add in the beef and sear for 2 to 3 minutes for each side until browned.

Add wine into the pot to deglaze, scrape the bottom to get rid of any browned beef bits.

Stir garlic powder, beef broth, onion powder, and oregano into the pot.

Seal the pressure lid, choose Pressure, set to High, and set the timer to 25 minutes. Press Start.

Release pressure naturally for 10 minutes. Spread each bread half with pesto, put beef on top, place pepperoncini slices over, add mozzarella cheese slices and cover with the second half of bread to serve.

Short Ribs with Mushroom and Asparagus Sauce

Servings: 6 | Ready in about: 1 hr 15 min

INGREDIENTS

3½ pounds boneless beef short ribs, cut into pieces
2 tsp salt
1 tsp ground black pepper
3 tbsp olive oil
1 onion, diced
1 cup dry red wine
1 tbsp tomato puree
2 carrots, peeled and chopped
2 garlic cloves, minced

5 sprigs parsley, chopped
2 sprigs rosemary, chopped
3 sprigs oregano, chopped
4 cups beef stock
10 ounces mushrooms, quartered
1 cup asparagus, trimmed and roughly chopped
1 tbsp cornstarch
¼ cup cold water

DIRECTIONS

Apply a seasoning of black pepper and salt to the ribs.

Warm oil on Sear/Sauté. In batches, add the short ribs to the oil and cook for 3 to 5 minutes each side until browned. Set aside on a bowl. Add onions to the hot oil and cook for 3 to 5 minutes until soft. Add tomato puree and red wine into the pot to deglaze, scrape the bottom to get rid of any browned beef bits. Cook for 2 minutes until wine reduces slightly.

Return the ribs to pot and top with carrots, oregano, rosemary, and garlic. Add in beef broth.

Seal the pressure lid, choose Pressure, set to High, and set the timer to 35 minutes. Press Start. Release pressure naturally for 10 minutes. Transfer ribs to a plate. Strain and get rid of herbs and vegetables, and return cooking broth to inner pot. Add mushrooms and asparagus to the broth.

Press Sear/Sauté and cook for 2 to 4 minutes until vegetables are soft.

In a bowl, mix water and cornstarch until cornstarch dissolves completely. Add the cornstarch mixture into the broth as you stir for 1 to 3 minutes until the broth thickens slightly. Season the sauce with black pepper and salt. Pour the sauce over ribs, add chopped parsley for garnish before serving.

The Crispiest Roast Pork

Servings: 4 | Ready in about: 50 min

INGREDIENTS:

4 pork tenderloins
1 tsp five spice seasoning
½ tsp white pepper

¾ tsp garlic powder
1 tsp salt
Cooking spray

DIRECTIONS:

Place the pork, white pepper, garlic powder, five seasoning, and salt into a bowl and toss to coat. Leave to marinate at room temperature for 30 minutes.

Place the pork into the Ninja Foodi basket, greased with cooking spray, close the crisping lid and cook for 20 minutes at 360 F. After 10 minutes, turn the tenderloins.

Serve hot.

Pork Tenderloin with Sweet Pepper Sauce & Potatoes

Servings: 4 | Ready in about: 35 min

INGREDIENTS

1 large (about 1¼-pound) beef tenderloin, cut into 2 pieces

2 tsp salt

¼ tsp freshly ground black pepper

2 tbsp olive oil

½ cup dry white wine

1 pound russet potatoes, quartered

¼ cup chicken stock

1 thyme sprig

2 medium garlic cloves, finely minced

1 small roasted red bell pepper, cut into strips

6 pickled pimientos, stemmed, seeded, and quartered

2 tsp pickling liquid from the peppers

2 tbsp unsalted butter

DIRECTIONS

Season the beef pieces with the salt and black pepper on all sides. On your Foodi, choose Sear/Sauté and adjust to Medium-High. Press Start to preheat the pot for 5 minutes.

Pour in the oil into the pot and heat until shimmering. Add the beef pieces, sear for 3 minutes or until browned. Turn and brown the other side. Remove the beef to a plate.

Pour in the wine into the pot and scrape off any browned bits at the bottom. Let the wine cook until reduced by one-third. Stir in the potatoes, chicken stock, thyme, and garlic. Return the beef to the pot.

Seal the pressure lid, choose Pressure; adjust the pressure to High and the cook time to 20 minutes; press Start. After cooking, perform a natural pressure release for 5 minutes, then a quick pressure release, and carefully open the pressure lid.

Remove the beef and allow resting while you finish the sauce. Remove and discard the thyme. Choose Sear/Sauté and adjust to Medium. Press Start to simmer the sauce.

Cook the potatoes for 2 to 4 minutes or until tender. Stir in the roasted pepper, pimiento, and the pickling liquid. Taste and adjust the seasoning.

Right before serving, turn off the heat and stir in the butter. Slice the tenderloin and lay the pieces on a platter. Ladle the peppers and potatoes around the pork and spoon the sauce over.

Philippine-Style Pork Chops

Servings: 6 | Ready in about: 2 hours 20 min

INGREDIENTS:

2 lb pork chops

2 bay leaves

2 tbsp soy sauce

5 garlic cloves, coarsely chopped

1 tbsp peppercorns

1 tbsp peanut oil

1 tsp salt

DIRECTIONS:

Combine the bay leaves, soy sauce, garlic, salt, peppercorns, and oil, in a bowl.

Rub the mixture onto meat. Wrap the pork with a plastic foil and refrigerate for 2h.

Place the pork in the Ninja Foodi, close the crisping lid and cook for 10 minutes on Air Crisp mode at 350 F. Increase the temperature to 370 F, flip the chops, and cook for another 10 minutes. Discard bay leaves before serving.

Honey Barbecue Pork Ribs

Servings: 2 | Ready in about: 4 h 35 min

INGREDIENTS:

1 lb pork ribs
½ tsp five spice powder
1 tsp salt
3 garlic cloves, chopped
1 tsp black pepper

1 tsp sesame oil
1 tbsp honey, plus more for brushing
4 tbsp barbecue sauce
1 tsp soy sauce

DIRECTIONS:

Chop the ribs into smaller pieces and place in a large bowl.

In a separate bowl, whisk together all of the other ingredients. Add to the bowl with the pork, and mix until the pork is thoroughly coated. Cover the bowl, place it in the fridge, and let it marinade for about 4 hours.

Place the ribs in the basket of the Ninja Foodi. Close the crisping lid and cook for 15 minutes on Air Crisp mode at 350 F. After, brush the ribs with some honey and cook for 15 more minutes.

Char Siew Pork Ribs

Servings: 6 | Ready in about: 4 hours 55 min

INGREDIENTS:

2 lb pork ribs
2 tbsp char siew sauce
2 tbsp minced ginger
2 tbsp hoisin sauce

2 tbsp sesame oil
1 tbsp honey
4 garlic cloves, minced
1 tbsp soy sauce

DIRECTIONS:

Whisk together all marinade ingredients, in a small bowl. Coat the ribs well with the mixture. Place in a container with a lid, and refrigerate for 4 hours.

Place the ribs in the basket but do not throw away the liquid from the container. Close the crisping lid and cook for 40 minutes on Air Crisp at 350 F. Stir in the liquid, increase the temperature to 350 F, and cook for 10 minutes.

Crunchy Cashew Lamb Rack

Servings: 4 | Ready in about: 30 min

INGREDIENTS:

3 oz chopped cashews
1 tbsp chopped rosemary
1 ½ lb rack of lamb
1 garlic clove, minced

1 tbsp breadcrumbs
1 egg, beaten
1 tbsp olive oil
Salt and pepper, to taste

DIRECTIONS:

Combine the olive oil with the garlic and brush this mixture onto the lamb. Combine the rosemary, cashews, and breadcrumbs, in a small bowl. Brush the egg over the lambs, and then coat it with the cashew mixture.

Place the lamb in the Ninja Foodi, close the crisping lid and cook for 25 minutes on Air Crisp at 320 F. Then increase to 390 degrees F, and cook for 5 more minutes. Cover with a foil and let sit for a couple of minutes before serving.

Pork Chops with Cremini Mushroom Sauce

Servings: 4 | Ready in about: 35 min

INGREDIENTS:

4 pork chops
1 tbsp olive oil
3 cloves garlic, minced
Salt and pepper, to taste
1 tsp garlic powder
1 (10 oz) can mushroom soup

8 oz Cremini mushrooms, sliced
1 small onion, chopped
1 cup beef broth
1 sprig fresh thyme
Chopped parsley to garnish

DIRECTIONS:

Select Sear/Sauté mode. Add oil, mushrooms, garlic, and onion. Sauté them, stirring occasionally with a spoon, until nice and translucent, for 3 minutes.

Season the pork chops with salt, garlic powder, and pepper, and add them to the pot followed by the thyme and broth. Seal the lid and select Pressure mode on High pressure for 10 minutes. Press Start/Stop to start cooking.

Once the timer has ended, do a natural pressure release for about 10 minutes, then a quick pressure release to let the remaining steam out.

Close the crisping lid and cook on Broil mode for 5 minutes.

When ready, add the mushroom soup. Stir it until the mixture thickens a little bit. Dish the pork and gravy into a serving bowl and garnish with parsley. Serve with a side of creamy sweet potato mash.

Ranch Flavored Pork Roast with Gravy

Servings: 4 | Ready in about: 25 min

INGREDIENTS:

2 lb pork roast, cut into 2-inch slabs
1 tbsp Italian Seasoning
1 tbsp Ranch Dressing
1 tsp red wine vinegar
2 cloves garlic, minced
Salt and pepper, to taste
1 small onion, chopped

1 tbsp olive oil
2 tsp onion powder
½ tsp paprika
2 cups vegetable broth
2 tbsp cornstarch
2 tbsp water
Chopped parsley to garnish

DIRECTIONS:

Season the pork roast with salt and pepper, and set aside.

In a bowl, add Italian seasoning, ranch dressing, red wine vinegar, garlic, onion powder, and paprika.

Open the pot, select Sear/Sauté mode, and heat the oil. Sauté the onion, until translucent. Pour the gravy mixture and broth over and add the pork. Close the lid, secure the pressure valve, and select Pressure mode on High pressure for 15 minutes. Press Start/Stop to start cooking.

Once the timer has ended, do a quick pressure release, and open the pot. Remove the pork roast with a slotted spoon onto a serving plate. Mix the cornstarch with the water in a small bowl and add it to the sauce. Select Sear/Sauté. Stir and cook the sauce for 4 minutes, until thickens.

Once the gravy is ready, turn off the pot and spoon the sauce over the pork.

Garnish with parsley and serve with a turnip mash.

Sweet-Garlic Pork Tenderloin

Servings: 4 | Ready in about: 30 min

INGREDIENTS:

2 lb pork tenderloin
2 tbsp olive oil
¼ cup honey
½ cup chicken broth
Salt and black pepper to taste
1 clove garlic, minced

1 tsp sage powder
1 tbsp Dijon mustard
¼ cup Balsamic vinegar
1 tbsp Worcestershire sauce
½ tbsp cornstarch
4 tbsp water

DIRECTIONS:

Put the pork on a clean flat surface and pat dry using paper towels. Season with salt and pepper. Select Sear/Sauté mode.

Heat the oil and brown the pork on both sides, for about 4 minutes in total. Remove the pork onto a plate and set aside. Add in honey, chicken broth, balsamic vinegar, garlic, Worcestershire sauce, mustard, and sage. Stir the ingredients and return the pork to the pot.

Close the lid, secure the pressure valve, and select Pressure mode on High for 15 minutes. Once the timer has ended, do a quick pressure release.

Remove the pork with tongs onto a plate and wrap it in aluminum foil.

Next, mix the cornstarch with water and pour it into the pot. Select Sear/Sauté mode, stir the mixture and cook until it thickens. Then, turn the pot off after the desired thickness is achieved.

Unwrap the pork and use a knife to slice it with 3 to 4-inch thickness. Arrange the slices on a serving platter and spoon the sauce all over it. Serve with a syrupy sautéed Brussels sprouts and red onion chunks.

Pork Tenderloin with Garlic and Ginger

Servings: 4 | Ready in about: 23 min

INGREDIENTS:

2 lb pork tenderloin
½ cup soy sauce
¼ cup sugar
½ cup water + 2 tbsp water
3 tbsp grated ginger

2 cloves garlic, minced
2 tbsp sesame oil
2 tsp cornstarch
Chopped scallions to garnish
Sesame seeds to garnish

DIRECTIONS:

In the Ninja Foodi's inner pot, add soy sauce, sugar, half cup of water, ginger, garlic, and sesame oil. Use a spoon to stir them. Then, add the pork.

Close the lid, secure the pressure valve, and select Pressure mode on High pressure for 12 minutes. Press Start/Stop.

Once the timer has ended, do a quick pressure release, and open the pot.

Remove the pork and set aside.

In a bowl, mix the cornstarch with the remaining water until smooth and pour it into the pot. Bring back the pork. Close the crisping lid and press Broil.

Cook for 5 minutes, until the sauce has thickened. Stir the sauce frequently, every 1-2 minutes, to avoid burning. Once the sauce is ready, serve the pork with a side endive salad or steamed veggies. Spoon the sauce all over it.

Pork Sandwiches with Slaw

Servings: 8 | Ready in about: 20 min

INGREDIENTS:

2 lb chuck roast
¼ cup sugar
1 tsp Spanish paprika
1 tsp garlic powder

Assembling:
4 Buns, halved
1 cup white Cheddar cheese, grated
4 tbsp mayonnaise

1 white onion, sliced
2 cups beef broth
Salt to taste
2 tbsp apple cider vinegar

1 cup red cabbage, shredded
1 cup white cabbage, shredded

DIRECTIONS:

Place the pork roast on a clean flat surface and sprinkle with paprika, garlic powder, sugar, and salt. Use your hands to rub the seasoning on the meat.

Open the Ninja Foodi, add beef broth, onions, pork, and apple cider vinegar.

Close the lid, secure the pressure valve, and select Pressure mode on High pressure for 12 minutes. Press Start/ Stop.

Once the timer has ended, do a quick pressure release. Remove the roast to a cutting board, and use two forks to shred them. Return to the pot, close the crisping lid, and cook for 3 minutes on Air Crisp at 300 F.

In the buns, spread the mayo, add the shredded pork, some cooked onions from the pot, and shredded red and white cabbage. Top with the cheese.

BBQ Pork Ribs

Servings: 2 | Ready in about: 45 min

INGREDIENTS:

½ lb rack baby back ribs
Salt and pepper to season
¼ cup beef broth

½ cup Barbecue sauce
3 tbsp apple cider vinegar

DIRECTIONS:

Select Sear/Sauté mode. Heat the oil into the pot. Meanwhile, season the ribs with salt and pepper. Cook them to brown, for 1 to 2 minutes per side.

Pour the barbecue sauce, broth, and apple cider vinegar over the ribs and use tongs to flip so they are well coated.

Close the lid and pressure valve and set to Pressure mode on High pressure for 30 minutes. Press Start/Stop to start cooking.

Once the timer goes off, do a natural pressure release for 12 minutes, then a quick pressure release to let out the remaining steam.

Close the crisping lid and set to Air Crisp mode for 5 minutes at 350 F. Make sure the sauce is thick enough.

Use a knife to slice the ribs and over the sauce all over it.

Serve the ribs with a generous side of steamed but crunchy green beans.

Italian Sausage with Potato Mash & Onion Gravy

Servings: 4 | Ready in about: 40 min

INGREDIENTS:

2 lb potatoes, peeled and halved
4 Italian sausages
1 cup water + 2 tbsp water
⅓ cup green onion, sliced
Salt and pepper, to taste
4 tbsp milk

¼ cup + 2 tbsp + 2 tbsp butter
1 tbsp cornstarch
3 tbsp balsamic vinegar
1 onion, sliced thinly
1 cup + 2 tbsp beef broth

DIRECTIONS:

Put the potatoes in the inner pot and pour the water over. Seal the lid; select Steam mode on High for 15 minutes and press Start/Stop.

Do a quick pressure release, and remove the potatoes to a bowl. Add in a quarter cup butter and use a masher to mash them until the butter is well mixed. Slowly add the milk and mix it using a spoon. Add the green onions, season with pepper and salt and fold it in with the spoon. Set aside.

Pour out the liquid in the Ninja Foodi, and use paper towels to wipe inside the pot dry. Select Sear/Sauté mode and melt two tablespoons of butter.

Brown the sausages on each side for 3 minutes. Remove to the potato mash and cover with aluminium foil to keep warm. Set aside Back into the pot, add the two tablespoons of the beef broth to deglaze the bottom of the pot while stirring and scraping the bottom with a spoon. Add the remaining butter and onions; sauté the onions until translucent, then pour in the balsamic vinegar. Stir for another minute.

In a bowl, mix the cornstarch with water and pour into the pot. Add the remaining beef broth. Allow the sauce to thicken and adjust the seasoning. Turn off the heat once a slurry is formed. Dish the mashed potatoes and sausages in serving plates. Spoon the gravy over it and serve immediately with steamed green beans.

Mediterranean Tender Pork Roast

Servings: 6 | Ready in about: 60 min

INGREDIENTS:

3 lb pork roast, cut into 3-inch pieces
3 tbsp Cavender's Greek Seasoning to taste
1 tsp onion powder
1 cup beef broth

½ cup Kalamata olives, pitted
¼ cup fresh lemon juice
Salt to taste

DIRECTIONS:

Put the pork chunks in the inner pot of the Ninja Foodi.

In a bowl, add greek seasoning, onion powder, beef broth, lemon juice, olives, and salt to taste. Mix using a spoon and pour the sauce over the pork.

Close the lid, secure the pressure valve, and select Pressure mode on High pressure for 35 minutes. Press Start/ Stop to start cooking.

Once the timer is off, do a natural pressure release for 10 minutes, then do a quick pressure release to let out any more steam, and open the pot.

Use two forks to shred the roast inside to pot and close the crisping lid. Cook on Broil mode for 10 minutes, until nice and tender. Serve with a green salad, potatoes or rice.

Garlicky Braised Pork Neck Bones

Servings: 6 | Ready in about: 40 min

INGREDIENTS:

3 lb pork neck bones

4 tbsp olive oil

Salt and black pepper to taste

2 cloves garlic, smashed

1 tbsp tomato paste

1 tsp dried thyme

1 white onion, sliced

½ cup red wine

1 cup beef broth

DIRECTIONS:

Open the lid and select Sear/Sauté mode. Warm the olive oil.

Meanwhile, season the pork neck bones with salt and pepper. After, place them in the oil to brown on all sides. Work in batches.

Each batch should cook in about 5 minutes. Then, remove them onto a plate.

Add the onion and season with salt to taste. Stir with a spoon and cook the onions until soft, for a few minutes.

Then, add garlic, thyme, pepper, and tomato paste. Cook them for 2 minutes, constant stirring to prevent the tomato paste from burning.

Next, pour the red wine into the pot to deglaze the bottom. Add the pork neck bones back to the pot and pour the beef broth over it.

Close the lid, secure the pressure valve, and select Pressure mode on High pressure for 10 minutes. Press Start/Stop to start cooking.

Once the timer has ended, let the pot sit for 10 minutes before doing a quick pressure release. Close the crisping lid and cook on Broil mode for 5 minutes, until nice and tender.

Dish the pork neck into a serving bowl and serve with the red wine sauce spooned over and a right amount of broccoli mash.

Hot Pork Carnitas Lettuce Cups

Servings: 6 | Ready in about: 30 min + overnight refrigerated

INGREDIENTS:

3 lb pork shoulder

2 tbsp olive oil

1 small head lettuce, leaves removed, washed and dried

2 Limes, cut in wedges

2 carrots, grated

1 ½ cup water

1 onion, chopped

½ tsp Cayenne pepper

½ tsp coriander powder

1 tsp cumin powder

1 tsp garlic powder

1 tsp white pepper

2 tsp dried oregano

1 tsp red pepper flakes

Salt to taste

DIRECTIONS:

In a bowl, add onion, cayenne, coriander, garlic, cumin, white pepper, dried oregano, red pepper flakes, and salt. Mix them well with a spoon.

Drizzle over the pork and rub to coat. Then, wrap the meat in plastic wrap and refrigerate overnight.

On the next day, open the Ninja Foodi lid, and select Sear/Sauté mode. Pour 2 tablespoons of olive oil in the pot and while heating, take the pork out from the fridge, remove the wraps and place it in the pot.

Brown it on both sides for 6 minutes and then pour the water.

Close the lid, secure the pressure valve, and select Pressure mode on High pressure for 15 minutes. Press Start/Stop to start cooking.

Once the timer has stopped, do a quick pressure release.Use two forks to shred the pork, inside the pot. Close the crisping lid, and select Bake/Roast mode. Set for 10 minutes at 350 F. When ready, turn off the heat and begin assembling.

Arrange double layers of lettuce leaves on a flat surface, make a bed of grated carrots in them, and spoon the pulled pork on them.

Drizzle a sauce of choice (I used mustardy sauce) over them, and serve with lime wedges for freshness.

Tomatillo & Sweet Potato pork Chili

Servings: 6 | Ready in about: 70 min

INGREDIENTS:

1 ½ lb pork roast, cut into 1-inch cubes
1 lb tomatillos, husks removed
2 tbsp olive oil, divided into 2
1 bulb garlic, tail sliced off, peeled
2 green chilies
3 cups chicken broth
1 green bell pepper, seeded and roughly chopped

Salt and pepper, to taste
½ tsp cumin powder
1 tsp dried oregano
1 bay leaf
1 bunch cilantro, chopped and divided into 2
2 sweet potatoes, peeled and cut into ½-inch cubes

DIRECTIONS:

Put the garlic bulb in a baking dish that fits in your reversible rack, inside the inner pot. Drizzle a bit of 1 portion of olive oil over the garlic bulb.

Place the green bell peppers, onion, green chilies, and tomatillos on the dish in a single layer.

Close the crisping lid and cook for 15 minutes at 400 F on Air Crisp mode.

Then, remove them, and set aside to cool. Wipe clean the pot if needed.

Place the garlic in a blender. Add green bell pepper, tomatillos, onions, and green chilies. Pulse for a few minutes not to be smooth but slightly chunky.

Now, open the lid of the Ninja Foodi, and select Sear/Sauté mode.

Pour in the remaining olive oil and while is heating, season the pork cubes with salt and pepper. Then, brown the pork, for about 5 minutes.

Stir in oregano, cumin, bay leaf, pour in the blended green sauce, potatoes, and add the chicken broth. Stir well.

Close the lid, secure the pressure valve, and select Pressure mode on High pressure for 25 minutes. Press Start/Stop to start cooking.

Once the timer has ended, let the pot sit closed for 10 minutes.

After, do a natural pressure release for 5 minutes, and then a quick pressure release to let the remaining steam out.

Open the pot. Remove and discard the bay leaf, add half of the cilantro, adjust with salt and pepper, and stir.

Close the crisping lid to give it nice and tender taste. Cook on Broil mode for 10 minutes.

Dish the chili into serving bowls and garnish it with the remaining chopped cilantro.

Serve topped with a side of chips or crusted bread.

Garlick & Ginger Pork with Coconut Sauce

Servings: 6 | Ready in about: 45 min

INGREDIENTS:

3 lb shoulder roast
1 tbsp olive oil
Salt and black pepper to season
2 cups coconut milk
1 tsp Coriander powder
1 tsp cumin powder

3 tbsp grated ginger
3 tsp minced garlic
½ cup beef broth
1 onion, peeled and quartered
Parsley leaves (unchopped), to garnish

DIRECTIONS:

In a bowl, add coriander, salt, pepper, and cumin. Use a spoon to mix them.

Season the pork with the spice mixture. Rub the spice onto meat, with hands. Open the lid of Ninja Foodi, add olive oil, pork, onions, ginger, garlic, broth and coconut milk.

Close the lid, secure the pressure valve, and select Pressure mode on High for 30 minutes. Press Start/Stop to start cooking.

Once the timer has stopped, do a quick pressure release. Give it a good stir and close the crisping lid. Cook for 10 minutes on Broil mode, until you perfect texture and creaminess.

Dish the meat with the sauce into a serving bowl, garnish it with the parsley and serve with a side of bread or cooked shrimp.

Savory Pork Loin with Carrot & Celery Sauce

Servings: 4 | Ready in about: 35 min

INGREDIENTS:

2 lb pork loin roast
Salt and pepper, to taste
3 cloves garlic, minced
1 medium onion, diced
2 tbsp butter
3 stalks celery, chopped
3 carrots, chopped
1 cup vegetable broth

2 tbsp Worcestershire sauce
½ tbsp sugar
1 tsp yellow mustard
2 tsp dried basil
2 tsp dried thyme
1 tbsp cornstarch
¼ cup water

DIRECTIONS:

Select Sear/Sauté mode, and heat oil. Season the pork with salt and pepper. Sear the pork to golden brown on both sides, about 4 minutes.

Then, add the garlic and onions, and cook them until soft, for about 4 minutes. Top with the celery, carrots, broth, Worcestershire sauce, mustard, thyme, basil, and sugar.

Close the lid, secure the pressure valve, and select Pressure mode on High pressure for 15 minutes. Press Start/Stop to start cooking.

Once the timer is off, do a quick pressure release. Next, add the cornstarch to the water, in a bowl, and mix with a spoon, until nice and smooth. Add it to the pot, close the crisping lid, and cook on Broil mode, for 3 - 5 minutes, until the sauce becomes a slurry with a bit of thickness, and the pork is nice and tender.

Adjust the seasoning, and ladle to a serving platter. Serve with a side of steamed almond garlicky rapini mix.

Spicy Pork Roast with Peanut Sauce

Servings: 6 | Ready in about: 30 min

INGREDIENTS:

3 lb pork roast
1 cup Hot water
1 large red bell pepper, seeded and sliced
Salt and pepper to taste
1 large white onion, sliced
½ cup soy sauce

1 tbsp plain vinegar
½ cup peanut butter
1 tbsp lime juice
1 tbsp garlic powder
1 tsp ginger puree
2 chilies, deseeded, chopped

To Garnish:
Chopped Peanuts
Chopped green onions

Lime Wedges

DIRECTIONS:

Add the soy sauce, vinegar, peanut butter, lime juice, garlic powder, chilies, and ginger puree, to a bowl. Whisk together and even. Add a few pinches of salt and pepper, and mix it.

Open the Ninja Foodi lid, and place the pork in the inner pot. Pour the hot water and peanut butter mixture over it.

Close the lid, secure the pressure valve, and select Pressure mode on High pressure for 15 minutes. Press Start/Stop to start cooking.

Once the timer has stopped, do a quick pressure release.

Use two forks to shred it, inside the pot, and close the crisping lid.

Cook on Broil mode for 4 - 5 minutes, until the sauce thickens.

On a bed of cooked rice, spoon the meat with some sauce and garnish it with the chopped peanuts, green onions, and the lemon wedges.

Tasty Ham with Collard Greens

Servings: 4 | Ready in about: 10 min

INGREDIENTS:

20 oz collard greens, washed and cut
2 cubes of chicken bouillon
4 cups water

½ cup diced sweet onion
2 ½ cups diced ham

DIRECTIONS:

Place the ham at the bottom of the inner pot. Add collard greens and onion.

Then, add chicken cubes to the water and dissolve it.

Pour the mixture into the pot. Close the lid, secure the pressure valve, to seal properly.

Select Steam mode on High pressure for 5 minutes. Press Start/Stop.

Once the timer has ended, do a quick pressure release, and open the lid.

Spoon the vegetables and the ham with sauce into a serving platter.

Serve with a side of steak dish of your choice.

Pulled Pork Tacos

Servings: 5 | Ready in about: 1 hr 25 min

INGREDIENTS

3 tbsp sugar
3 tsp taco seasoning
1 tsp ground black pepper
2 pounds pork shoulder, trimmed, cut into chunks
1 cup beer
1 cup vegetable broth

1/4 cup plus 2 tbsp lemon juice
1/4 cup mayonnaise
2 tbsp honey
2 tsp mustard
3 cups shredded cabbage
5 taco tortillas

DIRECTIONS

In a bowl, combine sugar, taco seasoning, and black pepper; rub the mixture onto pork pieces to coat well. Allow to settling for 30 minutes. Into the Foodi, add 1/4 cup lemon juice, broth, pork and beer.

Seal the pressure lid, choose Pressure, set to High, and set the timer to 50 minutes. Press Start. Meanwhile in a large bowl, mix mayonnaise, mustard, 2 tbsp lemon juice, cabbage and honey until well coated.

Release pressure naturally for 15 minutes before doing a quick release. Transfer the pork to a cutting board and Allow cooling before using two forks to shred. Skim and get rid of fat from liquid in the pressure cooker.

Return pork to the pot and mix with the liquid. Top the pork with slaw on taco tortillas before serving.

Pork Chops with Broccoli and Gravy

Servings: 6 | Ready in about: 45 min

INGREDIENTS

Pork Chops:
1 ½ tsp salt
1 tsp ground black pepper
1 tsp garlic powder
1 tsp onion powder
1 tsp red pepper flakes
6 boneless pork chops
1 broccoli head, broken into florets

1 cup chicken stock
¼ cup butter, melted
¼ cup milk
Gravy:
3 tbsp flour
½ cup heavy cream
salt and ground black pepper to taste

DIRECTIONS

Combine salt, garlic powder, red pepper flakes, onion powder, and black pepper; rub the mixture to the pork chops. Place stock and broccoli into the Foodi. Lay the pork chops on top.

Seal the pressure lid, choose Pressure, set to High, and set the timer to 15 minutes. Press Start.

When ready, release the pressure quickly.

Transfer the pork chops and broccoli to a plate. Press Sear/Sauté and simmer the liquid remaining in the pot.

Mix cream and flour; pour into the simmering liquid and cook for 5 to 7 minutes until thickened and bubbly; season with pepper and salt. Top the chops with gravy before, drizzle melted butter over broccoli and serve.

Cuban-Style Pork

Servings: 8 | Ready in about: 2 hr 30 min

INGREDIENTS

½ cup orange juice
¼ cup lime juice
¼ cup canola oil
¼ cup chopped fresh cilantro
1 tsp red pepper flakes
8 cloves garlic, minced

1 tbsp ground cumin
1 tbsp fresh oregano
2 tsp ground black pepper
1 tsp salt
3 pounds pork shoulder

DIRECTIONS

In a bowl, mix orange juice, olive oil, cumin, salt, pepper, oregano, lime juice, and garlic; add into a large plastic bag alongside the pork. Seal and massage the bag to ensure the marinade covers the pork completely.

Place in the refrigerator for an hour to overnight. In the Foodi, set your removed pork from bag.

Add the marinade on top. Seal the pressure lid, choose Pressure, set to High, and set the timer to 50 minutes. Press Start. Release pressure naturally for 15 minutes. Transfer the pork to a cutting board; use a fork to break into smaller pieces.

Skim and get rid of the fat from liquid in the cooker. Serve the liquid with pork and sprinkle with cilantro.

Baby Back Ribs with BBQ Sauce

Servings: 4 | Ready in about: 45 min

INGREDIENTS

2 pounds baby back pork ribs
4 cups orange juice
Juice from 1 lemon
For BBQ sauce:
2 tbsp honey
½ cup ketchup

Juice from ½ lemon
1 tbsp Worcestershire sauce
1tsp mustard
2 tsp paprika
½ tsp cayenne pepper
Salt to taste

DIRECTIONS

Mix all the BBQ sauce ingredients in a bowl until well incorporated. Set aside.

Place ribs in your Foodi pot; add in lemon juice and orange juice.

Seal the pressure lid, choose Pressure, set to High, and set the timer to 20 minutes. Press Start. Release pressure naturally for 15 minutes. Meanwhile, preheat oven to 400° F. Line the sheet pan with aluminum foil.

Transfer the ribs to the prepared sheet. Do away with the cooking liquid. Onto both sides of ribs, brush barbecue sauce. Bake ribs in the oven for 10 minutes until sauce is browned and caramelized; set the ribs aside and cut into individual bones to serve.

Italian Sausage and Cannellini Stew

Servings: 6 | Ready in about: 45 min

INGREDIENTS

1 tbsp olive oil
1 pound Italian sausages, halved
1 celery stalk, chopped
1 carrot, chopped
1 onion, chopped
1 sprig fresh sage

1 sprig fresh rosemary
1 bay leaf
1 cup Cannellini Beans, soaked and rinsed
2 cups vegetable stock
3 cups fresh spinach
1 tsp salt

DIRECTIONS

Warm oil on Sear/Sauté. Add in sausage pieces and sear for 5 minutes until browned; set aside on a plate.

To the pot, add celery, onion, bay leaf, sage, carrot, and rosemary; cook for 3 minutes to soften slightly.

Stir in vegetable stock and beans. Arrange seared sausage pieces on top of the beans.

Seal the pressure lid, choose Pressure, set to High, and set the timer to 10 minutes. Press Start. Release pressure naturally for 20 minutes,

Once ready, do a quick release. Get rid of bay leaf, rosemary and sage. Mix spinach into the mixture to serve.

Red Pork and Chickpea Stew

Servings: 6 | Ready in about: 40 min

INGREDIENTS

1 tbsp olive oil
1 (3 pounds) boneless pork shoulder, trimmed and cubed
1 white onion, chopped
15 ounces canned chickpeas, drained and rinsed
1½ cups water
½ cup sweet paprika

2 tsp salt
1 tbsp chilli powder
1 bay leaf
2 red bell peppers, chopped
6 cloves garlic, minced
1 tbsp cornstarch
1 tbsp water

DIRECTIONS

Set on Sear/Sauté, set to Medium High, and choose Start/Stop to preheat the pot; add pork and oil and allow cooking for 5 minutes until browned. Add in the onion, paprika, bay leaf, salt, water, chickpeas, and chili powder. Seal the pressure lid, choose Pressure, set to High, and set the timer to 8 minutes. Press Start.

Do a quick release and discard bay leaf. Remove 1 cup of cooking liquid from the Foodi; add to a blender alongside garlic, water, cornstarch, and red bell peppers; blend well until smooth.

Add the blended mixture into the stew and mix well.

Ranch Pork with Mushroom Sauce

Servings: 4 | Ready in about: 22 min

INGREDIENTS:

4 pork loin chops
1 (15 oz) can mushroom soup cream
1 oz Ranch Dressing and Seasoning mix

½ cup chicken broth
Chopped parsley to garnish

DIRECTIONS:

Add pork, mushroom soup cream, ranch dressing and seasoning mix, and chicken broth, inside the inner pot of your Ninja Foodi.

Close the lid, secure the pressure valve, and select Pressure mode on High pressure for 10 minutes. Press Start/Stop.

Once the timer has ended, do a natural pressure release for 10 minutes, then a quick pressure release to let the remaining steam out.

Close the crisping lid and cook for 5 minutes on Broil mode, until tender.

Serve with well-seasoned sautéed cremini mushrooms, and the sauce.

Beer-Braised Hot Dogs with Peppers

Servings: 6 | Ready in about: 15 min

INGREDIENTS

1 tbsp olive oil
6 sausages pork sausage links
1 green bell pepper, sliced into strips
1 red bell pepper, sliced into strips

1 yellow bell pepper, sliced into strips
2 spring onions, sliced
1 ½ cups beer
6 hot dog rolls

DIRECTIONS

Warm oil on Sear/Sauté. Add in sausage links and sear for 5 minutes until browned; set aside on a plate.

Into the Foodi, pile peppers. Lay the sausages on top. Add beer into the pot.

Seal the pressure lid, choose Pressure, set to High, and set the timer to 5 minutes. Press Start.

When ready, release the pressure quickly.

Serve sausages in buns topped with onions and peppers.

Pork Chops with Plum Sauce

Servings: 4 | Ready in about: 20 min

INGREDIENTS

4 pork chops
1 tsp cumin seeds
1 tsp salt
1 tsp ground black pepper

2 cups firm plums, pitted and sliced
1 tbsp vegetable oil
¾ cup vegetable stock

DIRECTIONS

Sprinkle salt, cumin, and pepper on the pork chops. Set your Foodi to Sear/Sauté, set to Medium High, and choose Start/Stop to preheat the pot. Warm oil. Add the chops and cook for 3 to 5 minutes until browned and set aside on a bowl.

Arrange plum slices on the bottom of your Foodi. Place the pork chops on top of the plumes. Add any juice from the plate over the pork and apply stock around the edges.

Seal lid and cook on High pressure for 8 minutes.

When ready, do a quick pressure release.

Transfer the pork chops to a serving plate and spoon over the plum sauce before serving.

Holiday Honey-Glazed Ham

Servings: 10 | Ready in about: 30 min

INGREDIENTS

½ cup apple cider
¼ cup honey
1 tbsp Dijon mustard
¼ cup brown sugar
2 tbsp orange juice

2 tbsp pineapple juice (optional)
½ tsp ground cinnamon
¼ tsp grated nutmeg
1 pinch ground cloves
1 (5 pounds) ham, bone-in

DIRECTIONS

Set on Sear/Sauté, set to Medium High, and choose Start/Stop to preheat the pot. Press Start. Mix in apple cider, mustard, pineapple juice, cloves, cinnamon, brown sugar, honey, orange juice, and nutmeg; cook until sauce becomes warm and the sugar and spices are completely dissolved.

Lay ham into the sauce. Seal the pressure lid, choose Pressure, set to High, and set the timer to 10 minutes; press Start. When ready, release the pressure quickly.

As the ham cooks, preheat the oven's broiler. Line aluminum foil to a baking sheet.

Transfer the ham to the prepared baking sheet. On Sear/Sauté, cook the remaining liquid for 4 to 6 minutes until you have a thick and syrupy glaze. Brush the glaze onto ham.

Set the glazed ham in the preheated broiler and bake for 3 to 5 minutes until the glaze is caramelized.

Place the ham on a cutting board and slice. Transfer to a serving bowl and drizzle glaze over the ham.

Jamaican Pulled Pork with Mango Sauce

Servings: 6 | Ready in about: 1 hr 15 min

INGREDIENTS

1 ½ tsp onion powder
1 tsp sea salt
1 tsp dried thyme
1 tsp ground black pepper
1 tsp cayenne pepper
1 tsp ground allspice
½ tsp ground nutmeg

½ tsp ground cinnamon
3 pounds pork shoulder
1 mango, cut into chunks
1 tbsp olive oil
½ cup water
2 tbsp fresh cilantro, finely minced

DIRECTIONS

In a bowl, combine onion powder, thyme, allspice, cinnamon, sugar, pepper, sea salt, cayenne, and nutmeg.

Coat the pork shoulder with olive oil; season with seasoning mixture. Warm oil on Sear/Sauté. Add in the pork and cook for 5 minutes until browned completely.

To the pot, add water and mango chunks. Seal the pressure lid, choose Pressure, set to High, and set the timer to 45 minutes. Press Start. Release pressure naturally for 15 minutes, then release the remaining pressure quickly.

Transfer the pork to a cutting board and allow cooling. To make the sauce, pour the cooking liquid in a food processor and pulse until smooth. Use two forks to shred the pork and arrange on a serving platter. Serve the pulled pork topped with mango salsa and fresh cilantro.

Crispy Pork Fajitas

Servings: 5 | Ready in about: 1 hr 30 min

INGREDIENTS

1 tbsp ground cumin
2 tsp dried oregano
1 tsp paprika
1 tsp onion powder
1 tsp salt
1 tsp ground black pepper
1/2 tsp ground cinnamon
3 pounds boneless pork shoulder

¾ cup vegetable broth
¼ cup pineapple juice
1 lime, juiced
4 cloves garlic, crushed
2 bay leaves
5 corn tortillas, warmed
½ cup queso Cotija, crumbled

DIRECTIONS

In a bowl, combine cumin, paprika, pepper, onion powder, oregano, salt, and cinnamon; toss in pork to coat. Place the pork in the Foodi and allow settling for 15 to 30 minutes.

Add in chicken broth, garlic, lime juice, bay leaves, and pineapple juice.

Seal the pressure lid, choose Pressure, set to High, and set the timer to 50 minutes; press Start. When ready, release pressure naturally for 15 minutes, then release the remaining pressure quickly.

Transfer the pork to a rimmed baking sheet and use two forks to shred the meat. Reserve the juices in a bowl.

Place the Cook & Crisp Basket into the inner pot. Close the crisping lid and choose Air Crisp; adjust the temperature to 380°F and the time to 4 minutes to preheat. Press Start.

Add the baking sheet to the Cook & Crisp basket. Close the crisping lid. Select Air Crisp; adjust the temperature to 375°F and the cook time to 10 minutes. Press Start. After 5 minutes, open the lid and toss the meat. Continue cooking until the pork is done. Skim and get rid of fat from the liquid remaining. Dispose of the bay leaves.

Over the pork, pour the liquid and serve alongside warm corn tortillas and queso fresco.

Sweet and Sour Pork

Servings: 4 | Ready in about: 40 min

INGREDIENTS

1 pound pork loin, cut into chunks
2 tbsp white wine
15 ounces canned peaches
¼ cup beef stock
2 tbsp sweet chili sauce

2 tbsp honey
2 tbsp soy sauce
2 tbsp cornstarch
¼ cup water

DIRECTIONS

Into the pot, mix soy sauce, beef stock, white wine, juice from the canned peaches, and sweet chili sauce; stir in pork to coat.

Seal the pressure lid, choose Pressure, set to High, and set the timer to 5 minutes. Press Start. Release pressure naturally for 10 minutes, then release the remaining pressure quickly. Remove the pork to a serving plate. Chop the peaches into small pieces.

In a bowl, mix water and cornstarch until cornstarch dissolves completely; stir the mixture into the pot. Press Sear/Sauté and cook for 5 more minutes until you obtain the desired thick consistency; add in the chopped peaches and stir well. Serve the pork topped with peach sauce and enjoy.

Sausage with Celeriac & Potato Mash

Servings: 4 | Ready in about: 45 min

INGREDIENTS

1 tbsp olive oil

4 pork sausages

1 onion

2 cups vegetable broth

½ cup water

4 potatoes, peeled and diced

1 cup celeriac, chopped

2 tbsp butter

¼ cup milk

salt and ground black pepper to taste

1 tbsp heavy cream

1 tsp Dijon mustard

½ tsp dry mustard powder

Fresh flat-leaf parsley, chopped

DIRECTIONS

Warm oil on Sear/Sauté. Add in sausages and cook for 1 to 2 minutes for each side until browned. Set the sausages to a plate. To the same pot, add onion and cook for 3 minutes until fragrant.

Add sausages on top of onions and pour water and broth over them. Place a trivet over onions and sausages. Put potatoes and celeriac in the steamer basket and transfer it to the trivet.

Seal the pressure lid, choose Pressure, set to High, and set the timer to 11 minutes. Press Start.

When ready, release the pressure quickly.

Transfer potatoes and celeriac to a bowl and set sausages on a plate and cover them with aluminum foil.

Using a potato masher, mash potatoes and celeriac together with black pepper, milk, salt and butter until mash becomes creamy and fluffy. Adjust the seasonings.

Set your Foodi to Sear/Sauté. Add the onion mixture and bring to a boil. Cook for 5 to 10 minutes until the mixture is reduced and thickened. Into the gravy, stir in dry mustard, salt, pepper, mustard and cream.

Place the mash in 4 bowls in equal parts, top with a sausage or two, and gravy. Add parsley for garnishing.

Pork Carnitas Wraps

Servings: 12 | Ready in about: 1 hr 15 min

INGREDIENTS

2 tsp grapeseed oil

1 (4 to 5 pounds) boneless pork shoulder

1 onion, sliced

2 garlic cloves, minced

2 oranges, juiced

2 limes, juiced

2 tbsp sweet smoked paprika

1 tbsp dried oregano

1 tbsp salt

2 jalapeños, sliced

1 avocado, sliced

Fresh cilantro leaves, chopped

2 tsp ground black pepper

12 corn tortillas, warmed

DIRECTIONS

Warm oil on Sear/Sauté. Add in pork and cook for 5 minutes until golden brown. Transfer the pork to a plate.

Add garlic and onions to the inner pot and cook for 2 to 3 minutes until soft.

Add lime and orange juices into the pot to deglaze, scrape the bottom to get rid of any browned bits of food.

Stir in pepper, paprika, salt and oregano. Return the pork to pot; stir to coat in seasoning and liquid.

Seal the pressure lid, choose Pressure, set to High, and set the timer to 35 minutes. Press Start.

When ready, release the pressure quickly.

Press Sear/Sauté. When the liquid starts to simmer, use two forks to shred the pork. Cook for 10 more minutes until liquid is reduced by half. Serve in warmed tortillas topped with jalapeños, avocado slices and cilantro.

Holiday Apricot-Lemon Ham

Servings: 12 | Ready in about: 1 hr

INGREDIENTS

¼ cup water
5 pounds smoked ham
¾ cup apricot jam
½ cup brown sugar
Juice from 1 Lime

2 tsp mustard
½ tsp ground cardamom
¼ tsp ground nutmeg
freshly ground black pepper to taste

DIRECTIONS

Into the pot, add water and ham to the steel pot of a pressure cooker.

In a bowl, combine jam, lemon juice, cardamom, pepper, nutmeg, mustard, and brown sugar; pour the mixture over the ham. Seal the pressure lid, choose Pressure, set to High, and set the timer to 10 minutes. Press Start.

When ready, release the pressure quickly.

Transfer the ham to a cutting board; allow to sit for 10 minutes. Press Sear/Sauté.

Simmer the liquid and cook for 4 to 6 minutes until thickened into a sauce. Slice ham and place onto a serving bowl. Drizzle with sauce before serving.

Pork Chops with Squash Purée & Mushroom Gravy

Servings: 4 | Ready in about: 45 min

INGREDIENTS

2 tbsp olive oil
2 sprigs thyme, leaves removed and chopped
2 sprigs rosemary, leaves removed and chopped
4 pork chops
1 cup mushrooms, chopped
4 cloves garlic, minced

1 cup chicken broth
1 tbsp soy sauce
1 pound butternut squash, cubed
1 tbsp olive oil
1 tsp cornstarch

DIRECTIONS

Set on Sear/Sauté, set to Medium High, and choose Start/Stop to preheat the pot and heat rosemary, thyme and 1 tbsp of olive oil. Add the pork chops and sear for 1 minute for each side until lightly browned.

Sauté garlic and mushrooms in the pressure cooker for 5-6 minutes until mushrooms are tender. Add soy sauce and chicken broth. Transfer pork chops to a wire trivet and place it into the pressure cooker. Over the chops, place a cake pan. Add butternut squash in the pot and drizzle with 1 tbsp olive oil.

Seal the pressure lid, choose Pressure, set to High, and set the timer to 10 minutes. Press Start.

When ready, release the pressure quickly. Remove the pan and trivet fromthe pot. Stir cornstarch into the mushroom mixture for 2 to 3 minutes until the sauce thickens.

Transfer the mushroom sauce to an immersion blender and blend until you attain the desired consistency. Scoop sauce into a cup with a pour spout. Smash the squash into a purée.

Set pork chops on a plate and ladle squash puree next to them. Top the pork chops with gravy.

Lamb Chops and Creamy Potato Mash

Servings: 8 | Ready in about: 40 min

INGREDIENTS

8 lamb cutlets
salt to taste
3 sprigs rosemary leaves, chopped
3 tbsp butter, softened
1 tbsp olive oil
1 tbsp tomato puree

1 green onion, chopped
1 cup beef stock
5 potatoes, peeled and chopped
⅓ cup milk
4 cilantro leaves, for garnish

DIRECTIONS

Rub rosemary leaves and salt to the lamb chops. Warm oil and 2 tbsp of butter on Sear/Sauté.

Add in the lamb chops and cook for 1 minute for each side until browned; set aside on a plate.

In the pot, mix tomato puree and green onion; cook for 2-3 minutes.

Add beef stock into the pot to deglaze, scrape the bottom to get rid of any browned bits of food.

Return lamb cutlets alongside any accumulated juices to the pot.

Set a reversible rack on lamb cutlets. Place steamer basket on the reversible rack. Arrange potatoes in the steamer basket.

Seal the pressure lid, choose Pressure, set to High, and set the timer to 4 minutes. Press Start.

When ready, release the pressure quickly.

Remove trivet and steamer basket from pot. In a high speed blender, add potatoes, milk, salt, and remaining tbsp butter. Blend well until you obtain a smooth consistency.

Divide the potato mash between serving dishes. Lay lamb chops on the mash. Drizzle with cooking liquid obtained from pressure cooker; apply cilantro sprigs for garnish.

DESSERTS & BEVERAGES

Wheat Flour Cinnamon Balls

Servings: 4 | Ready in about: 20 min

INGREDIENTS

⅓ cup whole-wheat flour
⅓ cup all-purpose flour
½ teaspoon baking powder
3 tablespoons sugar, divided
¼ teaspoon ground cinnamon, plus ½ tablespoon

¼ teaspoon sea salt
2 tablespoons cold unsalted butter, cut into small pieces
¼ cup plus 1½ tablespoons whole milk
Cooking spray

DIRECTIONS

Mix the whole-wheat flour, all-purpose flour, baking powder, 1 tablespoon of sugar, ¼ teaspoon of cinnamon, and the salt in a medium bowl.

Add the butter and use a pastry cutter to cut into the butter to be broken into little pieces until resembling cornmeal. Pour in the milk and mix until the dough forms into a ball.

Knead the dough on a flat surface until a smooth both is achieved. Divide the dough into 8 pieces and roll each piece into a ball.

Put the crisping basket in the pot, close, select Air Crisp, set the temperature to 350°F, and the time to 3 minutes. Press Start/Stop to preheat the basket.

Coat the preheated Crisping Basket with cooking spray. Put the balls in the basket with space in between each ball and oil the balls with cooking spray.

Close the crisping lid. Choose Air Crisp, set the temperature to 350°F, and set the time to 10 minutes. Press Start/Stop to begin.

In a medium mixing bowl, combine the remaining sugar and cinnamon. When done baking, toss the dough balls in the cinnamon and sugar mixture.

White Filling Coconut and Oat Cookies

Servings: 4 | Ready in about: 30 min

INGREDIENTS:

5 ½ oz flour
1 tsp vanilla extract
3 oz sugar

½ cup oats
1 small egg, beaten
¼ cup coconut flakes

Filling:
1 oz white chocolate, melted
2 oz butter

4 oz powdered sugar
1 tsp vanilla extract

DIRECTIONS:

Beat all cookie ingredients, with an electric mixer, except the flour. When smooth, fold in the flour. Drop spoonfuls of the batter onto a prepared cookie sheet. Close the crisping lid and cook in the Ninja Foodi at 350 F for about 18 minutes on Air Crisp mode; let cool.

Prepare the filling by beating all ingredients together. Spread the mixture on half of the cookies. Top with the other halves to make cookie sandwiches.

Apple Vanilla Hand Pies

Servings: 8 | Ready in about: 40 min

INGREDIENTS

2 apples, peeled, cored, and diced
3 tablespoons sugar
1 lemon, juiced
¼ teaspoon salt
1 teaspoon vanilla extract

1 teaspoon corn-starch
1 (2-crust) package refrigerated piecrusts, at room temperature
Cooking spray

DIRECTIONS

In a large mixing bowl, combine the apples, sugar, lemon juice, salt, and vanilla. Allow the mixture to stand for 10 minutes, then drain, and reserve 1 tablespoon of the liquid.

In a small bowl, whisk the corn-starch into the reserved liquid and then, mix with the apple mixture. Put the crisping basket in the pot and close the crisping lid. Choose Air Crisp, set the temperature to 350°F, and the time to 5 minutes. Press Start/Stop to preheat.

Put the piecrusts on a lightly floured surface and cut into 8 (4-inch- diameter) circles. Spoon a tablespoon of apple mixture in the center of the circle, with ½ an inch's border around the dough. Brush the edges with water and fold the dough over the filling. Press the edges with a fork to seal.

Cut 3 small slits on top of each pie and oil with cooking spray. Arrange the pies in a single layer in the preheated basket. Close the crisping lid. Choose Air Crisp, set the temperature to 350°F, and set the time to 12 minutes. Press Start/Stop to begin baking.

Once done baking, remove, and place the pies on a wire rack to cool. Repeat with the remaining hand pies.

Raspberry Crumble

Servings: 6 | Ready in about: 40 min

INGREDIENTS

1 (16-ounce) package frozen raspberries
2 tablespoons arrowroot starch
½ cup water, plus 1 tablespoon
1 teaspoon freshly squeezed lemon juice
5 tablespoons sugar, divided

½ cup all-purpose flour
⅔ cup brown sugar
½ cup rolled oats
⅓ cup cold unsalted butter, cut into pieces
1 teaspoon cinnamon powder

DIRECTIONS

Place the raspberries in the baking pan. In a small mixing bowl, combine the arrowroot starch, 1 tablespoon of water, lemon juice, and 3 tablespoons of sugar. Pour the mixture all over the raspberries.

Put the reversible rack in the lower position of the pot. Cover the pan with foil and pour the remaining water into the pot. Put the pan on the rack in the pot. Put the pressure lid together, and lock in the Seal position. Choose Pressure, set to High, and set the time to 10 minutes, then Choose Start/Stop to begin.

In a bowl, mix the flour, brown sugar, oats, butter, cinnamon, and remaining sugar until crumble forms. When done pressure-cooking, do a quick release and carefully open the lid.

Remove the foil and stir the fruit mixture. After, spread the crumble evenly on the berries.

Close the crisping lid; choose Air Crisp, set the temperature to 400°F, and the time to 10 minutes. Choose Start/Stop to begin crisping. Cook until the top has browned and the fruit is bubbling. When done baking, remove the rack with the pan from the pot, and serve.

Simple Vanilla Cheesecake

Servings: 6 | Ready in about: 60 min

INGREDIENTS

Cooking spray
1½ cups finely crushed graham crackers
2 tablespoons sugar
4 tablespoons unsalted butter, melted
16 ounces cream cheese, at room temperature
½ cup brown sugar

¼ cup sour cream
1 tablespoon all-purpose flour
1½ teaspoons vanilla extract
½ teaspoon salt
2 eggs
1 cup water

DIRECTIONS

Grease a spring form pan with cooking spray, then line the pan with parchment paper, grease with cooking spray again, and line with aluminium foil. This is to ensure that there are no air gaps in the pan.

In a medium mixing bowl, mix the graham cracker crumbs, sugar, and butter. Spoon the mixture into the pan and press firmly into with a spoon.

In a deep bowl and with a hand mixer, beat the beat the cream cheese and brown sugar until well-mixed. Whisk in the sour cream to be smooth and stir in the flour, vanilla, and salt.

Crack the eggs in and beat but not to be overly smooth. Pour the mixture into the pan over the crumbs. Next, pour the water into the pot. Put the spring form pan on the reversible rack and put the rack in the lower positon of the pot.

Seal the pressure lid, choose Pressure, set to High, and set the time to 35 minutes. Choose Start/Stop to begin.

Once done baking, perform a natural pressure release for 10 minutes, then a quick pressure release to let out any remaining pressure. Carefully open the lid.

Remove the pan from the rack and allow the cheesecake to cool for 1 hour. Cover the cheesecake with foil and chill in the refrigerator for 4 hours.

Dark Chocolate Brownies

Servings: 6 | Ready in about: 40 min

INGREDIENTS

1 cup water
2 eggs
⅓ cup granulated sugar
¼ cup olive oil
⅓ cup flour
⅓ cup cocoa powder

⅓ cup dark chocolate chips
⅓ cup chopped Walnuts
1 tbsp milk
½ tsp baking powder
1 tbsp vanilla extract
A pinch salt

DIRECTIONS

In the Foodi, add water and set in the reversible rack. Line a parchment paper on. a springform pan.

In a bowl, beat eggs and sugar to mix until smooth; stir in olive oil, cocoa powder, milk, salt baking powder, chocolate chips, flour, walnuts, vanilla, and sea salt.

Transfer the batter to the prepared springform pan and place the pan in the pot on the rack. Close the crisping lid and select Bake/Roast; adjust the temperature to 250°F and the cook time to 20 minutes. Press Start.

When the time is up, open the lid and. and allow the brownie to cool for 10 minutes before cutting. Use powdered sugar to dust the brownies before serving lightly.

Mixed Berry Cobbler

Servings: 4 | Ready in about: 40 min

INGREDIENTS

2 bags frozen mixed berries

3 tablespoons arrowroot starch

1 cup sugar

For the topping

1 cup self-rising flour

¼ teaspoon cinnamon powder

5 tablespoons powdered sugar, divided

⅔ cup crème fraiche, plus more as needed

1 tablespoon melted unsalted butter

1 tablespoon whipping cream

DIRECTIONS

To make the base, pour the blackberries into the inner pot along with the arrowroot starch and sugar. Mix to combine. Seal the pressure lid, choose Pressure; adjust the pressure to High and the cook time to 3 minutes; press Start.

After cooking, perform a quick pressure release and carefully open the lid.

To make the topping, in a small bowl, whisk the flour, cinnamon powder, and 3 tablespoons of sugar. In a separate small bowl, whisk the crème fraiche with the melted butter. Pour the cream mixture on the dry ingredients and combine evenly. If the mixture is too dry, mix in 1 tablespoon of crème fraiche at a time until the mixture is soft.

Spoon 2 to 3 tablespoons of dough on top over the peaches and spread out slightly on top. Brush the topping with the whipping cream and sprinkle with the remaining sugar.

Close the crisping lid and Choose Bake/Roast; adjust the temperature to 325°F and the cook time to 12 minutes. Press Start. Check after 8 minutes; if the dough isn't cooking evenly, rotate the pot about 90 degrees, and continue cooking.

When ready, the topping should be cooked through and lightly browned. Allow cooling before slicing. Serve warm.

Chocolate Vanilla Swirl Cheesecake

Servings: 8 | Ready in about: 60 min + Chilling time

INGREDIENTS

4 ounces chocolate wafer cookies, crushed into crumbs

2 tablespoons unsalted butter, melted

16 ounces cream cheese, at room temperature

½ cup sugar

2 tablespoons heavy cream

2 teaspoons vanilla extract

2 tablespoons sour cream

2 large eggs

3 ounces sweet chocolate chips, melted

DIRECTIONS

In a small bowl, mix the cookie crumbs and butter. Spoon the crumbs into a spring form pan and press all around with a spoon.

Place the reversible rack in the lower position of the inner pot and put the spring form pan on top. Close the crisping lid and Choose Air Crisp; adjust the temperature to 350°F and the cook time to 6 minutes. Press Start and bake until fragrant and set. Remove the pan and let the crumbs cool.

In a medium bowl and using a hand mixer, beat the cream cheese until smooth, add the sugar, and beat further until smooth. Pour in the heavy cream, vanilla extract, and sour cream. Whisk again and crack the eggs into the bowl one after the other while whisking after each egg is added.

Spoon ½ cup of the cream mixture into a bowl and mix in the chocolate chips.

Pour the remaining cream mixture into the spring form pan, drop spoonfuls of the chocolate mixture with even distance on the filling and run the tip of a skewer through each chocolate drop to marbleize the top of the filling. Cover the filling with aluminium foil.

Pour 1 cup of water into the inner pot. Fix in the reversible rack in the lower position of the pot and put the spring form pan on top.

Seal the pressure lid, choose Pressure; adjust the pressure to High and the cook time to 25 minutes; press Start.

After cooking, do a natural pressure release for 10 minutes, and then a quick pressure release to let out any remaining pressure.

Carefully open the lid and remove the cheesecake from the pot. Take off the foil. Let the cheesecake rest for 15 to 20 minutes and then refrigerate the cooled cake for 3 to 4 hours to chill through.

Vanilla Hot Lava Cake

Servings: 8 | Ready in about: 40 min

INGREDIENTS:

1 cup butter
4 tbsp milk
4 tsp vanilla extract
1 ½ cups chocolate chips
1 ½ cups sugar

Powdered sugar to garnish
7 tbsp flour
5 eggs
1 cup water

DIRECTIONS:

Grease the cake pan with cooking spray and set aside. Open the Ninja Foodi, fit the reversible rack at the bottom of it, and pour in the water.

In a medium heatproof bowl, add the butter and chocolate and melt them in the microwave for about 2 minutes. Remove it from the microwave.

Add sugar and use a spatula to stir it well. Add the eggs, milk, and vanilla extract and stir again. Finally, add the flour and stir it until even and smooth.

Pour the batter into the greased cake pan and use the spatula to level it.

Place the pan on the trivet in the pot, close the lid, secure the pressure valve, and select Pressure on High for 15 minutes. Press Start/Stop.

Once the timer has gone off, do a natural pressure release for 10 minutes, then a quick pressure release, and open the lid.

Remove the rack with the pan on it and place the pan on a flat surface. Put a plate over the pan and flip the cake over into the plate. Pour the powdered sugar in a fine sieve and sift it over the cake. Use a knife to cut the cake into 8 slices and serve immediately (while warm).

Raspberry Cream Tart

Servings: 4 | Ready in about: 55 min+ Chilling time

INGREDIENTS

1 refrigerated piecrust, for the raspberries
2½ cups fresh raspberries, divided
1 tablespoon arrowroot starch
2 tablespoons water

¼ cup sugar
¼ teaspoon grated lemon zest
1 teaspoon lemon juice
Pinch salt

For The Filling

1 teaspoon vanilla extract
8 ounces cream cheese, at room temperature

½ cup confectioners' sugar
¼ cup heavy cream

DIRECTIONS

Roll out the pie crust and fit into a tart pan. Do not stretch the dough to prevent shrinking when cooking. Use a fork to prick all over the bottom of the dough.

Place the reversible rack in the pot in the lower position of the pot and put the tart pan on top.

Close the crisping lid, choose Bake/Roast; adjust the temperature to 250°F, and the cook time to 15 minutes. Press Start. When done baking, open the lid and check the crust. It should be set and lightly brown around the edges.

Close the crisping lid again. Adjust the temperature to 375°F and the cook time to 4 minutes. Press Start to begin baking.

After 3 minutes, check the crust, which should be a deep golden brown color by now. If not, cook for the remaining 1 minute. Remove the rack and set the crust aside to cool.

Fetch out 1 cup of berries into the inner pot. In a small bowl, whisk the arrowroot starch and water until smoothly mixed. Pour the slurry on the raspberries along with the sugar, lemon zest, lemon juice, and salt. Mix to distribute the slurry among the raspberries.

Seal the pressure lid, choose Pressure; adjust the pressure to High and the cook time to 2 minutes. Press Start.

Once done cooking, perform a quick pressure release and carefully open the lid. The raspberries will have softened. Add the remaining 1½ cups of raspberries, stirring to coat with the cooked mixture. Then, allow cooling.

To make the cream filling, in a bowl and with a hand mixer, whisk the vanilla extract and cream cheese until evenly combined and smooth. Mix in the confectioners' sugar and whisk again until the sugar has fully incorporated and the mixture is light and smooth.

With clean whisks and in another bowl, beat the heavy cream until soft peaks form. Fold the heavy cream into the vanilla mixture until both are evenly combined.

To assemble, spoon the cream filling into the piecrust and scatter the remaining raspberries on the cream. Chill for 30 minutes before cutting and serving.

Classic Caramel-Walnut Brownies

Servings: 4 | Ready in about: 60 min+ cooling time

INGREDIENTS

8 ounces white chocolate
8 tablespoons unsalted butter
1 cup sugar
2 teaspoons almond extract
A pinch of salt

2 large eggs, at room temperature
¾ cup all-purpose flour
Cooking spray
½ cup caramel sauce
½ cup toasted walnuts

DIRECTIONS

Put the white chocolate and butter in a small bowl and pour 1 cup of water into the inner pot. Place the reversible rack in the lower position of the pot and put the bowl on top.

Close the crisping lid. Choose Bake/Roast; adjust the temperature to 375°F and the cook time to 10 minutes to melt the white chocolate and butter. Press Start. Check after 5 minutes and stir. As soon as the chocolate has melted, remove the bowl from the pot.

Use a small spatula to transfer the chocolate mixture into a medium and stir in the almond extract, sugar, and salt. One after another, crack each egg into the bowl and whisk after each addition. Mix in the flour until smooth, about 1 minute.

Grease a round cake pan with cooking spray or line the pan with parchment paper. Pour the batter into the prepared pan and place on the rack.

Close the crisping lid and Choose Bake/Roast; adjust the temperature to 250°F and the cook time to 25 minutes. Press Start. Once the time is up, open the lid and check the brownies. The top should be just set. Blot out the butter that may pool to the top using a paper towel.

Close the crisping lid again and adjust the temperature to 300°F and the cook time to 15 minutes. Press Start.

Once the time is up, open the lid and check the brownies. A toothpick inserted into the center should come out with crumbs sticking to it but no raw batter.

Generously drizzle the caramel sauce on top of the brownies and scatter the walnuts on top. Close the crisping lid again and adjust the temperature to 325°F and the cook time to 8 minutes; press Start.

When the nuts are brown and the caramel is bubbling, take out the brownies, and allow cooling for at least 30 minutes and cut into squares.

Tasty Créme Brulee

Servings: 4 | Ready in about: 30 min + 6 hours of cooling

INGREDIENTS:

3 cups heavy whipping cream
6 tbsp sugar
7 large egg yolks

2 tbsp vanilla extract
2 cups water

DIRECTIONS:

In a mixing bowl, add the yolks, vanilla, whipping cream, and half of the swerve sugar. Use a whisk to mix them until they are well combined.

Pour the mixture into the ramekins and cover them with aluminium foil.

Open the Ninja Foodi, fit the reversible rack into the pot, and pour in the water.

Place 3 ramekins on the rack and place the remaining ramekins to sit on the edges of the ramekins below.

Close the lid, secure the pressure valve, and select Pressure mode on High for 8 minutes. Press Start/Stop.

Once the timer has stopped, do a natural pressure release for 10 minutes, then a quick pressure release to let out the remaining pressure.

With a napkin in hand, remove the ramekins onto a flat surface and then into a refrigerator to chill for at least 6 hours.

After refrigeration, remove the ramekins and remove the aluminium foil.

Equally, sprinkle the remaining sugar on it and return to the pot. Close the csisping lid, select Bake/Roast mode, set the timer to 4 minutes on 380 degrees F. Serve the crème brulee chilled with whipped cream.

Strawberry & Lemon Ricotta Cheesecake

Servings: 6 | Ready in about: 35 min

INGREDIENTS:

10 oz cream cheese
¼ cup sugar
½ cup Ricotta cheese
One lemon, zested and juiced
2 eggs, cracked into a bowl

1 tsp lemon extract
3 tbsp sour cream
1 ½ cups water
10 strawberries, halved to decorate

DIRECTIONS:

In the electric mixer, add the cream cheese, quarter cup of sugar, ricotta cheese, lemon zest, lemon juice, and lemon extract. Turn on the mixer and mix the ingredients until a smooth consistency is formed. Adjust the sweet taste to liking with more sugar.

Reduce the speed of the mixer and add the eggs. Fold it in at low speed until it is fully incorporated. Make sure not to fold the eggs in high speed to prevent a cracker crust. Grease the spring form pan with cooking spray and use a spatula to spoon the mixture into the pan. Level the top with the spatula and cover it with foil.

Open the Ninja Foodi, fit in the reversible rack, and pour in the water. Place the cake pan on the rack. Close the lid, secure the pressure valve, and select Pressure mode on High pressure for 15 minutes. Press Start/Stop.

Meanwhile, mix the sour cream and one tablespoon of sugar. Set aside.

Once the timer has gone off, do a natural pressure release for 10 minutes, then a quick pressure release to let out any extra steam, and open the lid.

Remove the rack with pan, place the spring form pan on a flat surface, and open it. Use a spatula to spread the sour cream mixture on the warm cake. Refrigerate the cake for 8 hours. Top with strawberries; slice it into 6 pieces and serve while firming.

Cheat Apple Pie

Servings: 9 | Ready in about: 30 min

INGREDIENTS:

4 apples, diced
2 oz butter, melted
2 oz sugar
1 oz brown sugar

2 tsp cinnamon
1 egg, beaten
3 large puff pastry sheets
¼ tsp salt

DIRECTIONS:

Whisk the white sugar, brown sugar, cinnamon, salt, and butter together.

Place the apples in a baking dish and coat them with the mixture.

Slide the dish into the Ninja Foodi and cook for 10 minutes on Roast at 350 F.

Meanwhile, roll out the pastry on a floured flat surface, and cut each sheet into 6 equal pieces. Divide the apple filling between the parts.

Brush the edges of the pastry squares with the egg. Fold and seal the edges with a fork.

Place on a lined baking sheet and cook in the fryer at 350 F for 8 minutes on Roast. Flip over, increase the temperature to 390 F, and cook for 2 more minutes.

Berry Vanilla Pudding

Servings: 4 | Ready in about: 35 min + 6h for refrigeration

INGREDIENTS:

1 cup heavy cream
4 egg yolks
4 tbsp water + 1 ½ cups water
½ cup milk

1 tsp vanilla extract
½ cup sugar
4 raspberries
4 blueberries

DIRECTIONS:

Turn on your Ninja Foodi and select Sear/Sauté mode on Medium. Add four tablespoons for water and the sugar. Stir it constantly until it dissolves. Press Stop. Add milk, heavy cream, and vanilla. Stir it with a whisk until evenly combined.

Crack the eggs into a bowl and add a tablespoon of the cream mixture. Whisk it and then very slowly add the remaining cream mixture while whisking.

Fit the reversible rack at the bottom of the pot, and pour one and a half cup of water in it. Pour the mixture into four ramekins and place them on the rack.

Close the lid of the pot, secure the pressure valve, and select Pressure mode on High Pressure for 4 minutes. Press Start/Stop. Once the timer has gone off, do a quick pressure release, and open the lid.

With a napkin in hand, carefully remove the ramekins onto a flat surface. Let cool for about 15 minutes and then refrigerate them for 6 hours.

After 6 hours, remove them from the refrigerator and garnish them with the raspberries and blueberries.

Enjoy immediately or refrigerate further until dessert time is ready.

Cinnamon Apple Crisp

Servings: 5 | Ready in about: 30 min

INGREDIENTS

Topping:
½ cup oat flour
½ cup old-fashioned rolled oats

½ cup granulated sugar
¼ cup olive oil

Filling:
5 apples, peeled, cored, and halved
2 tbsp arrowroot powder
½ cup water

1 tsp ground cinnamon
¼ tsp ground nutmeg
½ tsp vanilla paste

DIRECTIONS

In a bowl, combine sugar, oat flour, rolled oats, and olive oil to form coarse crumbs. Ladle the apples into the pressure cooker. Mix water with arrowroot powder in a small bowl; stir in salt, nutmeg, cinnamon, and vanilla and toss in the apples to coat.

Apply oat topping to the apples. Seal the pressure lid, choose Pressure, set to High, and set the timer to 10 minutes. Press Start. Release pressure naturally for 5 minutes, then release the remaining pressure quickly.

New York Cheesecake

Servings: 12 | Ready in about: 1 hr

INGREDIENTS

For the Crust:
1 cup graham crackers crumbs
2 tbsp butter, melted

1 tsp sugar
1/8 tsp salt

For the Filling:
2 cups cream cheese, at room temperature
½ cup sugar
1 tsp vanilla extract

Zest from 1 orange
1 pinch salt
2 eggs, at room temperature

DIRECTIONS

Fold a 20-inch piece of aluminum foil in half lengthwise twice and set on the pressure cooker.

Spray a parchment paper with cooking spray and line to the base of a 7-inch springform pan.

In a bowl, combine melted butter, salt, sugar and graham crackers crumbs; press into the bottom and about ⅓ up the sides of the pan. Transfer the pan to the freezer as you prepare the filling.

In a separate bowl, beat sugar, cream cheese, salt, orange zest, and vanilla until smooth. Beat eggs into the filling, one at a time. Stir until combined. Add the filling over the chilled crust in the pan.

To the Foodi, add 1 cup water and set the reversible rack into the pot. Carefully center the springform pan on the prepared foil sling. Lower pan into the inner pot using sling and place on steam reversible rack.

Close the crisping lid and select Bake/Roast; adjust the temperature to 250°F and the cook time to 40 minutes. Press Start.

Let cool the cheesecake before transferring to a refrigerator for 2 hours or overnight.

Use a paring knife to run along the edges between the pan and cheesecake to remove the cheesecake and set to the plate.

White Chocolate Chip Cookies

Servings: 8 | Ready in about: 30 min

INGREDIENTS:

6 oz self-rising flour
3 oz brown sugar
2 oz white chocolate chips

1 tbsp honey
1 ½ tbsp milk
4 oz butter

DIRECTIONS:

Beat the butter and sugar until fluffy.

Then, beat in the honey, milk, and flour. Gently fold in the chocolate chips.

Drop spoonfuls of the mixture onto a prepared cookie sheet.

Close the crisping lid and cook for 18 minutes on Air Crisp mode at 350 F.

Once the timer beeps, make sure the cookies are just set.

Holiday Cranberry Cheesecake

Servings: 8 | Ready in about: 1 hr

INGREDIENTS

1 cup coarsely crumbled cookies

2 tbsp butter, melted

1 cup mascarpone cheese, room temperature

½ cup sugar

2 tbsp sour cream

½ tsp vanilla extract

2 eggs, room temperature

1/3 cup dried cranberries

1 cup water

DIRECTIONS

Fold a 20-inch piece of aluminum foil in half lengthwise twice and set on the pressure cooker.

In a bowl, combine melted butter and crushed cookies; press firmly to the bottom and about 1/3 of the way up the sides of a 7-inch springform pan. Freeze the crust while the filling is being prepared.

In a separate bowl, beat together mascarpone cheese and sugar to obtain a smooth consistency; stir in vanilla extract and sour cream.

Beat one egg and add into the cheese mixture to combine well; do the same with the second egg.

Stir cranberries into the filling. Transfer the filling into the crust. Into the pot, add water and set the reversible rack at the bottom. Center the springform pan onto the prepared foil sling. Use the sling to lower the pan onto the reversible rack.

Fold foil strips out of the way of the lid.

Close the crisping lid and select Bake/Roast; adjust the temperature to 250°F and the cook time to 40 minutes. Press Start.

When the time is up, open the lid and let to cool the cheesecake. When, transfer the cheesecake to a refrigerator for 2 hours or overnight.

Use a paring knife to run along the edges between the pan and cheesecake to remove the cheesecake and set to the plate.

Blueberry Muffins

Servings: 10 | Ready in about: 30 min

INGREDIENTS:

1 ½ cup flour

½ tsp salt

½ cup sugar

¼ cup vegetable oil

2 tsp vanilla extract

1 cup blueberries

1 egg

2 tsp baking powder

Yogurt, as needed

DIRECTIONS:

Combine all the flour, salt and baking powder in a bowl.

In a bowl, place the oil, vanilla extract, and egg. Fill the rest of the bowl with yogurt.

Whisk the mixture until fully incorporated. Combine the wet and dry ingredients.

Gently fold in the blueberries. Divide the mixture between 10 muffin cups.

You may need to cook in batches. Close the crisping lid and cook for 10 minutes on Air Crisp mode at 350 F, until nice and crispy.

Pumpkin Cake

Servings: 8 | Ready in about: 1 hr 30 min

INGREDIENTS

3 eggs

⅔ cup sugar

1 cup flour

½ cup half-and-half

¼ cup olive oil

1 tsp baking powder

1 tsp vanilla extract

1 tsp ground cinnamon

½ tsp ground nutmeg

1 cup packed shredded pumpkin, plus more for topping

½ cup chopped walnuts

2 cups water

Frosting:

4 ounces cream cheese, room temperature

8 tbsp butter

½ cup confectioners sugar

½ tsp vanilla extract

⅛ tsp salt

DIRECTIONS

In a bowl, beat eggs and sugar to get a smooth mixture; mix in oil, flour, vanilla extract, cinnamon, half-and-half, baking powder, and nutmeg. Stir well to obtain a fluffy batter; fold walnuts and pumpkin through the batter. Add batter into a 6-inch cake pan and cover with aluminum foil.

Into the pot, add water and set the reversible rack over the water. Lay cake pan gently onto the trivet.

Close the crisping lid and select Bake/Roast; adjust the temperature to 250°F and the cook time to 40 minutes. Press Start.

Beat cream cheese, confectioners' sugar, salt, vanilla extract, and butter in a mixing bowl until smooth; place in the refrigerator until needed for use.

Remove cake from the pan and transfer to the cooking wire rack to cool.

Over the cake, spread frosting and apply a topping of shredded carrots, as desired.

Lemon Cheesecake with Strawberries

Servings: 8 | Ready in about: 3 hr

INGREDIENTS

Crust:

4 ounces graham crackers

1 tsp ground cinnamon

3 tbsp butter, melted

Filling:

1 pound mascarpone cheese, at room temperature

¾ cup sugar

¼ cup sour cream, at room temperature

2 eggs, at room temperature

1 tsp vanilla extract

1 tsp lemon zest

1 tbsp lemon juice

1 pinch salt

2 cups water

1 cup strawberries, halved

DIRECTIONS

In a food processor, beat cinnamon and graham crackers to attain a texture almost same as sand; mix in melted butter. Press the crumbs into the bottom of a 7-inch springform pan in an even layer.

In a stand mixer, beat sugar, mascarpone cheese, and sour cream for 3 minutes to combine well and have a fluffy and smooth mixture. Scrape the bowl's sides and add eggs, lemon zest, salt, lemon juice, and vanilla extract. Carry on to beat the mixture until you obtain a consistent color and all ingredients are completely combined. Pour filling over crust.

Into the inner pot of your Foodi, add water and set in the reversible rack. Insert the springform pan on the rack.

Close the crisping lid and select Bake/Roast; adjust the temperature to 250°F and the cook time to 40 minutes. Press Start.

Remove cheesecake and let cool for 1 hour.

Refrigerate for 2 hours. Transfer to a serving plate and garnish with strawberry halves on top. Use a paring knife to run along the edges between the pan and cheesecake to remove the cheesecake and set to the plate.

The Most Chocolaty Fudge

Servings: 8 | Ready in about: 55 min

INGREDIENTS:

1 cup sugar
7 oz flour, sifted
1 tbsp honey
¼ cup milk
1 tsp vanilla extract

1 oz cocoa powder
2 eggs
4 oz butter
1 orange, juice and zest

Icing:

1 oz butter, melted
4 oz powdered sugar
1 tbsp brown sugar

1 tbsp milk
2 tsp honey

DIRECTIONS:

In a bowl, mix the dry ingredients for the fudge. Mix the wet ingredients separately. Combine the two mixtures gently.

Transfer the batter to a prepared Ninja Foodi basket.

Close the crisping lid and cook for about 35 minutes on Roast mode at 350 F.

Once the timer beeps, check to ensure the cake is cooked.

For the Topping: whisk together all of the icing ingredients.

When the cake is cooled, coat it with the icing. Let set before slicing the fudge.

No Flour Lime Muffins

Servings: 6 | Ready in about: 30 min

INGREDIENTS:

2 eggs plus 1 yolk
Juice and zest of 2 limes
1 cup yogurt

¼ cup superfine sugar
8 oz cream cheese
1 tsp vanilla extract

DIRECTIONS:

With a spatula, gently combine the yogurt and cheese.

In another bowl, beat together the rest of the ingredients.

Gently fold the lime with the cheese mixture.

Divide the batter between 6 lined muffin tins.

Close the crisping lid and cook in the Ninja Foodi for 10 minutes on Air Crisp mode at 330 F.

Molten Lava Cake

Servings: 4 | Ready in about: 20 min

INGREDIENTS:

3 ½ oz butter, melted
3 ½ tbsp sugar
1 ½ tbsp self-rising flour

3 ½ oz dark chocolate, melted
2 eggs

DIRECTIONS:

Grease 4 ramekins with butter.

Beat the eggs and sugar until frothy. Stir in the butter and chocolate.

Gently fold in the flour. Divide the mixture between the ramekins and bake in the Ninja Foodi for 10 minutes on Air Crisp mode at 370 F.

Let cool for 2 minutes before turning the lava cakes upside down onto serving plates.

Air Fried Doughnuts

Servings: 4 | Ready in about: 25 min

INGREDIENTS:

8 oz self-rising flour
1 tsp baking powder
½ cup milk

2 ½ tbsp butter
1 egg
2 oz brown sugar

DIRECTIONS:

Beat the butter with the sugar, until smooth; beat in eggs, and milk.

In a bowl, combine the flour with the baking powder.

Gently fold the flour into the butter mixture.

Form donut shapes and cut off the center with cookie cutters.

Arrange on a lined baking sheet and cook in the Ninja Foodi for 15 minutes on Air Crisp mode at 350 F. Serve with whipped cream.

Air Fried Snickerdoodle Poppers

Servings: 6 | Ready in about: 30 min

INGREDIENTS:

1 box instant vanilla Jell-O
1 can of Pillsbury Grands Flaky Layers Biscuits

1 ½ cups cinnamon sugar
Melted butter, for brushing

DIRECTIONS:

Unroll the flaky biscuits and cut them into fourths. Roll each ¼ into a ball.

Arrange the balls on a lined baking sheet, and cook in the Ninja Foodi for 7 minutes, or until golden, on Air Crisp mode at 350 F.

Prepare the Jell-O following the package's instructions. Using an injector, inject some of the vanilla pudding into each ball. Brush the balls with melted butter and then coat them with cinnamon sugar.

Pineapple Cake

Servings: 4 | Ready in about: 50 min

INGREDIENTS:

2 oz dark chocolate, grated
8 oz self-rising flour
4 oz butter
7 oz pineapple chunks

½ cup pineapple juice
1 egg
2 tbsp milk
½ cup sugar

DIRECTIONS:

Preheat the Ninja Foodi to 390 F. Place the butter and flour into a bowl and rub the mixture with your fingers until crumbed.

Stir in the pineapple, sugar, chocolate, and juice.

Beat the eggs and milk separately, and then add them to the batter.

Transfer the batter to a previously prepared (greased or lined) cake pan, and cook for 40 minutes on Roast mode. Let cool for at least 10 minutes before serving.

Chocolate Soufflé

Servings: 2 | Ready in about: 25 min

INGREDIENTS:

2 eggs, whites and yolks separated
¼ cup butter, melted
2 tbsp flour

3 tbsp sugar
3 oz chocolate, melted
½ tsp vanilla extract

DIRECTIONS:

Beat the yolks along with the sugar and vanilla extract.

Stir in butter, chocolate, and flour. Whisk the whites until a stiff peak forms.

Working in batches, gently combine the egg whites with the chocolate mixture.

Divide the batter between two greased ramekins. Close the crisping lid and cook for 14 minutes on Roast at 330 F.

Cinnamon Mulled Red Wine

Servings: 6 | Ready in about: 30 min

INGREDIENTS

3 cups red wine
2 tangerines, sliced
1/4 cup honey
6 whole cloves
6 whole black peppercorns

2 cardamom pods
8 cinnamon sticks
1 tsp fresh ginger, sliced
1 tsp ground cinnamon
6 tangerine wedges

DIRECTIONS

In the Foodi, combine red wine, honey, cardamom pods, 2 cinnamon sticks, cloves, tangerines slices, ginger, and peppercorns. Seal the pressure lid, choose Pressure, set to High, and set the timer to 5 minutes. Press Start. Release pressure naturally for 20 minutes. Press Start. Using a fine mesh strainer, strain your wine. Discard spices. Divide the warm wine into glasses and add tangerine wedges and a cinnamon stick for garnishing before serving.

Homemade Apple Cider

Servings: 6 | Ready in about: 45 min

INGREDIENTS

6 green apples, cored and chopped
3 cups water

1/4 cup orange juice
2 cinnamon sticks

DIRECTIONS

In a blender, add orange juice, apples, and water and blend until smooth; use a fine-mesh strainer to strain and press using a spoon. Get rid of the pulp.

In the cooker, mix the strained apple puree, and cinnamon sticks.

Seal the pressure lid, choose Pressure, set to High, and set the timer to 10 minutes. Press Start. Release the pressure naturally for 15 minutes, then quick release the remaining pressure. Strain again and do away with the solids.

Valencian Horchata

Servings: 6 | Ready in about: 20 min

INGREDIENTS

2 cups water
1 cup chufa seed, overnight soak
¼ stick cinnamon

Zest from 1 lemon
2 tbsp sugar
4 cups cold water

DIRECTIONS

In the pot, combine cinnamon, chufa seed and 4 cups water.

Seal the pressure lid, choose Pressure, set to High, and set the timer to 1 minute. Press Start. Release pressure naturally for 10 minutes, then release the remaining pressure quickly. In a blender, add chufa seed mixture, lemon zest and sugar. Blend well to form a paste.

Add 2 cups cold water into a large container. Strain the blended chufa mixture into the water. Mix well and place in the refrigerator until ready for serving. Add cinnamon stick for garnishing.

Moon Milk

Servings: 2 | Ready in about: 10 min

INGREDIENTS

1 cup milk
1 tsp coconut oil
1/2 tsp ground cinnamon, plus more for garnish
1/2 tsp ground turmeric
1/4 cup hemp hearts
1/2 tsp maca powder

1/8 tsp ground cardamom
1 pinch ground nutmeg
1 pinch ground ginger
1 pinch freshly ground black pepper
1 tsp honey

DIRECTIONS

To the Foodi, add milk. Press Sear/Sauté and heat the milk for 3-4 minutes until the point of starting to bubble; stir in coconut oil, turmeric, nutmeg, pepper, ginger, hemp hearts, maca powder, cinnamon, and cardamom.

Press Start/Stop and allow mixture to cool for about a minute; whisk in honey.

Transfer the mixture into a mug. Add more cinnamon for garnishing!

Almond Milk

Servings: 4 | Ready in about: 20 min

INGREDIENTS

1 cup raw almonds, soaked overnight, rinsed and peeled
1 cup cold water
2 dried apricots, chopped

2 tbsp honey
4 cups water
1 vanilla bean

DIRECTIONS

In the pot, mix a cup of cold water with almonds and apricots. Seal the pressure lid, choose Pressure, set to High, and set the timer to 1 minute.

When ready, release the pressure quickly. Open the lid. The almonds should be soft and plump, and the water should be brown and murky. Use a strainer to drain almonds; rinse with cold water for 1 minute.

To a high-speed blender, add the rinsed almonds, vanilla bean, honey, and 4 cups water. Blend for 2 minutes until well combined and frothy. Line a cheesecloth to the strainer.

Place the strainer over a bowl and strain the milk. Use a wooden spoon to press milk through the cheesecloth and get rid of solids. Place almond milk in an airtight container and refrigerate.

Tiramisu Cheesecake

Servings: 12 | Ready in about: 1 hour + chilling time | Serves: 12

INGREDIENTS

1 tbsp Kahlua Liquor
1 ½ cups Ladyfingers, crushed
1 tbsp Granulated Espresso
1 tbsp Butter, melted
16 ounces Cream Cheese, softened
8 ounces Mascarpone Cheese, softened

2 Eggs
2 tbsp Powdered Sugar
½ cup White Sugar
1 tbsp Cocoa Powder
1 tsp Vanilla Extract

DIRECTIONS

In a bowl beat the cream cheese, mascarpone, and white sugar. Gradually beat in the eggs, the powdered sugar and vanilla. Combine the first 4 ingredients, in another bowl.

Spray a springform pan with cooking spray. Press the ladyfinger crust at the bottom. Pour the filling over. Cover the pan with a paper towel and then close it with aluminum foil.

Pour 1 cup of water in your Foodi and lower the reversible rack. Place the pan inside and seal the pressure lid. Select Pressure and set time to 35 minutes at High pressure. Press Start. Press Start.

Wait for about 10 minutes before releasing the pressure quickly. Allow to cool completely before refrigerating the cheesecake for 4 hours.

Chocolate and Banana Squares

Servings: 6 | Ready in about about: 25 min

INGREDIENTS

½ cup Butter
3 Bananas
2 tbsp Cocoa Powder

1 ½ cups Water
Cooking spray, to grease

DIRECTIONS

Place the bananas and butter in a bowl and mash finely with a fork. Add the cocoa powder and stir until well combined. Grease a baking dish that fits into the Foodi.

Pour the banana and almond batter into the dish. Pour the water in the Foodi and lower the reversible rack. Place the baking dish on top of the reversible rack and seal the pressure lid.

Select Pressure, set the timer to 15 minutes at High pressure. Press Start. Press Start. When it goes off, do a quick release. Let cool for a few minutes before cutting into squares

Coconut Pear Delight

Servings: 2 | Ready in about about: 15 min

INGREDIENTS

¼ cup Flour
1 cup Coconut Milk

2 Large Pears, peeled and diced
¼ cup Shredded Coconut, unsweetened

DIRECTIONS

Combine all ingredients in your Foodi. Seal the pressure lid, select Pressureand set the timer to 5 minutes at High pressure. Press Start. When ready, do a quick pressure release. Divide the mixture between two bowls.

Raspberry Cheesecake

Servings: 6 | Ready in about about: 30 min

INGREDIENTS

1 ½ cups Graham Cracker Crust
1 cup Raspberries
3 cups Cream Cheese
1 tbsp fresh Orange Juice
3 Eggs

½ stick Butter, melted
¾ cup Sugar
1 tsp Vanilla Paste
1 tsp finely grated Orange Zest
1 ½ cups Water

DIRECTIONS

Insert the reversible rack into the Foodi, and add 1 ½ cups of water. Grease a spring form. Mix in graham cracker crust with sugar and butter, in a bowl. Press the mixture to form a crust at the bottom.

Blend the raspberries and cream cheese with an electric mixer. Crack in the eggs and keep mixing until well combined. Mix in the remaining ingredients, and give it a good stir.

Pour this mixture into the pan, and cover the pan with aluminium foil. Lay the spring form on the tray.

Select Pressure and set the time to 20 minutes at High pressure. Press Start. Once the cooking is complete, do a quick pressure release. Refrigerate the cheesecake for at least 2 hours.

Lemon & Blueberries Compote

Servings: 4 | Ready in about about: 10 min + chilling time

INGREDIENTS

2 cups Blueberries
2 tbsp Cornstarch
¾ cups Coconut Sugar

Juice of ½ Lemon
½ cup Water + 2 tbsp

DIRECTIONS

Place blueberries, lemon juice, 1/2 cup water, and coconut sugar in your cooker. Seal the pressure lid, choose Steam and set the timer to 3 minutes at High pressure. Press Start. Once done, do a quick pressure.

Meanwhile, combine the cornstarch and water, in a bowl. Stir in the mixture into the blueberries and cook until the mixture thickens, pressure lid off, on Sear/Sauté. Transfer the compote to a bowl and let cool completely before refrigerating for 2 hours.

Tasty Coconut Cake

Servings: 4 | Ready in about about: 55 min

INGREDIENTS

3 Eggs, Yolks and Whites separated
¾ cup Coconut Flour
½ tsp Coconut Extract
1 ½ cups warm Coconut Milk

½ cup Coconut Sugar
2 tbsp Coconut Oil, melted
1 cup Water

DIRECTIONS

In a bowl, beat in the egg yolks along with the coconut sugar. In a separate bowl, beat the whites until soft form peaks. Stir in coconut extract and coconut oil. Gently fold in the coconut flour. Line a baking dish and pour the batter inside. Cover with aluminum foil.

Pour the water in your Foodi and add a reversible rack. Lower the dish onto the rack. Seal the pressure lid, choose Pressure, set to High, and set the time to 35 minutes. Press Start. Do a quick pressure release, and serve.

Brown Sugar & Butter Bars

Servings: 6 | Ready in about about: 55 min

INGREDIENTS

1 cup Flour
1 ½ cups Water
1 Egg
½ cup Peanut Butter, softened
½ cup Butter, softened

1 cup Oats
½ cup Sugar
½ tsp Baking Soda
½ tsp Salt
½ cup Brown Sugar

DIRECTIONS

Grease a springform pan and line it with parchment paper. Set aside. Beat together the eggs, peanut butter, butter, salt, white sugar, and brown sugar. Fold in the oats, flour, and baking soda.

Press the batter into the pan. Cover the pan with a paper towel and with a piece of foil. Pour the water into the Foodi and add a reversible rack. Lower the springform pan onto the rack. Seal the pressure lid, choose Pressure, set to High, and set the time to 35 minutes. Press Start. When ready, do a quick release. Wait for 15 minutes before inverting onto a plate and cutting into bars.

Milk Dumplings in Sweet Sauce

Servings: 20 | Ready in about about: 30 min

INGREDIENTS

6 cups Water
2 ½ cups Sugar
3 tbsp Lime Juice

6 cups Milk
1 tsp ground Cardamom

DIRECTIONS

Bring to a boil the milk, on Sear/Sauté, and stir in the lime juice. The solids should start to separate. Pour milk through a cheesecloth-lined colander. Drain as much liquid as you can. Place the paneer on a smooth surface. Form a ball and divide into 20 equal pieces.

Pour water in the Foofi and bring to a boil on Sear/Sauté. Add in sugar and cardamom and cook until dissolved. Shape the dumplings into balls, and place them in the syrup. Seal the pressure lid and choose Pressure, set to High, and set the time to 5 minutes. Press Start.

Once done, do a quick pressure release. Let cool and refrigerate for at least 2 hours.

Poached Peaches

Servings: | Ready in about about: 15 min | Serves: 4 | Per serving: Calories 140; Carbs 15g; Fat 1g; Protein 1g

INGREDIENTS

½ cup Black Currants
4 Peaches, peeled, pits removed

1 cup Freshly Squeezed Orange Juice
1 Cinnamon Stick

DIRECTIONS

Place black currants and orange juice in a blender. Blend until the mixture becomes smooth. Pour the mixture in your Foodi, and add the cinnamon stick.

Add the peaches to the steamer basket and then insert the basket into the pot. Seal the pressure lid, select Pressure, and set to 5 minutes at High pressure.

When done, do a quick pressure release. Serve the peaches drizzled with sauce, to enjoy!

Ninja Pear Wedges

Servings: 3 | Ready in about about: 15 min

INGREDIENTS

2 Large Pears, peeled and cut into wedges
3 tbsp Almond Butter

2 tbsp Olive Oil

DIRECTIONS

Pour 1 cup of water in the Foodi. Place the pear wedges in a steamer basket and then lower the basket at the bottom. Seal the pressure lid, and cook for 2 minutes on High pressure.

When the timer goes off, do a quick pressure release. Remove the basket, discard the water and wipe clean the cooker. Press the Sear/Sauté and heat the oil. Add the pears and cook until browned. Top them with almond butter, to serve.

Almond and Apple Delight

Servings: 4 | Ready in about about: 14 min

INGREDIENTS

3 Apples, peeled and diced
½ cup Almonds, chopped or slivered

½ cup Milk
¼ tsp Cinnamon

DIRECTIONS

Place all ingredients in the Foodi. Stir well to combine and seal the pressure lid. Cook on Pressure for 4 minutes at High. Release the pressure quickly. Divide the mixture among 4 serving bowls.

Ninja Cherry Pie

Servings: 6 | Ready in about about: 45 min

INGREDIENTS

1 9-inch double Pie Crust
2 cups Water
½ tsp Vanilla Extract
4 cups Cherries, pitted

¼ tsp Almond Extract
4 tbsp Quick Tapioca
1 cup Sugar
A pinch of Salt

DIRECTIONS

Pour water inside your cooker and add the reversible rack. Combine the cherries with tapioca, sugar, extracts, and salt, in a bowl. Place one pie crust at the bottom of a lined springform pan.

Spread the cherries mixture and top with the other crust. Lower the pan onto the reversible rack. Seal the pressure lid, choose Pressure, set to High, and set the time to 18 minutes. Press Start. Once cooking is completed, do a quick pressure release. Let cool the pie on a cooling rack. Slice to serve.

Cinnamon Butternut Squash Pie

Servings: 4 | Ready in about about: 30 min

INGREDIENTS

1 pound Butternut Squash, diced
1 Egg
¼ cup Honey
½ cup Milk

½ tsp Cinnamon
½ tbsp Cornstarch
1 cup Water
A pinch of Sea Salt

DIRECTIONS

Pour the water inside your Foodi and add a reversible rack. Lower the butternut squash onto the reversible rack. Seal the pressure lid, and cook on Pressure for 4 minutes at High pressure.

Meanwhile, whisk all remaining ingredients in a bowl. Do a quick pressure. Drain the squash and add it to the milk mixture. Pour the batter into a greased baking dish. Place in the cooker, and seal the pressure lid.

Choose Pressure, set to High, and set the time to 10 minutes. Press Start. Do a quick pressure release. Transfer pie to wire rack to cool.

Gingery Chocolate Pudding

Servings: 4 | Ready in about about: 20 min

INGREDIENTS

Zest and Juice from ½ Lime
2 oz chocolate, coarsely chopped
¼ cup Sugar
2 tbsp Butter, softened
3 Eggs, separated into whites and yolks

¼ cup Cornstarch
1 cup Almond Milk
A pinch of Salt
½ tsp Ginger, caramelized
1 ½ cups of Water

DIRECTIONS

Combine together the sugar, cornstarch, salt, and softened butter, in a bowl. Mix in lime juice and grated lime zest. Add in the egg yolks, ginger, almond milk, and whisk to mix well.

Mix in egg whites. Pour this mixture into custard cups and cover with aluminium foil. Add 1 ½ cups of water to the Foodi. Place a reversible rack into the Foodi, and lower the cups onto the rack.

Seal the pressure lid, choose Pressure, set to High, and set the time to 25 minutes. Press Start. Once the cooking is complete, do a quick pressure release. Carefully open the pressure lid, and stir in the chocolate. Serve chilled.

Orange Banana Bread

Servings: 12 | Ready in about about: 45 min

INGREDIENTS

3 ripe Bananas, mashed
1 ¼ cups Sugar
1 cup Milk
2 cups all-purpose Flour
1 tsp Baking Soda
1 tsp Baking Powder

1 tbsp Orange Juice
1 stick Butter, room temperature
A pinch of Salt
¼ tsp Cinnamon
½ tsp Pure Vanilla Extract

DIRECTIONS

In a bowl, mix together the flour, baking powder, baking soda, sugar, vanilla, and salt. Add in the bananas, cinnamon, and orange juice. Slowly stir in the butter and milk.

Give it a good stir until everything is well combined. Pour the batter into a medium-sized round pan.

Place the reversible rack at the bottom of the Foodi and fill with 2 cups of water. Place the pan on the reversible rack. Seal the pressure lid, select Pressure and and set the time to 40 minutes at High. Press Start. Do a quick pressure release.

Delicious Pecan Stuffed Apples

Servings: 6 | Ready in about about: 20 min

INGREDIENTS

3 ½ pounds Apples, cored
½ cup dried Apricots, chopped
¼ cup Sugar
¼ cup Pecans, chopped
¼ cup Graham Cracker Crumbs
¼ tsp Cardamom

½ tsp grated Nutmeg
½ tsp ground Cinnamon
1 ¼ cups Red Wine

DIRECTIONS

Lay the apples at the bottom of your cooker, and pour in the red wine. Combine the other ingredients, except the crumbs. Seal the pressure lid, and cook at High pressure for 15 minutes. Once ready, do a quick pressure release. Top with graham cracker crumbs and serve!

Fruity Sauce

Servings: 2 | Ready in about about: 15 min

INGREDIENTS

1 cup Pineapple Chunks
1 cup Berry Mix
2 Apples, peeled and diced

¼ cup Almonds, chopped
¼ cup Fresh Orange Juice
1 tbsp Olive Oil

DIRECTIONS

Pour ½ cup of water, orange juice, and fruits, in the Foodi. Give it a good stir and seal the pressure lid. Press Pressure and set the timer to 5 minutes at High. Press Start.

When it goes off, release the pressure quickly. Blend the mixture with a hand blender and immediately stir in the coconut oil. Serve sprinkled with chopped almonds. Enjoy!

Savory Peaches with Chocolate Biscuits

Servings: 4 | Ready in about about: 20 min

INGREDIENTS

4 small Peaches, halved lengthwise and pitted
8 dried Dates, chopped
4 tbsp Walnuts, chopped
1 cup Coarsely Crumbled Cookies

1 tsp Cinnamon Powder
¼ tsp grated nutmeg
¼ tsp ground Cloves

DIRECTIONS

Pour 2 cups of water into the Foodi and add a reversible rack. Arrange the peaches on a greased baking dish cut-side-up. To prepare the filling, mix all of the remaining ingredients.

Stuff the peaches with the mixture. Cover with aluminium foil and lower it onto the reversible rack.

Seal the lid, choose Pressure, set to High, and set the time to 15 minutes. Press Start. Do a quick pressure release.

Vanilla Chocolate Spread

Servings: 16 | Ready in about about: 25 min

INGREDIENTS

1 ¼ pounds Hazelnuts, halved
½ cup Cocoa Powder
½ cups icing Sugar, sifted
1 tsp Vanilla Extract

¼ tsp Cardamom, grated
¼ tsp Cinnamon powder
½ tsp grated Nutmeg
10 ounces Water

DIRECTIONS

Place the hazelnut in a blender and blend until you obtain a paste. Place in the cooker along with the remaining ingredients. Seal the pressure lid, choose Pressure, set to High, and set the time to 15 minutes. Press Start.

Once the cooking is over, allow for a natural pressure release, for 10 minutes.

Apricots with Honey Sauce

Servings: 4 | Ready in about about: 15 min

INGREDIENTS

8 Apricots, pitted and halved
2 cups Blueberries
¼ cup Honey
1 ½ tbsp Cornstarch

½ Vanilla Bean, sliced lengthwise
¼ tsp ground Cardamom
½ Cinnamon stick
1 ¼ cups Water

DIRECTIONS

Add all ingredients, except for the honey and the cornstarch, to your Foodi. Seal the pressure lid, choose Pressure, set to High, and set the time to s 8 minutes. Press Start. Do a quick pressure release and open the pressure lid.

Remove the apricots with a slotted spoon. Choose Sear/Sauté, add the honey and cornstarch, then let simmer until the sauce thickens, for about 5 minutes.

Split up the apricots among serving plates and top with the blueberry sauce, to serve.

Coconut Milk Crème Caramel

Servings: 4 | Ready in about about: 20 min

INGREDIENTS

2 Eggs
7 ounces Condensed Coconut Milk
½ cup Coconut Milk

1 ½ cups Water
½ tsp Vanilla
4 tbsp Caramel Syrup

DIRECTIONS

Divide the caramel syrup between 4 small ramekins. Pour water in the Foodi and add the reversible rack. In a bowl, beat the rest of the ingredients. Divide them between the ramekins.Cover them with aluminum foil and lower onto the reversible rack.

Seal the pressure lid, and choose Pressure, set to High, and set the time to 15 minutes. Press Start. Once cooking is completed, do a quick pressure release. Let cool completely. To unmold the flan, insert a spatula along the ramekin' sides and flip onto a dish.

Chocolate Fondue

Servings: 12 | Ready in about about: 5 min

INGREDIENTS

10 ounces Milk Chocolate, chopped into small pieces
2 tsp Coconut Liqueur
8 ounces Heavy Whipping Cream

¼ tsp Cinnamon Powder
1 ½ cups Lukewarm Water
A pinch of Salt

DIRECTIONS

Melt the chocolate in a heat-proof recipient. Add the remaining ingredients, except for the liqueur. Transfer this recipient to the metal reversible rack. Pour 1 ½ cups of water into the cooker, and place a reversible rack inside.

Seal the pressure lid, choose Pressure, set to High, and set the time to 5 minutes. Press Start.

Once the cooking is complete, do a quick pressure release. Pull out the container with tongs. Mix in the coconut liqueur and serve right now with fresh fruits. Enjoy!

Homemade Egg Custard

Servings: 4 | Ready in about about: 20 min

INGREDIENTS

1 Egg plus 2 Egg yolks
½ cup Sugar
½ cups Milk

2 cups Heavy Cream
½ tsp pure rum extract
2 cups Water

DIRECTIONS

Beat the egg and the egg yolks in a bowl. Gently add pure rum extract. Mix in the milk and heavy cream. Give it a good, and add the sugar. Pour this mixture into 4 ramekins.

Add 2 cups of water, insert the reversible rack, and lay the ramekins on the reversible rack. Choose Pressure, set to High, and set the time to 10 minutes. Press Start. Do a quick pressure release. Wait a bit before removing from ramekins.

Almond Banana Dessert

Servings: 1 | Ready in about about: 8 min

INGREDIENTS

1 Banana, sliced
1 tbsp Coconut oil

2 tbsp Almond Butter
½ tsp Cinnamon

DIRECTIONS

Melt oil on Sear/Sauté mode. Add banana slices and fry them for a couple of minutes, or until golden on both sides.

Top the fried bananas with almond butter and sprinkle with cinnamon.

Made in the USA
Lexington, KY
09 February 2019